A Cochrane Pocketbook:
Pregnancy and Childbirth

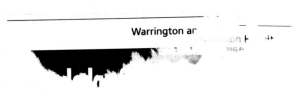

Warrington ar ... on H ...
NHS F...

A Cochrane Pocketbook: Pregnancy and Childbirth

G Justus Hofmeyr

James P Neilson

Zarko Alfirevic

Caroline A Crowther

A Metin Gülmezoglu

Ellen D Hodnett

Gillian ML Gyte

Lelia Duley

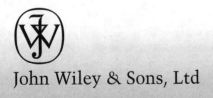

John Wiley & Sons, Ltd

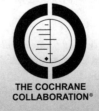

THE COCHRANE
COLLABORATION®

This work is a co-publication between The Cochrane Collaboration and John Wiley & Sons Ltd.

Published by John Wiley & Sons Ltd, The Atrium, Southern Gate, Chichester, West Sussex PO19 8SQ, England   Telephone   (+44) 1243 779777

Email (for orders and customer service enquiries): cs-books@wiley.co.uk
Visit our Home Page on www.wiley.com

Other Wiley Editorial Offices

John Wiley & Sons Inc., 111 River Street, Hoboken, NJ 07030, USA

Jossey-Bass, 989 Market Street, San Francisco, CA 94103-1741, USA

Wiley-VCH Verlag GmbH, Boschstr. 12, D-69469, Weinheim , Germany

John Wiley & Sons Australia Ltd, 42 McDougall Street, Milton, Queensland 4064, Australia

John Wiley & Sons (Asia) Pte Ltd, 2 Clementi Loop #02-01, Jin Xing Distripark, Singapore 129809

John Wiley & Sons Canada Ltd, 6045 Freemont Blvd, Mississauga Ontario, L5R 4J3, Canada

Wiley also publishes its books in a variety of electronic formats. Some content that appears in print may not be available in electronic books.

Library of Congress Cataloging-in-Publication Data

A Cochrane pocketbook. Pregnancy and childbirth / G. Justus Hofmeyr ... [et al.].
    p. ; cm.
  Includes bibliographical references and index.
  ISBN 978-0-470-51845-8 (alk. paper)
1. Maternal health services--Handbooks, manuals, etc.
2. Pregnancy--Handbooks, manuals, etc.
3. Pregnancy--Complications--Handbooks, manuals, etc.
4. Childbirth--Handbooks, manuals, etc. I. Hofmeyr, G. Justus. II. Title: Pregnancy & childbirth.
  [DNLM: 1. Pregnancy--Handbooks. 2. Maternal Health Services--methods--Handbooks.
  3. Parturition--Handbooks. 4. Pregnancy Complications--Handbooks. WQ 39 C668 2008]
  RG940.C58 2008
  362.198'2--dc22   2007050501

British Library Cataloguing in Publication Data

A catalogue record for this book is available from the British Library

ISBN   978-0-470-51845-8

Typeset in 10/13 pt Optima by Thomson Digital
Printed and bound in Great Britain by T.J. International Ltd, Padstow, Cornwall.

Contents

Foreword

The Cochrane Handbook: Pregnancy and Childbirth

For most people the day a child is born is a time of joy and celebration. It is a moment when families are afforded a brief glimpse into the future, and it is filled with hope and promise. In much of the world, however, this vision is far from reality. For women in many countries in the developing world, the day when she gives birth is a life-threatening event. For want of basic, known technologies and care over half a million women die unnecessarily in childbirth each year. The facts are stark: a woman in Sweden faces a one in 30,000 chance of dying in childbirth, while a woman in Sierra Leone faces chances of dying as high as one in six. When a mother dies, her newborn baby has much less chance of surviving the first weeks. These gross inequities underscore the fact that the right to health of childbearing women and their babies globally is far from being assured.

What does it mean, precisely, to say that health is a human right? In 2002, during my tenure as UN High Commissioner for Human Rights, I welcomed the appointment of a Special Rapporteur on the Right to Health, Paul Hunt, who has defined the right to health in the following way:

> "The right to health can be understood as a right to an effective and integrated health system encompassing health care and the underlying determinants of health, which is responsive to national and local priorities, and accessible to all. In other words, the health system must encompass both health care and the underlying determinants of health, such as adequate sanitation and safe drinking water. It must be accessible to all. Not just the wealthy, but those living in poverty. Not just majority ethnic groups, but minorities and indigenous peoples too. Not just those living

in urban areas, but also remote villagers. The health system has to be accessible to all disadvantaged individuals and communities."

To address the right to safe motherhood will require both strong political will and practical interventions based on evidence of effectiveness.

The Cochrane Pocketbook on Pregnancy and Childbirth aims to put the best evidence of effectiveness of pregnancy and childbirth interventions in the hands of those who can advocate for change—public and private decision makers, as well as health workers responsible for the care of childbearing women. The Cochrane Pocketbook authors and editors are concerned both with ensuring that health-preserving procedures are accessible to women as well as the elimination of ineffective and humiliating traditional procedures.

This book provides user-friendly access both to the Cochrane Library and to the World Health Organization Reproductive Health Library, which is distributed free of charge to health workers in low income countries globally in English, Spanish, French and Chinese.

It would be a great achievement to put these Cochrane Pocketbooks in the hands of health workers the world over. Let us join together to ensure that for every woman, anywhere in the world, the day she gives birth is one of the most hopeful days of her life.

Mary Robinson
President
Realizing Rights
Former President of Ireland,
    former UN High Commissioner for Human Rights
December 18, 2007

Preface

Care for pregnant women differs fundamentally from most other medical endeavours. 'Routine' care during pregnancy and birth interferes in the lives of healthy people, and in a process which has the potential to be an important life experience. It is difficult to measure the extent to which our efforts may, for example, disturb the development of a confident, nurturing relationship between mother and baby. The harmful effects we measure in randomised trials are limited to those we have predicted may occur. Sometimes after many years unexpected harmful effects surface only because they are relatively common, or striking in their presentation. Many unanticipated harmful effects probably never come to light.

For these reasons, interventions in pregnancy and childbirth need to be subjected to special scrutiny. Our guiding principle is to advise no interference in the process of pregnancy and childbirth unless there is compelling evidence that the intervention has worthwhile benefits for the mother and/or her baby – only then is there a good chance that benefits will outweigh both known adverse effects and those which may not have been thought of.

All pregnant women deserve the best possible care and advice founded on the best available evidence of effectiveness, applied with understanding, empathy and a philosophy of respect for the process of normal pregnancy and birth.

The Cochrane Library is the leading source of healthcare effectiveness reviews. This pocketbook provides quick access to evidence from Cochrane systematic reviews. We have arranged the contents in a logical sequence of chapters, making it easy for users to locate a topic and browse the available evidence. Users of *The Cochrane Library* will find it a convenient way to locate reviews of interest, and then use the 'CD' code provided to pick up the full electronic review in *The Cochrane Library*.

Where no Cochrane reviews of effectiveness are currently available, we have described, for completeness, options for care which are in common use. It is clear from the text that these measures are referred to without adequate evidence of effectiveness or hazards.

We have kept references to a minimum, as the original Cochrane reviews are extensively referenced.

Chapter introductions and linking paragraphs provide context and flow, but we have purposefully kept them brief to avoid detracting from the primary objective of the book: providing evidence summaries based on Cochrane reviews in a compact, accessible format.

The information in this book is a distillation of 3 decades of work by hundreds of collaborators from every corner of the globe. The spirit of collaboration which has made this possible has indeed been remarkable. We trust that readers will find it a valuable contribution to the personal health choices of those in their care, or themselves.

How to Use This Book

What is evidence?

> Then Daniel said to the steward.... "test your servants for ten days; let us be given vegetables to eat and water to drink. Then let our appearance and the appearance of the youths who eat the king's rich food be observed by you...." So he hearkened to them in this matter, and tested them for ten days. At the end of ten days it was seen that they were better in appearance and fatter in flesh than all the youths who ate the king's rich food. Daniel 1: 11–15.

The results of David's experiment were impressive. However, the wellbeing of those eating vegetables and water may have been due to factors other than their diet. This uncertainty could have been reduced by allocating the alternative diets at random rather than to a preselected group.

Random allocation is the only known method of ensuring that different outcomes in groups of women receiving a particular treatment are the result of the treatment, rather than some pre-existing characteristic.

The focus of this pocketbook is the effect of interventions on the health and wellbeing of pregnant women and their babies, derived from Cochrane systematic reviews. These are based almost entirely on evidence from randomised controlled trials (RCTs). Our purpose is not to recommend specific methods of care, but to provide easy access to high-quality evidence which can contribute to clinical decision-making and the development of management guidelines and protocols.

We have taken care to ensure the quality of information in this book. However, the responsibility for use of this information for clinical care or other purposes rests with the reader.

The Cochrane Pregnancy and Childbirth Group

The foundations upon which the Cochrane Collaboration is based were laid by Iain Chalmers and colleagues in Oxford in the late 1970s. These incorporated the following principles:

- Randomisation is the most reliable method of evaluating alternative forms of care.
- To avoid bias, reviews of randomised trials must follow a pre-specified protocol and include all trials on the topic conducted globally which meet quality criteria specified in the protocol.
- Reviews need to be updated regularly and disseminated quickly.
- Global collaboration is necessary to achieve these goals.

Handsearching of journals to identify all randomised trials was an essential basis for this work, and was commenced with a grant from WHO in 1978. Some subsequent landmarks were:

- A classified bibliography of more than 3000 trials, prepared by the National Perinatal Epidemiology Unit in Oxford, was published in 1985. This formed the basis for an electronic database, the 'Oxford Database of Perinatal Trials'.
- 'Effective Care in Pregnancy and Childbirth', a two-volume book edited by Iain Chalmers, Murray Enkin and Marc Keirse, was published in 1989.
- The Cochrane Collaboration was formed in 1992. The Oxford Database of Perinatal Trials became the 'Cochrane Pregnancy and Childbirth Database', edited by Murray Enkin, Marc Keirse, Mary Renfrew and Jim Neilson.
- In 1995, the administrative base of the Pregnancy and Childbirth Review Group, led by Jim Neilson, moved from Oxford to Liverpool. The administrative support is ably led by Sonja Henderson. The Group's systematic reviews are published in *The Cochrane Library*.
- Current editors are: Jim Neilson (UK), Zarko Alfirevic (UK), Caroline Crowther (Australia), Lelia Duley (UK), Metin Gulmezoglu (Switzerland), Ellen Hodnett (Canada) and Justus Hofmeyr (South Africa).
- Selected reviews with commentaries providing a low-income country context and video teaching aids are published in parallel in the World Health Organization 'Reproductive Health Library' and distributed globally in English, Spanish, French and Chinese (RHL@who.int; http://www.rhlibrary.com).

Scope of this book

The focus of this book is care, based on best evidence. For more details of aetiology, pathophysiology, diagnosis and epidemiology, please consult the background sections of the relevant Cochrane reviews, and standard textbooks. We have included the abstracts of Cochrane reviews relevant to the care of women and their babies before, during and after pregnancy. These include the Cochrane Pregnancy and Childbirth Group's reviews, as well as selected reviews from the following Cochrane Review Groups: Anaesthesia; Consumers and Communication; Depression, Anxiety and Neurosis; Developmental, Psychosocial and Learning Problems; Drugs and Alcohol; Effective Practice and Organisation of Care; Epilepsy; Fertility Regulation; Gynaecological Cancer; HIV/AIDS; Infectious Diseases; Neonatal; Oral Health; Schizophrenia; and Wounds. We acknowledge with thanks the contribution of these Cochrane Review Groups.

Methods for the Cochrane Pregnancy and Childbirth Group reviews

The Cochrane Pregnancy and Childbirth Group assembles, maintains and administers a register of trials, containing more than 12 000 reports of controlled trials relevant to the care of pregnant women and their babies. About 800 new records are added annually. Review authors conduct additional searches such as electronic searches, reference lists in key papers, and by personal contact with experts in the field.

Review authors set the quality criteria for inclusion of trials in the review (limited to randomised and sometimes quasi-randomised trials) and follow the methods described in the Cochrane Handbook of Systematic Reviews of Interventions (http://www.cochrane.org/resources/handbook/) and additional methods advised by the Review Group as described in the 'Methods used in reviews' section of the information about the Pregnancy and Childbirth Group in *The Cochrane Library*. The authors pre-specify outcomes in the protocol. They extract data and analyse them using Review Manager software. Generally, for dichotomous outcomes, they use relative risks (risk ratios) and sometimes odds ratios, with 95% confidence intervals. For continuous outcomes, they use weighted mean difference or standardised mean difference, with 95% confidence intervals.

For more detail, please consult the Cochrane Pregnancy and Childbirth Group's section in 'About the Cochrane Collaboration (About; Cochrane Groups)' in *The Cochrane Library*. An explanation of common statistical terms appears on page xxi.

Abridgement of the Cochrane Pregnancy and Childbirth abstracts in this book

To avoid repetition, we have abridged the methods of the abstracts as described by the authors of the individual reviews. The following elements are common to many abstracts:

'Search strategy
We searched the Cochrane Pregnancy and Childbirth Group's Trials Register [date].

Selection criteria
Randomised trials of [the study interventions].

Data collection and analysis
We independently assessed trial quality and extracted data. We performed double-data entry. If necessary, we contacted study authors to request additional information.'

In this book we have abridged the above three headings and descriptions as:

'***Methods:*** 'Standard PCG methods (see page xvii). Search date ….'

(This is followed, if necessary, by additional methods specific to the review).

Systematic review protocols

We have included abridged background and objectives of protocols published in *The Cochrane Library* for reviews which are still in progress. Please consult *The Cochrane Library* (using the CD number to search), as these reviews may have been completed since going to press with this book.

Effectiveness icons

To highlight reviews with clear evidence of benefit or harm, we have adapted the system of icons used by the WOMBAT collaboration (**www. wombatcollaboration.net**).

☺ - Benefits likely to outweigh harms in at least some circumstances
☹ - Likely to be ineffective or harmful
☺ - Benefits versus harms equivocal

How to locate the original review

In *The Cochrane Library:*
Each review or protocol has a 'CD' number. Enter the 'CD......' number in the search window of *The Cochrane Library* and 'Search all text', to get directly to the review or protocol.

The Cochrane Library is available on CD-ROM, as well as online through Wiley InterScience at http://www.interscience.wiley.com/cgi-bin/mrwhome/106568753/HOME or through the Cochrane Collaboration's website at http://www.cochrane.org/index.htm.

In *the WHO Reproductive Health Library:*
If the 'CD' number is followed by '(in RHL11)', the review is also available in the WHO Reproductive Health Library issue 11. Search the RHL using the title, or part of it. Subsequent issues of the RHL will include additional reviews (RHL@who.int; http://www.rhlibrary.com).

A brief guide to the format of results in Cochrane reviews

- This figure shows the rates of pre-eclampsia in all the included trials comparing calcium supplementation during pregnancy with placebo.
- In the trial by Crowther et al (1999), pre-eclampsia occurred in 10 out of 227 women who received calcium, compared with 23 out of 229 who received placebo.
- In this trial the **relative risk** (RR) of developing pre-eclampsia in the calcium group compared with the placebo group was (10/227 ÷ 23/229) = 0.44 (44%). This is a **risk reduction** of (1 − 0.44) = 56%.
- We are 95% certain that the 'true' relative risk lies somewhere between 0.21 and 0.90 (the 95% **confidence interval** (CI)).
- The whole range of the 95% confidence interval is <1. The bar representing the CI does not cross the '**no effect**' line (RR = 1 = no effect). This indicates that the reduction in pre-eclampsia with calcium is statistically significant.

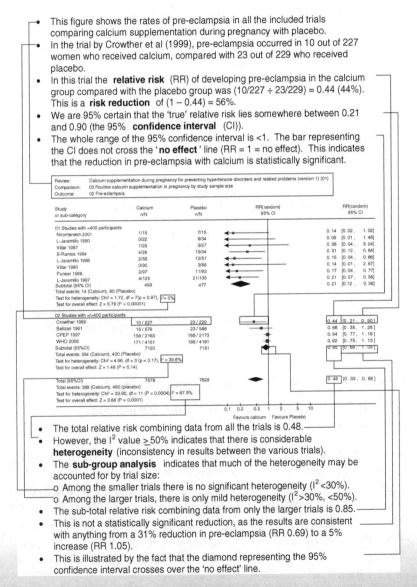

Review: Calcium supplementation during pregnancy for preventing hypertensive disorders and related problems (version 1) (01)
Comparison: 03 Routine calcium supplementation in pregnancy by study sample size
Outcome: 02 Pre-eclampsia

Study or sub-category	Calcium n/N	Placebo n/N	RR(random) 95% CI	RR(random) 95% CI
01 Studies with <400 participants				
Niromanesh 2001	1/15	7/15		0.14 [0.02, 1.02]
L-Jaramillo 1990	0/22	8/34		0.09 [0.01, 1.48]
Villar 1987	1/25	3/27		0.36 [0.04, 3.24]
S-Ramos 1994	4/29	15/34		0.31 [0.12, 0.84]
L-Jaramillo 1989	2/55	12/51		0.15 [0.04, 0.66]
Villar 1990	0/90	3/88		0.14 [0.01, 2.67]
Purwar 1996	2/97	11/93		0.17 [0.04, 0.77]
L-Jaramillo 1997	4/125	21/135		0.21 [0.07, 0.58]
Subtotal (95% CI)	458	477		0.21 [0.12, 0.36]
Total events: 14 (Calcium), 80 (Placebo)				
Test for heterogeneity: Chi² = 1.72, df = 7(p = 0.97), I²= 0%				
Test for overall effect: Z = 5.78 (P < 0.00001)				
02 Studies with =/>400 participants				
Crowther 1999	10 / 227	23 / 229		0.44 [0.21, 0.90]
Belizan 1991	15 / 579	23 / 588		0.66 [0.35, 1.26]
CPEP 1997	158 / 2163	168 / 2173		0.94 [0.77, 1.16]
WHO 2006	171 / 4151	186 / 4161		0.92 [0.75, 1.13]
Subtotal (95%CI)	7120	7151		0.85 [0.69, 1.05]
Total events: 354 (Calcium), 400 (Placebo)				
Test for heterogeneity: Chi² = 4.96, df = 3 (p = 0.17), I²= 39.6%				
Test for overall effect: Z = 1.48 (P = 0.14)				
Total (95%CI)	7578	7628		0.48 [0.33, 0.69]
Total events: 368 (Calcium), 480 (placebo)				
Test for heterogeneity: Chi² = 33.90, df = 11 (P = 0.0004) I² = 67.5%				
Test for overall effect: Z = 3.88 (P = 0.0001)				

0.1 0.2 0.5 1 2 5 10
Favours calcium   Favours Placebo

- The total relative risk combining data from all the trials is 0.48.
- However, the I² value $\geq$ 50% indicates that there is considerable **heterogeneity** (inconsistency in results between the various trials).
- The **sub-group analysis** indicates that much of the heterogeneity may be accounted for by trial size:
  - Among the smaller trials there is no significant heterogeneity (I² <30%).
  - Among the larger trials, there is only mild heterogeneity (I² >30%, <50%).
- The sub-total relative risk combining data from only the larger trials is 0.85.
- This is not a statistically significant reduction, as the results are consistent with anything from a 31% reduction in pre-eclampsia (RR 0.69) to a 5% increase (RR 1.05).
- This is illustrated by the fact that the diamond representing the 95% confidence interval crosses over the 'no effect' line.

Figure 1: Displaying categorical data

- This figure shows the average haematocrit of preterm babies randomly allocated to early cord clamping, compared with delayed cord clamping.
- In the trial by McDonnelll (1997), 23 babies with early cord clamping had an average haematocrit of 52.9% (standard deviation 7.1); another 23 who received delayed cord clamping had an average haematocrit of 55.0% (standard deviation 7.7).
- The difference between these means (early minus delayed) was −2.1%.

Review: Early Versus delayed umbilical cord clamping in Preterm infants
Comparison: 01 Early versus delayed cord clamping
Outcome: 05 Haematocrit at birth or 1 hour (%)

Study	Early N	Mean(SD)	Delayed N	Mean(SD)	Weighted Mean Difference (Fixed) 95% CI	Weight (%)	Weighted Mean Difference (fixed) 95% CI
Mc Donnell 1997	23	52.90 (7.10)	23	55.00 (7.70)		31.8	−2.10 [−6.38, 2.18]
Oh 2002	14	39.00 (5.60)	13	44.00 (7.10)		24.8	−5.00 [−9.85, −0.15]
Rabe 2000	20	48.00 (6.35)	19	51.10 (5.30)		43.4	−3.00 [−6.66, 0.66]
Total (95% CI)	57		55			100.0	−3.21 [−5.62, −0.80]

Test for heterogeneity chi-square=0.79 df=2 p=0.67 P =0.0%
Test for overall effect z=2.61 p=0.009

−10.0   −5.0   0   5.0   10.0
Favours early clamp   Favours delayed

- There was no heterogeneity between the trials ($I^2 = 0\%$).
- Thus the trials were combined using a fixed effects model.
- The combined difference between the means for all three trials, weighted for the trial sizes, was −3.21%.
- We can be 95% certain that the true difference in the means lies somewhere between −5.62 and −0.80.
- As the whole range of the 95% confidence interval lies in the same direction (−ve) (the diamond representing the confidence interval does not cross the zero or no effect line), this difference is statistically significant at the 5% level.

Figure 2: Continuous data (measurements, as opposed to either–or outcomes)

Notes on the orientation of the analysis figures

Which intervention is chosen as the 'treatment' intervention?

The 'treatment' or experimental intervention is listed in the first columns (to the left). In the example above, it may be argued that since early clamping of the umbilical cord is current routine practice, delayed clamping should be regarded as the experimental intervention. However, we prefer to regard the intervention which deviates most from the 'normal' as the experimental one, consistent with the philosophy that in childbirth any deviation from the normal requires justification.

How is the outcome defined?

Where possible, we prefer to define the outcome as an adverse health event. Thus beneficial effects of the experimental intervention will appear to the left of the 'no effect' line, and harms to the right. In some cases, this may result in somewhat cumbersome outcomes. For example, in reviews of methods of labour induction, the simpler outcome 'vaginal delivery in 24 hours' is rather presented as the reciprocal 'vaginal delivery not achieved in 24 hours'.

Acknowledgements

We acknowledge the commitment and administrative support of Sonja Henderson, Lynn Hampson, Denise Atherton and Jill Hampson (Cochrane Pregnancy and Childbirth Group editorial office, UK); Simon Gates (Statistical Adviser, UK); Dell Horey (Australasian Consumer Panel Co-ordinator, Australia); Carol Sakala (North American Consumer Panel Co-ordinator, USA); Philippa Middleton (Co-ordinator, Australian Review Authors' Group, Australia); and the review authors, expert reviewers and consumer panel members who have produced the original reviews.

Authors

Professor Zarko Alfirevic
Professor of Fetal and Maternal Medicine, Division of Perinatal and Reproductive Medicine, The University of Liverpool, First Floor, Liverpool Women's NHS Foundation Trust, Crown Street, Liverpool L8 7SS,UK

Professor Caroline A Crowther
Professor, Discipline of Obstetrics and Gynaecology, The University of Adelaide, Women's and Children's Hospital, 72 King William Road, Adelaide, South Australia 5006, Australia

Dr Lelia Duley
Obstetric Epidemiologist, Nuffield Department of Medicine, University of Oxford, Room 5609, Level 5, John Radcliffe Hospital, Headington, Oxford OX3 9DU, UK

Dr A Metin Gülmezoglu
Scientist, UNDP/UNFPA/WHO/World Bank Special Programme of Research, Development and Research Training in Human Reproduction (HRP), Department of Reproductive Health and Research, World Health Organization, 1211 Geneva 27, Switzerland

Mrs Gillian ML Gyte
Research Associate (formerly Consumer Panel Co-ordinator), Cochrane Pregnancy and Childbirth Group, Division of Perinatal and Reproductive Medicine, The University of Liverpool, First Floor, Liverpool Women's NHS Foundation Trust, Crown Street, Liverpool L8 7SS, UK

Professor Ellen D Hodnett
Professor, Faculty of Nursing, University of Toronto, 155 College Street, Suite 130, Toronto, Ontario M5T 1P8, Canada

Professor G Justus Hofmeyr
Director/Hon. Professor, Effective Care Research Unit, University of the Witwatersrand, University of Fort Hare, Eastern Cape Department of Health , Frere and Cecilia Makiwane Hospitals, Private Bag X 9047, 5200 East London, Eastern Cape, South Africa

Professor James P Neilson
Professor of Obstetrics and Gynaecology/ Head of School of Reproductive and Developmental Medicine, Division of Perinatal and Reproductive Medicine, The University of Liverpool, Liverpool Women's NHS Foundation Trust, Crown Street, Liverpool L8 7SS, UK

Chapter 1: The Context of Care for Pregnant Women

How care is provided to childbearing women and by whom varies considerably between countries, and between health sectors within countries.

> ☺ **CONTINUITY OF CAREGIVERS FOR CARE DURING PREGNANCY AND CHILDBIRTH:** reduced: hospital admission; use of pain relief in labour; resuscitation in newborns; and increased satisfaction with their care. (Hodnett ED) CD000062

BACKGROUND: Care during pregnancy, childbirth and the postnatal period is often provided by multiple caregivers, many of whom work only in the antenatal clinic, labour ward or postnatal unit. However, continuity of care is provided by the same caregiver or a small group from pregnancy through the postnatal period.

OBJECTIVES: To assess continuity of care during pregnancy and childbirth and the puerperium with usual care by multiple caregivers.

METHODS: Standard PCG methods (see page xvii). Search date: April 2000.

MAIN RESULTS: Two studies, involving 1815 women, were included. Both trials compared continuity of care by midwives with non-continuity of care by a combination of physicians and midwives. The trials were of good quality. Compared to usual care, women who had continuity of care from a team of midwives were less likely to be admitted to hospital antenatally (odds ratio (OR) 0.79, 95% confidence interval (CI) 0.64 to 0.97) and more likely to attend antenatal education programmes (OR 0.58, 95% CI 0.41 to 0.81). They were also less likely to have drugs for pain relief during labour (OR 0.53, 95% CI 0.44 to 0.64) and their newborns were less likely

A Cochrane Pocketbook: Pregnancy and Childbirth   G.J. Hofmeyr et al.
Copyright © 2008, Z. Alfiervic, C. A. Crowther, L. Duley, A. M. Gulmezoglu, G. ML. Gyte , E. D. Hodnett, G. J. Hofmeyr, J. P. Neilson

to require resuscitation (OR 0.66, 95% CI 0.52 to 0.83). No differences were detected in Apgar scores, low birthweight and stillbirths or neonatal deaths. While they were less likely to have an episiotomy (OR 0.75, 95% CI 0.60 to 0.94), women receiving continuity of care were more likely to have either a vaginal or perineal tear (OR 1.28, 95% CI 1.05 to 1.56). They were more likely to be pleased with their antenatal, intrapartum and postnatal care.

AUTHOR'S CONCLUSIONS: Studies of continuity of care show beneficial effects. It is not clear whether these are due to greater continuity of care or to midwifery care.

> **GIVING WOMEN THEIR OWN CASE NOTES TO CARRY DURING PREGNANCY:** increased women's sense of control; but also increased operative births. (Brown HC, Smith HJ) CD002856

BACKGROUND: In many countries women are given their own case notes to carry during pregnancy so as to increase their sense of control and satisfaction with their care.

OBJECTIVES: To evaluate the effects of giving women their own case notes to carry during pregnancy.

METHODS: Standard PCG methods (see page xvii). Search date: June 2007.

MAIN RESULTS: Three trials were included (n = 675 women). Women carrying their own notes were more likely to feel in control (relative risk (RR) 1.56, 95% confidence interval (CI) 1.18 to 2.06). Women's satisfaction: one trial reported more women in the case notes group (66/95) were satisfied with their care than the control group (58/102) (RR 1.22, 95% CI 0.99 to 1.52); two trials reported no difference in women's satisfaction (one trial provided no data and one trial used a 17 point satisfaction scale). More women in the case notes group wanted to carry their own notes in a subsequent pregnancy (RR 1.79, 95% CI 1.43 to 2.24). Overall, the pooled estimate of the two trials (n = 347) that reported on the risk of notes lost or left at home was not significant (RR 0.38, 95% CI 0.04 to 3.84). There was no difference for health related behaviours (cigarette smoking and breastfeeding), analgesia needs during labour, miscarriage, stillbirth and neonatal deaths. More women in the case notes group had operative deliveries (RR 1.83, 95% CI 1.08 to 3.12).

AUTHORS' CONCLUSIONS: The three trials are small, and not all of them reported on all outcomes. The results suggest that there are

both potential benefits (increased maternal control and satisfaction during pregnancy, increased availability of antenatal records during hospital attendance) and harms (more operative deliveries). Importantly, all of the trials report that more women in the case notes group would prefer to hold their antenatal records in another pregnancy. There is insufficient evidence on health related behaviours (smoking and breastfeeding) and clinical outcomes. It is important to emphasise that this review shows a lack of evidence of benefit rather than evidence of no benefit.

MIDWIFERY-LED VERSUS OTHER MODELS OF CARE DELIVERY FOR CHILDBEARING WOMEN: (Hatem M, Hodnett ED, Devane D, Fraser WD, Sandall J, Soltani H) Protocol [see page xviii] CD004667

ABRIDGED BACKGROUND: In many parts of the world, midwives are the primary providers of care for childbearing women. There are, however, considerable variations in the organization of midwifery services and in the education and role of midwives. Furthermore in some countries, e.g. in North America, medical doctors are the primary care providers for the vast majority of childbearing women, while in other countries, e.g. Australia, the UK, and Ireland, various combinations of midwifery-led, medical doctor-led, and shared care models are available, and childbearing women may be faced with many different options and conflicting advice as to which option is best for them.

OBJECTIVES: The primary objective of this review is to compare midwifery-led models of care with other models of care for childbearing women and their infants.

CRITICAL INCIDENT AUDIT AND FEEDBACK TO IMPROVE PERINATAL AND MATERNAL MORTALITY AND MORBIDITY: found no randomised trials. (Pattinson RC, Say L, Makin JD, Bastos MH) CD002961

BACKGROUND: Audit and feedback of critical incidents is an established part of obstetric practice. However, the effect on perinatal and maternal mortality is unclear. The potential harmful effects and costs are unknown.

OBJECTIVES: Is critical incident audit and feedback effective in reducing the perinatal mortality rate, the maternal mortality ratio and severe neonatal and maternal morbidity?

METHODS: Standard PCG methods (see page xvii). Search date: January 2005.
MAIN RESULTS: None.

AUTHORS' CONCLUSIONS: The necessity of recording the number and cause of deaths is not in question. Mortality rates are essential in identifying problems within the healthcare system. Maternal and perinatal death reviews should continue to be held, until further information is available. The evidence from serial data clearly suggests more benefit than harm. Feedback is essential in any audit system. The most effective mechanisms for this are unknown, but it must be directed at the relevant people.

TRADITIONAL BIRTH ATTENDANT TRAINING FOR IMPROVING HEALTH BEHAVIOURS AND PREGNANCY OUTCOMES: reduced perinatal complications; more research needed. (Sibley LM, Sipe TA, Brown CM, Diallo MM, McNatt K, Habarta N) CD005460 (in RHL 11)

BACKGROUND: Between the 1970s and 1990s, the World Health Organization promoted traditional birth attendant (TBA) training as one strategy to reduce maternal and neonatal mortality. To date, evidence in support of TBA training remains limited and conflicting.
OBJECTIVES: To assess effects of TBA training on health behaviours and pregnancy outcomes.
METHODS: Standard PCG methods (see page xvii). Search date: June 2006.
MAIN RESULTS: Four studies, involving over 2000 TBAs and nearly 27 000 women, are included. One cluster-randomized trial found significantly lower rates in the intervention group regarding stillbirths (adjusted OR 0.69, 95% confidence interval (CI) 0.57 to 0.83, P < 0.001), perinatal death rate (adjusted OR 0.70, 95% CI 0.59 to 0.83, P < 0.001) and neonatal death rate (adjusted OR 0.71, 95% CI 0.61 to 0.82, P < 0.001). Maternal death rate was lower but not significant (adjusted OR 0.74, 95% CI 0.45 to 1.22, P = 0.24) while referral rates were significantly higher (adjusted OR 1.50, 95% CI 1.18 to 1.90, P < 0.001). A controlled before/after study among women who were referred to a health service found perinatal deaths decreased in both intervention and control groups with no significant difference between groups (OR 1.02, 95% CI 0.59 to 1.76, P = 0.95). Similarly, the mean number of monthly referrals did not differ between groups (P = 0.321). One RCT

found a significant difference in advice about introduction of complementary foods (OR 2.07, 95% CI 1.10 to 3.90, P = 0.02) but no significant difference for immediate feeding of colostrum (OR 1.37, 95% CI 0.62 to 3.03, P = 0.44). Another RCT found no significant differences in frequency of postpartum haemorrhage (OR 0.94, 95% CI 0.76 to 1.17, P = 0.60) among women cared for by trained versus TBAs.

AUTHORS' CONCLUSIONS: The potential of TBA training to reduce peri-neonatal mortality is promising when combined with improved health services. However, the number of studies meeting the inclusion criteria is insufficient to provide the evidence base needed to establish training effectiveness.

MATERNITY WAITING FACILITIES FOR IMPROVING MATERNAL AND NEONATAL OUTCOME IN LOW-RESOURCE COUNTRIES: (van Lonkhuijzen L, Stekelenburg J, van Roosmalen J) Protocol [*see* page xviii] CD006759

ABRIDGED BACKGROUND: Low utilisation of maternal health services is mainly a result of barriers to access, and leads to high maternal and perinatal mortality and morbidity. Differences in utilisation figures between high- and low-income countries are enormous. Access to maternity health services is a key indicator for maternal mortality. Therefore, reaching a health facility, which can provide emergency obstetric care, is the best tool for reducing maternal mortality, and will also lead to a significant reduction of perinatal morbidity and mortality. Since the 1960s, maternity waiting homes have been advocated to bridge the geographical gap and the difference in care received by women living in remote areas compared to the women living in urban areas. The maternity waiting home could be anything from a simple hut with a latrine where women would care for themselves, to a fully catered for building. Waiting homes may be provided by the health authorities or by the local community. As one component of a comprehensive package of essential obstetric services, maternity waiting homes may offer a cheaper and more effective way to bring women close to obstetric care, as compared to interventions that aim to bring women to a hospital only at the time of delivery or complication.

OBJECTIVES: To assess, using the best available evidence, the effects of a maternity waiting facility on maternal and perinatal health.

Chapter 2: Antenatal Care

2.1 Pre-pregnancy evaluation

Women are encouraged to consult a healthcare provider prior to pregnancy. Possible advantages include giving dietary advice, starting prophylactic supplementation such as folate, giving immunisations such as rubella, identifying genetic risks, screening for medical conditions, changing medication and optimising management of conditions such as diabetes and epilepsy.

Some pre-pregnancy interventions such as folate supplementation and lifestyle advice are covered in the antenatal section.

2.2 General antenatal care

Routine antenatal care for healthy women was introduced on the compelling assumption that early diagnosis of complications would improve outcomes. The conventional frequency of routine visits (four-weekly till 28 weeks, two-weekly till 36 weeks, then weekly) is an empirical schedule introduced in Europe in the 1920s. Women who failed to attend for antenatal care had worse pregnancy outcomes than those who did. They were labelled 'unbooked', and often held responsible for poor outcomes when they occurred. On the other hand, women who attend antenatal care may on average be those with lower risks. The effectiveness of routine antenatal care has been notoriously difficult to prove.

> ☺ **PATTERNS OF ROUTINE ANTENATAL CARE FOR LOW-RISK PREGNANCY:** reduced frequency of antenatal visits showed no change in pregnancy outcomes; some women preferred the more frequent visits. (Villar J, Carroli G, Khan-Neelofur D, Piaggio G, Gülmezoglu M) CD000934 (in RHL 11)

A Cochrane Pocketbook: Pregnancy and Childbirth   G.J. Hofmeyr et al.
Copyright © 2008, Z. Alfiervic, C. A. Crowther, L. Duley, A. M. Gulmezoglu, G. ML. Gyte , E. D. Hodnett, G. J. Hofmeyr, J. P. Neilson

BACKGROUND: It has been suggested that reduced antenatal care packages or prenatal care managed by providers other than obstetricians for low-risk women can be as effective as standard models of antenatal care.

OBJECTIVES: The objective of this review was to assess the effects of antenatal care programmes for low-risk women.

METHODS: Standard PCG methods (see page xvii). Search date: May 2001.

MAIN RESULTS: 10 trials involving over 60 000 women were included. Seven trials evaluated the number of antenatal clinic visits, and three trials evaluated the type of care provider. Most trials were of acceptable quality. A reduction in the number of antenatal visits was not associated with an increase in any of the negative maternal and perinatal outcomes reviewed. However, trials from developed countries suggest that women can be less satisfied with the reduced number of visits and feel that their expectations with care are not fulfilled. Antenatal care provided by a midwife/general practitioner was associated with improved perception of care by women. Clinical effectiveness of midwife/general practitioner managed care was similar to that of obstetrician/gynaecologist led shared care.

AUTHORS' CONCLUSIONS: A reduction in the number of antenatal care visits with or without an increased emphasis on the content of the visits could be implemented without any increase in adverse biological maternal and perinatal outcomes. Women can be less satisfied with reduced visits. Lower costs for the mothers and providers could be achieved. While clinical effectiveness seemed similar, women appeared to be slightly more satisfied with midwife/general practitioner managed care compared with obstetrician/gynaecologist led shared care.

SUPPORT DURING PREGNANCY FOR WOMEN AT INCREASED RISK OF LOW BIRTHWEIGHT BABIES: reduced caesarean sections; improved some psychosocial outcomes; increased elective pregnancy terminations and did not affect perinatal outcomes. (Hodnett ED, Fredericks S) CD000198 (in RHL 11)

BACKGROUND: Studies consistently show a relationship between social disadvantage and low birthweight. Many countries have programs offering special assistance to women thought to be at risk for giving birth to a low birthweight infant. These programs may include advice and counseling (about nutrition, rest, stress management, alcohol and recreational drug use), tangible assistance (e.g. transportation to clinic appointments, help with household responsibilities), and emotional support. The programs may be delivered by multidisciplinary teams of health professionals, by specially trained lay workers, or by a combination of lay and professional workers.

OBJECTIVES: The objective of this review was to assess the effects of programs offering additional social support for pregnant women who are believed to be at risk for giving birth to preterm or low birthweight babies.

METHODS: Standard PCG methods (see page xvii). Search date: September 2005. Additional support was defined as some form of emotional support (e.g. counseling, reassurance, sympathetic listening) and information or advice or both, either in home visits or during clinic appointments, and could include tangible assistance (e.g. transportation to clinic appointments, assistance with the care of other children at home)

MAIN RESULTS: 18 trials, involving 12 658 women, were included. The trials were generally of good to excellent quality, although three used an allocation method likely to introduce bias. Programs offering additional social support for at-risk pregnant women were not associated with improvements in any perinatal outcomes, but there was a reduction in the likelihood of caesarean birth and an increased likelihood of elective termination of pregnancy. Some improvements in immediate maternal psychosocial outcomes were found in individual trials.

AUTHORS' CONCLUSIONS: Pregnant women need the support of caring family members, friends, and health professionals. While programs which offer additional support during pregnancy are unlikely to prevent the pregnancy from resulting in a low birthweight or preterm baby, they may be helpful in reducing the likelihood of caesarean birth.

☺ **ANTENATAL DAY CARE UNITS VERSUS HOSPITAL ADMISSION FOR WOMEN WITH COMPLICATED PREGNANCY:** for women with non-proteinuric hypertension, reduced hospital admissions and labour inductions in one small trial. (Kröner C, Turnbull D, Wilkinson C) CD001803

BACKGROUND: The use of antenatal day care units is widely recognized as an alternative for inpatient care for women with complicated pregnancy. Objectives: To assess the clinical safety, plus maternal, perinatal and psychosocial consequences for the women and cost effectiveness of this type of care.

METHODS: Standard PCG methods (see page xvii). Search date: May 2001

MAIN RESULTS: One trial involving 54 women was included. This trial was of average quality. It was found that day care assessment for non-proteinuric hypertension can reduce inpatient stay (difference in mean stay: 4.0 days; 95% confidence interval (CI): 2.1 to 5.9 days). Also a significant increase in the rate of induction of labour in the control group was found (4.9 times more likely: 95% CI: 1.6 to 13.8). The other clinical outcomes did not show a statistically significant difference between the control and intervention group. No other significant differences were observed.

AUTHORS' CONCLUSIONS: Admission to day care for non-proteinuric hypertension reduces the amount of time spent in the hospital and proportion of women induced for labour. However, one trial of 54 women is not sufficient to draw sound conclusions. Additional studies are needed to give more solid evidence to confirm the advantages of antenatal day care units.

REPEAT DIGITAL CERVICAL ASSESSMENT IN PREGNANCY FOR IDENTIFYING WOMEN AT RISK OF PRETERM LABOUR: (Alexander S, Boulvain M, Ceysens G, Haelterman E, Zhang WH) Protocol [*see* page xviii] CD005940

OBJECTIVES: To assess the effect of repeat digital cervical assessment during pregnancy for the risk of preterm birth and other adverse effects for mother and baby.

HOME-BASED SUPPORT FOR DISADVANTAGED TEENAGE MOTHERS: limited evidence of improvement in certain outcomes. (G Macdonald, C Bennett, J Dennis, E Coren, J Patterson, M Astin, J Abbott) CD006723 (Developmental, Psychosocial and Learning Problems Group)

BACKGROUND: Babies born to socio-economically disadvantaged mothers are at higher risk of injury, abuse or neglect and health problems than babies born to more affluent mothers; disadvantaged teenage mothers are at particular risk of adverse outcomes. Home-visiting programmes are thought to improve outcomes for both mothers and children, largely through advice and support.

OBJECTIVES: To assess the effectiveness of home-visiting programmes for women who have recently given birth and who are socially or economically disadvantaged.

SEARCH STRATEGY: The following electronic databases were searched: CENTRAL (2006, Issue 3); MEDLINE (1966 to March 2006); EMBASE (1980 to week 12 2006); CINAHL (1982 to March week 4 2006); PsycINFO (1872 to March week 4 2006); ASSIA (1987 to March 2006); LILACS (1982 to March 2006); and Sociological Abstracts (1963 to March 2006). Grey literature was also searched using ZETOC (1993 to March 2006); Dissertation Abstracts International (late 1960s to 2006); and SIGLE (1980 to March 2006). Communication with published authors about ongoing or unpublished research was also undertaken.

SELECTION CRITERIA: Included studies were randomised controlled trials investigating the efficacy of home visiting directed at teenage mothers.

DATA COLLECTION AND ANALYSIS: Titles and abstracts identified in the search were independently assessed for eligibility by two review authors (EC and JP or CB). Data were extracted and entered into RevMan (EC, JP and CB), synthesised and presented in both written and graphical form (forest plots). Outcomes included in this review were established at the protocol stage by an international steering group. The review did not report on all outcomes reported in included studies.

MAIN RESULTS: Five studies with 1838 participants were included in this review. Data from single studies provided support for the effectiveness of home visiting on some outcomes, but the evidence overall provided only limited support for the effectiveness of home visiting as a means of improving the range of maternal and child outcomes considered in this review.

AUTHORS' CONCLUSIONS: This review suggests there is only limited evidence that home-visiting programmes of the kind described in this review can impact positively on the quality of parenting of teenage mothers or on child development outcomes for their offspring. For reasons discussed in the review, this does not amount to a conclusion that home-visiting programmes are ineffective but indicates a need to think carefully about the problems that home visiting might influence

and about improvements in the conduct and reporting of outcome studies in this area.

> **HOME-BASED SUPPORT FOR DISADVANTAGED ADULT MOTHERS:** no evidence of improved outcomes. (C Bennett, GM Macdonald, J Dennis, E Coren, J Patterson, M Astin, J Abbott) CD003759 (Developmental, Psychosocial and Learning Problems Group)

BACKGROUND: Babies born to socio-economically disadvantaged mothers at higher risk of a range of problems in infancy. Home visiting programmes are thought to improve outcomes, both for mothers and children, largely through advice and support.

OBJECTIVES: To assess the effectiveness of home visiting programmes for women who have recently given birth and who are socially or economically disadvantaged.

SEARCH STRATEGY: We searched the following electronic databases: The Cochrane Central Register of Controlled Trials (CENTRAL) (Issue 3, 2006); MEDLINE (1966 to March 2006); EMBASE (1980 to 2006 week 12); CINAHL (1982 to March week 4 2006); PsycINFO (1872 to March week 4 2006); ASSIA (1987 to March 2006); LILACS (1982 to March 2006); and Sociological Abstracts(1963 to March 2006). We searched grey literature using ZETOC (1993 to March 2006); Dissertation Abstracts International (late 1960s to 2006); and SIGLE (1980 to March 2006). We also undertook communication with published authors about ongoing or unpublished research.

SELECTION CRITERIA: Included studies were randomised controlled trials investigating the efficacy of home visiting directed at disadvantaged adult mothers.

DATA COLLECTION AND ANALYSIS: Two reviewers (EC and JP or CB) independently assessed titles and abstracts identified in the search for eligibility. Data were extracted and entered into RevMan (EC, JP and CB), synthesised and presented in both written and graphical form (forest plots). Outcomes included in this review were established at the protocol stage by an international steering group. The review does not report on all outcomes reported in included studies.

MAIN RESULTS: We included 11 studies with 4751 participants in this review. Data show no statistically significant differences for those receiving home visiting, either for maternal outcomes (maternal depression, anxiety, the stress associated with parenting, parenting skills, child abuse risk or potential or breastfeeding) or child outcomes (preventive health care visits, psychosocial health, language development, behaviour problems or accidental injuries. Evidence about uptake of immunisations is mixed, and the data on child maltreatment difficult to interpret.

AUTHORS' CONCLUSIONS: This review suggests that for disadvantaged adult women and their children, there is currently no evidence to support the adoption of home visiting as a means of improving maternal psychosocial health, parenting or outcomes for children. For reasons discussed in the review, this does not amount to a conclusion that home visiting programmes are ineffective, but indicates a need to think carefully about the problems that home visiting might influence, and improvements in the conduct of outcome studies in this area.

SOCIAL AND LIFESTYLE INTERVENTIONS FOR PREVENTING LOW BIRTHWEIGHT IN SOUTH ASIANS: (West J, Wright J, Tuffnell DJ, Farrar D, Watt I) Protocol [see page xviii] CD006500

ABRIDGED BACKGROUND: The potential causes of IUGR are considerable and complex.
OBJECTIVES: To assess the effectiveness of social and lifestyle interventions to prevent low birthweight in South Asians (India, Pakistan and Bangladesh).

2.3 Behaviour/advice during pregnancy

'Scaring people with disease and death is counterproductive and explains much of the failure of health promotion programmes.' Skrabanek P. Preventive Medicine and Morality. *Lancet* 1986; 1: 143–144.

This chapter highlights the potential of interpersonal interactions to do both good and harm. We need to evaluate 'soft' interventions just as stringently as we do medications or operations. For example, several studies aiming to reduce preterm births by information, advice and counselling, have found the opposite effect. Let us keep in mind that well-intentioned advice which creates guilt may be counterproductive. One of our most valuable and vulnerable assets is our self-esteem.

INDIVIDUAL OR GROUP ANTENATAL EDUCATION FOR CHILD-
BIRTH OR PARENTHOOD OR BOTH: did not reduce vaginal births
after caesarean sections; for other objectives evidence was inadequate.
(Gagnon AJ, Sandall J) CD002869

BACKGROUND: Structured antenatal education programs for childbirth
or parenthood, or both, are commonly recommended for pregnant
women and their partners by healthcare professionals in many parts
of the world. Such programs are usually offered to groups but may be
offered to individuals.

OBJECTIVES: To assess the effects of this education on knowledge
acquisition, anxiety, sense of control, pain, labour and birth support, breastfeeding, infant-care abilities, and psychological and social adjustment.

METHODS: Standard PCG methods (see page xvii). Search date:
April 2006.

MAIN RESULTS: Nine trials, involving 2284 women, were included.
37 studies were excluded. Educational interventions were the focus of
eight of the studies (combined n = 1009). Details of the randomization
procedure, allocation concealment, and/or participant accrual or loss
for these trials were not reported. No consistent results were found.
Sample sizes were very small to moderate, ranging from 10 to 318. No
data was reported concerning anxiety, breastfeeding success, or general
social support. Knowledge acquisition, sense of control, factors related
to infant-care competencies, and some labour and birth outcomes were
measured. The largest of the included studies (n = 1275) examined an
educational and social support intervention to increase vaginal birth
after caesarean section. This high-quality study showed similar rates of
vaginal birth after caesarean section in 'verbal' and 'document' groups
(relative risk 1.08, 95% confidence interval 0.97 to 1.21).

**AUTHORS' CONCLUSIONS: The effects of general antenatal education for
childbirth or parenthood, or both, remain largely unknown. Individual-
ized prenatal education directed toward avoidance of a repeat caesarean
birth does not increase the rate of vaginal birth after caesarean section.**

INFORMATION FOR PREGNANT WOMEN ABOUT CAESAREAN
BIRTH: not enough data to provide reliable evidence. (Horey D, Weaver
J, Russell H) CD003858 (Consumers and Communication Group)

BACKGROUND: Information is routinely given to pregnant women, but information about caesarean birth may be inadequate.

OBJECTIVES: To examine the effectiveness of information about caesarean birth.

SEARCH STRATEGY: We searched the Cochrane Pregnancy and Childbirth Register, CENTRAL (26 November 2002), MEDLINE [online via PubMed 1966–] and the Web of Science citation database [1995–] (20 September 2002), and reference lists of relevant articles.

SELECTION CRITERIA: Randomised controlled trials, non-randomised clinical trials and controlled before-and-after studies of information given to pregnant women about caesarean birth.

DATA COLLECTION AND ANALYSIS: Two reviewers independently assessed trial quality and extracted data. Missing and further data were sought from trial authors unsuccessfully. Analyses were based on 'intention to treat'. Relative risk and confidence intervals were calculated and reported.

Consumer reviewers commented on adequacy of information reported in each study.

MAIN RESULTS: Two randomised controlled trials involving 1451 women met the inclusion criteria. Both studies aimed to reduce caesarean births by encouraging women to attempt vaginal delivery. One used a programme of prenatal education and support, and the other cognitive therapy to reduce fear. Results were not combined because of differences in the study populations. Non-clinical outcomes were ascertained in both studies through questionnaires, but were subject to rates of loss to follow-up exceeding 10%. A number of important outcomes cannot be reported: knowledge or understanding; decisional conflict; and women's perceptions: of their ability to discuss care with clinicians or family/friends, of whether information needs were met, and of satisfaction with decision-making.

Neither study assessed women's perception of participation in decision-making about caesarean birth, but Fraser (1997), who examined the effect of study participation on decision-making, found that women in the intervention group were more likely to consider that attempting vaginal birth was easier (51% compared to 28% in control group), or more difficult (10% compared to 6%). These results could be affected by the attrition rate of 11%, and are possibly subject to bias.

Neither intervention used in these trials made any difference to clinical outcomes. About 70% or more women attempted vaginal delivery in both trials, yet caesarean delivery rates exceeded 40%, at least 10% higher than was hoped. There was no significant difference between control and intervention groups for any of the outcomes measured: vaginal birth, elective/scheduled caesarean, and attempted vaginal delivery.

Outcome data, although similar for both groups, were not sufficient to compare maternal and neonatal morbidity or neonatal mortality.

There was no difference in the psychological outcomes for the intervention and control groups reported by either of the included trials.

Consumer reviewers said information for women considering a vaginal birth after caesarean (VBAC) should include: risks of VBAC and elective caesarean; warning signs in labour; philosophy and policies of hospital and staff; strategies to improve chances of success; and information about probability of success with specific care givers.

AUTHORS' CONCLUSIONS: Research has focussed on encouraging women to attempt vaginal delivery. Trials of interventions to encourage women to attempt vaginal birth showed no effect, but shortcomings in study design mean that the evidence is inconclusive. Further research on this topic is urgently needed.

NON-CLINICAL INTERVENTIONS FOR REDUCING UNNECESSARY CAESAREAN SECTION: (Khunpradit S, Lumbiganon P, Jaipukdee J, Laopaiboon M) Protocol [see page xviii] CD005528 (Effective Practice and Organisation of Care Group)

ABRIDGED BACKGROUND: Medical technology and public health measures have been introduced to reduce childbirth complications and mortality. One intervention is caesarean section. Nevertheless, this procedure may lead to increased maternal morbidities such as infections, haemorrhage, transfusion, other organ injury, anaesthetic complications and psychological complications. Maternal mortality has been reported to be two to four times greater than that of vaginal birth in some settings. Reported rates of caesarean sections have varied, especially between developed and developing countries.

OBJECTIVES: To determine the effectiveness and safety of non-clinical interventions for reducing unnecessary caesarean section. Non-clinical interventions refer to those that are applied independent of patient care in a clinical encounter between a particular provider and a particular patient.

2.3.1 Alcohol in pregnancy; drug misuse (Cochrane Drugs and Alcohol Group)

Non-prescription drugs, including alcohol and caffeine, may affect the baby's growth and development, cause specific pregnancy complications and anomalies such as the fetal alcohol syndrome, and cause symptoms of withdrawal in the newborn.

HOME VISITS DURING PREGNANCY AND AFTER BIRTH FOR WOMEN WITH AN ALCOHOL OR DRUG PROBLEM: not enough high quality data to provide reliable evidence. (Doggett C, Burrett S, Osborn DA) CD004456

BACKGROUND: One potential method of improving outcome for pregnant or postpartum women with a drug or alcohol problem is with home visits.

OBJECTIVES: To determine the effects of home visits during pregnancy and/or after birth for pregnant women with a drug or alcohol problem.

METHODS: Standard PCG methods (see page xvii). Search date: April 2004.

MAIN RESULTS: Six studies (709 women) compared home visits after birth with no home visits. None provided a significant antenatal component of home visits. The visitors included community health nurses, paediatric nurses, trained counsellors, paraprofessional advocates, midwives and lay African-American women. Most studies had methodological limitations, particularly large losses to follow up. There were no significant differences in continued illicit drug use (two studies, 248 women; relative risk (RR) 0.95, 95% confidence interval (CI) 0.75 to 1.20), continued alcohol use (RR 1.08, 95% CI 0.83 to 1.41) or failure to enrol in a drug treatment programme (two studies, 211 women; RR 0.45, 95% CI 0.10 to 1.94). There was no significant difference in the Bayley MDI (three studies, 199 infants; weighted mean difference 2.89, 95% CI -1.17 to 6.95) or Psychomotor Index (WMD 3.14, 95% CI -0.03 to 6.32). Other outcomes reported by one study only included breastfeeding at six months (RR 1.00, 95% CI 0.81 to 1.23), incomplete six-month infant vaccination schedule (RR 1.07, 95% CI 0.58 to 1.96), non-accidental injury and non-voluntary foster care (RR 0.16, 95% CI 0.02 to 1.23), failure to use postpartum contraception (RR 0.41, 95% CI 0.20 to 0.82), child behavioural problems (RR 0.46, 95% CI 0.21 to 1.01), and involvement with child protective services (RR 0.38, 95% CI 0.20 to 0.74).

AUTHORS' CONCLUSIONS: There is insufficient evidence to recommend the routine use of home visits for women with a drug or alcohol problem. Further large, high-quality trials are needed, and women's views on home visiting need to be assessed.

MAINTENANCE TREATMENTS FOR OPIATE DEPENDENT PREGNANT WOMEN: (Minozzi S, Amato L, Vecchi S) Protocol [see page xviii] CD006318 (Cochrane Drugs and Alcohol Group)

ABRIDGED BACKGROUND: The estimated prevalence of opiate use among pregnant women ranges from 1% to 2% to as much as 21%. Heroin readily crosses the placenta and pregnant opiate dependent women experience a six fold increase in maternal obstetric complications and significant increase in neonatal complications.

OBJECTIVES: To assess the effectiveness of any maintenance treatment alone or in combination with psychosocial intervention compared to no intervention, other pharmacological intervention or psychosocial interventions on child health status, neonatal mortality, retaining pregnant women in treatment, and reducing the use of substances.

PSYCHOSOCIAL INTERVENTIONS FOR PREGNANT WOMEN IN OUTPATIENT ILLICIT DRUG TREATMENT PROGRAMS: contingency management improved retention of women in the programmes and transiently reduced illicit drug use; more research needed. (Terplan M, Grimes D) CD006037 (Cochrane Drugs and Alcohol Group)

BACKGROUND: Illicit drug use in pregnancy is a complex social and public health problem. It is important to develop and evaluate effective treatments. There is evidence for the effectiveness of psychosocial interventions in this population; however, to our knowledge, no systematic review on the subject has been undertaken.

OBJECTIVES: To evaluate the effectiveness of psychosocial interventions in pregnant women enrolled in illicit drug treatment programs on birth and neonatal outcomes, on attendance and retention in treatment, as well as on maternal and neonatal drug abstinence. In short, do psychosocial interventions translate into less illicit drug use, greater abstinence, better birth outcomes, or greater clinic attendance?

SEARCH STRATEGY: We searched the Cochrane Drugs and Alcohol Group's trial register (May 2006), the Cochrane Central Register of controlled Trials (CENTRAL, The Cochrane Library, Issue 3, 2005), MEDLINE (1.1996–8.2006), EMBASE (1.1996–8.2006), CINAHL (1.1982–8.2006), and reference lists of articles.

SELECTION CRITERIA: Randomized studies comparing any psychosocial intervention versus pharmacological interventions or placebo or non-intervention or another psychosocial intervention for treating illicit drug use in pregnancy.

DATA COLLECTION AND ANALYSIS: Two reviewers independently assessed trial quality and extracted data.

MAIN RESULTS: Nine trials involving 546 pregnant women were included. Five studies considered contingency management (CM), and four studies considered manual based interventions such as motivational interviewing (MI).

The main finding was that contingency management led to better study retention. There was only minimal effect of CM on illicit drug abstinence. In contrast, motivational interviewing led towards poorer study retention, although this did not approach statistical significance. For both, no difference in birth or neonatal outcomes was found, but this was an outcome rarely captured in the studies.

REVIEWERS' CONCLUSIONS: The present evidence suggests that CM strategies are effective in improving retention of pregnant women in illicit drug treatment programs as well as in transiently reducing illicit drug use. There is insufficient evidence to support the use of MI. Overall the available evidence has low numbers and, therefore, it is impossible to accurately assess the effect of psychosocial interventions on obstetric and neonatal outcomes.

It is important to develop a better evidence base to evaluate psychosocial modalities of treatment in this important population.

PSYCHOLOGICAL AND/OR EDUCATIONAL INTERVENTIONS FOR REDUCING PRENATAL ALCOHOL CONSUMPTION IN PREGNANT WOMEN AND WOMEN PLANNING PREGNANCY: (Stade B, Bailey C, Dzandoletas D, Sgro M) Protocol [see page xviii] CD004228

ABRIDGED BACKGROUND: It is estimated that over 20% of pregnant women worldwide consume alcohol. Current research suggests that alcohol intake of seven or more standard drinks (one standard drink = 13.6 grams of absolute alcohol) per week during pregnancy places the fetus at significant risk for the negative effects of ethanol.

The incidence of fetal alcohol syndrome and its milder variants is around nine per 1000 live births. Prenatal exposure is the leading cause of developmental and cognitive disabilities among the world's children and its effects are lifelong. Psychological and/or educational interventions for reducing alcohol use among heavy users have been described. They include educational sessions, motivational enhancement therapy, self-help groups, psychotherapeutic techniques and cognitive-behavioural interventions.

OBJECTIVES: The primary objective of this review is to determine the effectiveness of psychological and/or educational interventions for reducing prenatal consumption of alcohol among pregnant women, or women planning for pregnancy.

The secondary objectives are to describe any adverse effects to the mother and to the fetus when psychological and/or educational interventions are used to reduce prenatal alcohol consumption.

2.3.2 Smoking

> ☺ **INTERVENTIONS FOR PROMOTING SMOKING CESSATION DURING PREGNANCY:** reduced both smoking and harmful effects of smoking such as low birthweight and prematurity. A strategy of rewards plus social support was more effective than other strategies. (Lumley J, Oliver SS, Chamberlain C, Oakley L) CD001055

BACKGROUND: Smoking remains one of the few potentially preventable factors associated with low birthweight, preterm birth and perinatal death.

OBJECTIVES: To assess the effects of smoking cessation programme implemented during pregnancy on the health of the fetus, infant, mother, and family.

METHODS: Standard PCG methods (see page xvii). Search date: July 2003.

MAIN RESULTS: This review included 64 trials. 51 randomised controlled trials (20 931 women) and six cluster-randomised trials (over 7500 women) provided data on smoking cessation and/or perinatal outcomes. Despite substantial variation in the intensity of the intervention and the extent of reminders and reinforcement through pregnancy, there was an increase in the median intensity of both 'usual care' and interventions over time.

There was a significant reduction in smoking in the intervention groups of the 48 trials included (relative risk (RR) 0.94, 95% confidence interval (CI) 0.93 to 0.95), an absolute difference of six in 100 women continuing to smoke. The 36 trials with validated smoking cessation had a similar reduction (RR 0.94, 95% CI 0.92 to 0.95). Smoking cessation interventions reduced low birthweight (RR 0.81, 95% CI 0.70 to 0.94) and preterm birth (RR 0.84, 95% CI 0.72 to 0.98), and there was a 33 g (95% CI 11 g to 55 g) increase in mean birthweight. There were no statistically significant differences in very low birthweight, stillbirths, perinatal or neonatal mortality but these analyses had very limited power. One intervention strategy, rewards plus social support (two trials), resulted in a significantly greater smoking reduction than other strategies (RR 0.77, 95% CI 0.72 to 0.82). Five trials of smoking relapse prevention (over 800 women) showed no statistically significant reduction in relapse.

AUTHORS' CONCLUSIONS: Smoking cessation programme in pregnancy reduce the proportion of women who continue to smoke, and reduce low birthweight and preterm birth. The pooled trials have inadequate power to detect reductions in perinatal mortality or very low birthweight.

2.3.3   Work and physical activity

> **AEROBIC EXERCISE FOR WOMEN DURING PREGNANCY:** improved women's fitness; there were not enough data to infer adverse or beneficial effects on the pregnancy. (Kramer MS, McDonald SW) CD000180

BACKGROUND: Physiological responses of the fetus (especially increase in heart rate) to single, brief bouts of maternal exercise have been documented frequently. Many pregnant women wish to engage in aerobic exercise during pregnancy but are concerned about possible adverse effects on the outcome of pregnancy.

OBJECTIVES: The objective of this review was to assess the effects of advising healthy pregnant women to engage in regular aerobic exercise (at least two to three times per week), or to increase or reduce the intensity, duration, or frequency of such exercise, on physical fitness, the course of labour and delivery, and the outcome of pregnancy.

METHODS: Standard PCG methods (see page xvii). Search date: June 2005.

MAIN RESULTS: 11 trials involving 472 women were included. The trials were small and not of high methodologic quality. Five trials reported significant improvement in physical fitness in the exercise group, although inconsistencies in summary statistics and measures used to assess fitness prevented quantitative pooling of results. Seven trials reported on pregnancy outcomes. A pooled increased risk of preterm birth (relative risk 1.82, 95% confidence interval (CI) 0.35 to 9.57) with exercise, albeit statistically nonsignificant, does not cohere with the absence of effect on mean gestational age (weighted mean difference +0.3, 95% CI −0.2 to +0.9 weeks), while the results bearing on growth of the fetus are inconsistent. One small trial reported that physically fit women who increased the duration of exercise bouts in early pregnancy and then reduced that duration in later pregnancy gave birth to larger infants with larger placentas.

AUTHORS' CONCLUSIONS: Regular aerobic exercise during pregnancy appears to improve (or maintain) physical fitness. Available data are insufficient to infer important risks or benefits for the mother or infant. Larger and better trials are needed before confident recommendations can be made about the benefits and risk of aerobic exercise in pregnancy.

2.4 Nutrition during pregnancy

The striking reduction of birthweight during the Dutch famine at the end of World War Two stimulated interest in mothers' diets and their babies' growth. However, the response of babies to the effects of less extreme dietary variations seems to be variable and at times unexpected.

2.4.1 Pre/periconceptional nutrition

☺PERICONCEPTIONAL SUPPLEMENTATION WITH FOLATE AND/OR MULTIVITAMINS FOR PREVENTING NEURAL TUBE DEFECTS: reduced the risk of neural tube defects. (Lumley J, Watson L, Watson M, Bower C) CD001056 (in RHL 11)

BACKGROUND: Neural tube defects arise during the development of the brain and spinal cord.

OBJECTIVES: To assess the effects of increased consumption of folate or multivitamins on the prevalence of neural tube defects periconceptionally (that is before pregnancy and in the first two months of pregnancy). **METHODS**: Standard PCG methods (see page xvii). Search date: April 2001. Trials both of supplementation and of advice to increase vitamin intake were included. **MAIN RESULTS**: Four trials of supplementation involving 6425 women were included. The trials all addressed the question of supplementation and they were of variable quality. Periconceptional folate supplementation reduced the incidence of neural tube defects (relative risk 0.28, 95% confidence interval 0.13 to 0.58). Folate supplementation did not significantly increase miscarriage, ectopic pregnancy or stillbirth, although there was a possible increase in multiple gestation. Multivitamins alone were not associated with prevention of neural tube defects and did not produce additional preventive effects when given with folate.

One dissemination trial, a community randomised trial, was identified involving six communities, matched in pairs, and where 1206 women of child-bearing age were interviewed following the dissemination intervention. This showed that the provision of printed material increased the awareness of the folate/neural tube defects association by 4% (odds ratio 1.37, 95% confidence interval 1.33 to 1.42).

AUTHORS' CONCLUSIONS: Periconceptional folate supplementation has a strong protective effect against neural tube defects. Information about folate should be made more widely available throughout the health and education systems. Women whose fetuses or babies have neural tube defects should be advised of the risk of recurrence in a subsequent pregnancy and offered continuing folate supplementation. The benefits and risks of fortifying basic food stuffs, such as flour, with added folate remain unresolved.

2.4.2   Energy/protein intake

ENERGY AND PROTEIN INTAKE IN PREGNANCY: balanced energy/protein supplementation improved fetal growth and may reduce perinatal mortality; high-protein or balanced protein supplementation, and protein/energy restriction of pregnant women who are overweight, may be harmful to the baby. (Kramer MS, Kakuma R) CD000032 (in RHL 11)

BACKGROUND: Gestational weight gain is positively associated with fetal growth, and observational studies of food supplementation in pregnancy have reported increases in gestational weight gain and fetal growth.

OBJECTIVES: To assess the effects of advice to increase or reduce energy or protein intake, or of actual energy or protein supplementation or restriction, during pregnancy on energy and protein intakes, gestational weight gain, and the outcome of pregnancy.

METHODS: Standard PCG methods (see page xvii). Search date: November 2006.

MAIN RESULTS: In five trials (1134 women), nutritional advice to increase energy and protein intakes was successful in achieving those goals, but no consistent benefit was observed on pregnancy outcomes.

In 13 trials (4665 women), balanced energy/protein supplementation was associated with modest increases in maternal weight gain and in mean birthweight, and a substantial reduction in risk of small-for-gestational-age (SGA) birth. These effects did not appear greater in undernourished women. No significant effects were detected on preterm birth, but significantly reduced risks were observed for stillbirth and neonatal death.

In two trials (529 women), high-protein supplementation was associated with a small, nonsignificant increase in maternal weight gain but a nonsignificant reduction in mean birthweight, a significantly increased risk of SGA birth, and a nonsignificantly increased risk of neonatal death. In three trials, involving 966 women, isocaloric protein supplementation was also associated with an increased risk of SGA birth.

In three trials (384 women), energy/protein restriction of pregnant women who were overweight, or exhibited high weight gain, significantly reduced weekly maternal weight gain and mean birthweight but had no effect on pregnancy-induced hypertension or pre-eclampsia.

AUTHORS' CONCLUSIONS: Dietary advice appears effective in increasing pregnant women's energy and protein intakes but is unlikely to confer major benefits on infant or maternal health.

Balanced energy/protein supplementation improves fetal growth and may reduce the risk of fetal and neonatal death. High-protein or balanced-protein supplementation alone is not beneficial and may be harmful to the fetus.

Protein/energy restriction of pregnant women who are overweight, or exhibit high weight gain, is unlikely to be beneficial and may be harmful to the fetus.

2.4.3 Vitamins/minerals

> **FOLATE SUPPLEMENTATION IN PREGNANCY:** (Haider BA, Humayun Q, Bhutta ZA) Protocol [see page xviii] CD006896.

ABRIDGED BACKGROUND: During pregnancy, fetal growth causes an increase in the total number of rapidly dividing cells, which leads to increased requirements for folate. If inadequate folate intake is sustained during pregnancy, megaloblastic anaemia develops. An increased folate intake might delay the diagnosis of vitamin B-12 deficiency by correcting the anaemia, or even exacerbate its neurologic and neuropsychiatric effects. Plasma total homocysteine (tHcy) is regulated by folate status, and hyperhomocysteinaemia is linked to vaso-occlusive disease. Impaired placental perfusion due to hyperhomocysteinaemia is implicated in having a negative effect on pregnancy outcome, as are inadequate folate intake and low serum folate concentrations. Periconceptional supplementation with folate has been shown to reduce the risk of neural tube defects by almost three-quarters.

OBJECTIVES: To assess the effectiveness of oral folate supplementation alone during pregnancy on haemotological and biochemical parameters during pregnancy and on pregnancy outcomes.

> **ZINC SUPPLEMENTATION FOR IMPROVING PREGNANCY AND INFANT OUTCOME:** reduced preterm birth but not other measures; results may reflect poor nutrition in the participants. (Mahomed K, Bhutta Z, Middleton P) CD000230

BACKGROUND: It has been suggested that low serum zinc levels may be associated with suboptimal outcomes of pregnancy such as prolonged labour, atonic postpartum haemorrhage, pregnancy-induced hypertension, preterm labour and post-term pregnancies, although many of these associations have not yet been established.

OBJECTIVES: To assess the effects of zinc supplementation in pregnancy on maternal, fetal, neonatal and infant outcomes.

METHODS: Standard PCG methods (see page xvii). Search date: February 2007.

MAIN RESULTS: We included 17 randomized controlled trials (RCTs) involving over 9000 women and their babies. Zinc supplementation resulted in a small but significant reduction in preterm birth (relative risk (RR) 0.86, 95% confidence interval (CI) 0.76 to 0.98 in 13 RCTs; 6854 women). This was not accompanied by a similar reduction in numbers of babies with low birthweight (RR 1.05, 95% CI 0.94 to 1.17; 11 studies of 4941 women). No significant differences were seen between the zinc and no zinc groups for any of the other primary maternal or neonatal outcomes, except for a small effect favouring zinc for caesarean section (four trials with high heterogeneity) and for induction of labour in a single trial. No differing patterns were evident in the subgroups of women with low versus normal zinc and nutrition levels or in women who complied with their treatment versus those who did not.

AUTHORS' CONCLUSIONS: The 14% relative reduction in preterm birth for zinc compared with placebo was primarily in the group of studies involving women of low income and this has some relevance in areas of high perinatal mortality. There was no convincing evidence that zinc supplementation during pregnancy results in other useful and important benefits. Since the preterm association could well reflect poor nutrition, studies to address ways of improving the overall nutritional status of populations in impoverished areas, rather than focusing on micronutrient and/or zinc supplementation in isolation, should be an urgent priority.

MAGNESIUM SUPPLEMENTATION IN PREGNANCY: reduced the risk of preterm birth and low birth weight in a cluster randomised trial; this was not confirmed in several individually randomised trials. (Makrides M, Crowther CA) CD000937

BACKGROUND: Many women, especially those from disadvantaged backgrounds, have intakes of magnesium below recommended levels. Magnesium supplementation during pregnancy may be able to reduce fetal growth retardation and pre-eclampsia, and increase birth weight.

OBJECTIVES: To assess the effects of magnesium supplementation during pregnancy on maternal, neonatal and paediatric outcomes.

METHODS: Standard PCG methods (see page xvii). Search date: June 2001.

MAIN RESULTS: Seven trials involving 2689 women were included. Six of these trials randomly allocated women to either an oral magnesium supplement or a control group, whilst the largest trial with 985 women had a cluster design where randomisation was according to study centre. The analysis was conducted with and without the cluster trial.

In the analysis of all trials, oral magnesium treatment from before the 25th week of gestation was associated with a lower frequency of preterm birth, (relative risk (RR) 0.73, 95% confidence interval (CI) 0.57 to 0.94), a lower frequency of low birth weight (RR 0.67, 95% CI 0.46 to 0.96) and fewer small for gestational age infants (RR 0.70, 95% CI 0.53 to 0.93) compared with placebo. In addition, magnesium treated women had less hospitalisations during pregnancy (RR 0.66, 95% CI 0.49 to 0.89) and fewer cases of antepartum haemorrhage (RR 0.38, 95% CI 0.16 to 0.90) than placebo treated women.

In the analysis excluding the cluster randomised trial, the effects of magnesium treatment on the frequencies of preterm birth, low birth weight and small for gestational age were not different from placebo.

Of the seven trials included in the review, only one was judged to be of high quality. Poor quality trials are likely to have resulted in a bias favouring magnesium supplementation.

AUTHORS' CONCLUSIONS: There is not enough high quality evidence to show that dietary magnesium supplementation during pregnancy is beneficial.

PYRIDOXINE (VITAMIN B6) SUPPLEMENTATION IN PREGNANCY: reduced maternal caries; there was not enough data to infer any impact on other perinatal outcomes. (Thaver D, Saeed MA, Bhutta ZA) CD000179

BACKGROUND: Vitamin B6 plays vital roles in numerous metabolic processes in the human body, such as nervous system development and functioning. It has been associated with some benefits in non-randomised studies, such as higher Apgar scores, higher birthweights, and reduced incidence of pre-eclampsia and preterm birth. Recent studies also suggest a protection against certain congenital malformations.

OBJECTIVES: To evaluate the clinical effects of vitamin B6 supplementation during pregnancy and/or labour.

METHODS: Standard PCG methods (see page xvii). Search date: December 2005.

MAIN RESULTS: Five trials (1646 women) were included. Four trials used blinding. One had an adequate method of randomisation and allocation concealment; four did not report this. Three trials had large losses to follow up. Vitamin B6 as oral capsules or lozenges resulted in decreased risk of dental decay in pregnant women (capsules: relative risk (RR) 0.84; 95% confidence interval (CI) 0.71 to 0.98; one trial, n = 371; lozenges: RR 0.68; 95% CI 0.56 to 0.83; one trial, n = 342). A small trial showed reduced mean birthweights with vitamin B6 supplementation (weighted mean difference −0.23 kg; 95% CI −0.42 to −0.04; n = 33; one trial). We did not find any statistically significant differences in the risk of eclampsia (capsules: n = 1242; three trials; lozenges: n = 944; one trial), pre-eclampsia (capsules: n = 1197; two trials; lozenges: n = 944; one trial) or low Apgar scores at one minute (oral pyridoxine: n = 45; one trial), between supplemented and non-supplemented groups. No differences were found in Apgar scores at one or five minutes, or breastmilk production between controls and women receiving oral (n = 24; one trial) or intramuscular (n = 24; one trial) loading doses of pyridoxine at labour.

AUTHORS' CONCLUSIONS: There were few trials, reporting few clinical outcomes and mostly with unclear trial methodology and inadequate follow up. There is not enough evidence to detect clinical benefits of vitamin B6 supplementation in pregnancy and/or labour other than one trial suggesting protection against dental decay. Future trials assessing this and other outcomes such as orofacial clefts, cardiovascular malformations, neurological development, preterm birth, pre-eclampsia and adverse events are required.

VITAMIN A SUPPLEMENTATION DURING PREGNANCY: appeared to reduce maternal deaths, night blindness and anaemia in one of three trials in women at increased risk through poor dietary intake; there was no evidence on routine intake. (van den Broek N, Kulier R, Gülmezoglu AM, Villar J) CD001996 (in RHL 11)

BACKGROUND: Vitamin A supplements have been recommended in pregnancy to improve outcomes that include maternal mortality and morbidity.

OBJECTIVES: To review the effectiveness of vitamin A supplementation during pregnancy, alone or in combination with other supplements, on maternal and newborn clinical and laboratory outcomes.

METHODS: Standard PCG methods (see page xvii). Search date: April 2002.

MAIN RESULTS: Five trials involving 23426 women were included. Because the trials were heterogeneous with regard to type of supplement given, duration of supplement use and outcomes measured, pooled results using meta analysis could not be performed. One large population based trial in Nepal showed a possible beneficial effect on maternal mortality after weekly vitamin A supplements. In this study a reduction was noted in all cause maternal mortality up to 12 weeks postpartum with vitamin A supplementation (RR 0.60, 95% CI 0.37–0.97). Nightblindness was assessed in a nested case-control study within this trial and found to be reduced but not eliminated. Three trials examined the effect of vitamin A supplementation on haemoglobin levels. The trial from Indonesia showed a beneficial effect in women who were anaemic ([Hb] <11.0 g/dl). After supplementation, the proportion of women who became non-anaemic was 35% in the vitamin A supplemented group, 68% in the iron-supplemented group, 97% in the group supplemented with both vitamin A and iron and 16% in the placebo group. The two trials from Malawi did not corroborate these positive findings.

AUTHORS' CONCLUSIONS: Although the two trials from Nepal and Indonesia suggested beneficial effects of vitamin A supplementation, further trials are needed to determine whether vitamin A supplements can reduce maternal mortality and morbidity and by what mechanism.

> **VITAMIN C SUPPLEMENTATION IN PREGNANCY:** had no clear benefits; appeared to increase preterm birth. (Rumbold A, Crowther CA) CD004072

BACKGROUND: Vitamin C supplementation may help reduce the risk of pregnancy complications like pre-eclampsia, intrauterine growth restriction and maternal anaemia. There is a need to evaluate the efficacy and safety of vitamin C supplementation in pregnancy.

OBJECTIVES: To evaluate the effects of vitamin C supplementation, alone or in combination with other separate supplements on pregnancy outcomes, adverse events, side-effects and use of health resources.

METHODS: Standard PCG methods (see page xvii). Search date: June 2004.

MAIN RESULTS: Five trials involving 766 women are included in this review. No difference was seen between women supplemented with vitamin C alone or in combination with other supplements compared with placebo for the risk of stillbirth (relative risk (RR) 0.87, 95% confidence interval (CI) 0.41 to 1.87, three trials, 539 women), perinatal death (RR 1.16, 95% CI 0.61 to 2.18, two trials, 238 women), birthweight (weighted mean difference (WMD) −139.00 g, 95% CI −517.68 to 239.68, one trial, 100 women) or intrauterine growth restriction (RR 0.72, 95% CI 0.49 to 1.04, two trials, 383 women). Women supplemented with vitamin C compared with placebo were at increased risk of giving birth preterm (RR 1.38, 95% CI 1.04 to 1.82, three trials, 583 women). Significant heterogeneity was found for neonatal death and pre-eclampsia. No difference was seen between women supplemented with vitamin C compared with placebo for the risk of neonatal death (RR 1.73, 95% CI 0.25 to 12.12, two trials, 221 women), using a random-effects model. For pre-eclampsia, women supplemented with vitamin C were at decreased risk when using a fixed-effect model (RR 0.47, 95% CI 0.30 to 0.75, four trials, 710 women), however this difference could not be demonstrated when using a random-effects model (RR 0.52, 95% CI 0.23 to 1.20, four trials, 710 women).

AUTHORS' CONCLUSIONS: The data are too few to say if vitamin C supplementation either alone or in combination with other supplements is beneficial during pregnancy. Preterm birth may have been increased with vitamin C supplementation.

> **VITAMIN D SUPPLEMENTATION IN PREGNANCY:** not enough data to provide reliable evidence. (Mahomed K, Gulmezoglu AM) CD000228

BACKGROUND: Vitamin D deficiency can occur in people whose diet is relatively low in the vitamin and those who are not exposed to much sunlight.

OBJECTIVES: To assess the effects of vitamin D supplementation on pregnancy outcome.

METHODS: Standard PCG methods (see page xvii). Search date: October 2001.

MAIN RESULTS: Two trials involving 232 women were included. In one trial the mothers had higher mean daily weight gain and lower number of low birthweight infants. In the other trial the supplemented group had lower birthweights.

AUTHORS' CONCLUSIONS: There is not enough evidence to evaluate the effects of vitamin D supplementation during pregnancy.

VITAMIN E SUPPLEMENTATION IN PREGNANCY: not enough data to provide reliable evidence in women with, or at increased risk of, pre-eclampsia. (Rumbold A, Crowther CA) CD004069

BACKGROUND: Vitamin E supplementation may help reduce the risk of pregnancy complications involving oxidative stress, such as pre-eclampsia. There is a need to evaluate the efficacy and safety of vitamin E supplementation in pregnancy.

OBJECTIVES: To assess the effects of vitamin E supplementation, alone or in combination with other separate supplements, on pregnancy outcomes, adverse events, side-effects and use of health services.

METHODS: Standard PCG methods (see page xvii). Search date: June 2004.

MAIN RESULTS: Four trials, involving 566 women either at high risk of pre-eclampsia or with established pre-eclampsia, were eligible for this review. All trials assessed vitamin E in combination with other supplements and two trials were published in abstract form only. No difference was found between women supplemented with vitamin E in combination with other supplements during pregnancy compared with placebo for the risk of stillbirth (relative risk (RR) was 0.77, 95% confidence interval (CI) 0.35 to 1.71, two trials, 339 women), neonatal death (RR 5.00, 95% CI 0.64 to 39.06, one trial, 40 women), perinatal death (RR 1.29, 95% CI 0.67 to 2.48, one trial, 56 women), preterm birth (RR 1.29, 95% CI 0.78 to 2.15, two trials, 383 women), intrauterine growth restriction (RR 0.72, 95% CI 0.49 to 1.04, two trials, 383 women) or birthweight (weighted mean difference −139.00 g, 95% CI −517.68 to 239.68, one trial, 100 women), using fixed-effect models.

Substantial heterogeneity was found for pre-eclampsia. Women supplemented with vitamin E in combination with other supplements compared with placebo were at decreased risk of developing clinical pre-eclampsia (RR 0.44, 95% CI 0.27 to 0.71, three trials, 510 women) using fixed-effect models; however, this difference could not be demonstrated when using random-effects models (RR 0.44, 95% CI 0.16 to 1.22, three trials, 510 women). There were no differences between women supplemented with vitamin E compared with placebo for any of the secondary outcomes.

AUTHORS' CONCLUSIONS: The data are too few to say if vitamin E supplementation either alone or in combination with other supplements is beneficial during pregnancy.

MULTIPLE-MICRONUTRIENT SUPPLEMENTATION FOR WOMEN DURING PREGNANCY: showed no benefits over iron and folate supplementation. (Haider BA, Bhutta ZA) CD004905 (in RHL 11)

BACKGROUND: Multiple-micronutrient deficiencies often coexist in low- to middle-income countries. They are exacerbated in pregnancy due to the increased demands, leading to potentially adverse effects on the mother. Substantive evidence regarding the effectiveness of multiple-micronutrient supplements (MMS) during pregnancy is not available.

OBJECTIVES: To evaluate the benefits to mother and infant of multiple-micronutrient supplements in pregnancy and assess the risk of excess supplementation and potential adverse interactions between micronutrients.

METHODS: Standard PCG methods (see page xvii). Search date: December 2005.

MAIN RESULTS: Nine trials (15 378 women) are included. When compared with supplementation of two or less micronutrients or no supplementation or a placebo, multiple-micronutrient supplementation resulted in a statistically significant decrease in the number of low birthweight babies (relative risk (RR) 0.83; 95% confidence interval (CI) 0.76 to 0.91), small-for-gestational-age babies (RR 0.92; 95% CI 0.86 to 0.99) and in maternal anaemia (RR 0.61; CI 0.52 to 0.71). However, these differences lost statistical significance when multiple-micronutrient supplementation was compared with iron folic acid supplementation alone. No statistically significant differences were shown for the outcomes of preterm births and perinatal mortality in any of the comparisons.

A number of prespecified clinically important outcomes could not be assessed due to insufficient or non-available data from the included trials. These include placental abruption, congenital anomalies including neural tube defects, premature rupture of membranes, pre-eclampsia, miscarriage, maternal mortality, neurodevelopmental delay, very preterm births, cost of supplementation, side-effects of supplements, maternal wellbeing or satisfaction and nutritional status of children.

AUTHORS' CONCLUSIONS: The evidence provided in this review is insufficient to suggest replacement of iron and folate supplementation with a multiple-micronutrient supplement. A reduction in the number of low birthweight and small-for-gestational-age babies and maternal anaemia has been found with a multiple-micronutrient supplement against supplementation with two or less micronutrients or none or a placebo, but analyses revealed no added benefit of multiple-micronutrient supplements compared with iron folic acid supplementation. These results are limited by the small number of studies available. There is also insufficient evidence to identify adverse effects and to say that excess multiple-micronutrient supplementation during pregnancy is harmful to the mother or the fetus.

Further research is needed to find out the beneficial maternal or fetal effects and to assess the risk of excess supplementation and potential adverse interactions between the micronutrients.

2.5 Weight gain in pregnancy

In the past, dietary restrictions have been used to limit excessive weight gain in pregnancy. However, the association between excessive weight gain and poor pregnancy outcome may be related to weight increase from oedema rather than dietary weight gain. The value of dietary restriction and repeatedly weighing pregnant women has been questioned.

There are no Cochrane reviews of this topic.

2.6 Symptoms during pregnancy

Some women experience an increased sense of wellbeing during pregnancy. However, women's experiences of pregnancy may be marred by considerable discomfort and distress caused by 'minor' symptoms of pregnancy. These symptoms may include nausea, vomiting, heartburn, constipation, faintness (syncope), low blood pressure when lying on one's back (supine hypotension), varicose veins, haemorrhoids, swelling (oedema), backache, cramps and frequency of emptying the bladder. Less common symptoms include inflammation of the gums (gingivitis), craving for unusual foods (pica), diarrhoea, flatulence, rapid heart beats (palpitations), nose bleeds (epistaxis), separation of the pubic bones at the front of the pelvis (symphyseal separation), urinary incontinence, headache, insomnia, tiredness, difficulty with breathing (dyspnoea), skin and hair changes, pain in the breasts (mastalgia), restless leg syndrome, heat intolerance and hand discomfort.

As these symptoms may not be related to serious illness, health workers tend to reassure the women without providing relief from the symptoms themselves. Providing relief is often not easy. This section evaluates the effectiveness of interventions to relieve such symptoms.

> ☺ **INTERVENTIONS FOR NAUSEA AND VOMITING IN EARLY PREGNANCY:** morning sickness was relieved by antihistamines; by ginger; and possibly by vitamin B6 and acupuncture. (Jewell D, Young G) CD000145

BACKGROUND: Nausea and vomiting are the most common symptoms experienced in early pregnancy, with nausea affecting between 70 and 85% of women. About half of pregnant women experience vomiting.

OBJECTIVES: To assess the effects of different methods of treating nausea and vomiting in early pregnancy.

METHODS: Standard PCG methods (see page xvii). Search date: December 2002.

MAIN RESULTS: 28 trials met the inclusion criteria. For milder degrees of nausea and vomiting, 21 trials were included. These trials were of variable quality. Nausea treatments were: different antihistamine medications, vitamin B6 (pyridoxine), the combination tablet Debendox (Bendectin), P6 acupressure and ginger. For hyperemesis gravidarum, seven trials were identified testing treatments with oral ginger root extract, oral or injected corticosteroids or injected adrenocorticotrophic hormone (ACTH), intravenous diazepam and acupuncture. Based on 12 trials, there was an overall reduction in nausea from anti-emetic medication (odds ratio 0.16, 95% confidence interval 0.08 to 0.33).

AUTHORS' CONCLUSIONS: Anti-emetic medication appears to reduce the frequency of nausea in early pregnancy. There is some evidence of adverse effects, but there is very little information on effects on fetal outcomes from randomised controlled trials. Of newer treatments, pyridoxine (vitamin B6) appears to be more effective in reducing the severity of nausea. The results from trials of P6 acupressure are equivocal. No trials of treatments for hyperemesis gravidarum show any evidence of benefit. Evidence from observational studies suggests no evidence of teratogenicity from any of these treatments.

ANTIHISTAMINES VERSUS ASPIRIN FOR ITCHING IN LATE PREGNANCY: chlorpheniramine relieved itching better than aspirin when a rash was present; aspirin relieved itching better than chlorpheniramine when there was no rash. (Young GL, Jewell D) CD000027

BACKGROUND: While not common, itching in pregnancy (not due to liver disease) can be distressing.

OBJECTIVES: To assess the effects of treatment for itching in late pregnancy.

METHODS: Standard PCG methods (see page xvii). Search date: January 2007.

DATA COLLECTION AND ANALYSIS: Two review authors independently assessed trial quality and extracted data.

MAIN RESULTS: One study of 38 women was included. This was a small crossover trial, using alternate allocation. The trial compared a histamine, chlorpheniramine, with aspirin. Aspirin was more effective than chlorpheniramine in relieving itching (odds ratio 2.39, 95% confidence interval 1.25 to 4.57). However, chlorpheniramine was more effective than aspirin when a rash was present.

AUTHORS' CONCLUSIONS: Aspirin appears to be more effective than chlorpheniramine for relief of itching in pregnancy when no rash is present. If there is a rash, chlorpheniramine may be more effective.

☺ **CREAMS FOR PREVENTING STRETCH MARKS IN PREGNANCY:** certain topical creams appear to prevent abdominal stretch marks. (Young GL, Jewell D) CD000066

BACKGROUND: Striae gravidarum (stretch marks developing during pregnancy) occur in over 50% of women. There is no evidence that any treatment removes striae once they have appeared. Some women are upset about the change in the appearance of their skin.

OBJECTIVES: To assess the effects of topical treatments in preventing the development of stretch marks.

METHODS: Standard PCG methods (see page xvii). Search date: April 2004.

MAIN RESULTS: Two studies, involving 130 women in total, were included.

One study, involving 80 women, indicated that, compared to placebo, massage with a cream (Trofolastin) containing Centella asiatica extract, alpha tocopherol and collagen–elastin hydrolysates was associated with less women developing stretch marks (odds ratio (OR) 0.41, 95% confidence interval (CI) 0.17 to 0.99). A second study of 50 women compared massage using an ointment (Verum) containing tocopherol, panthenol, hyaluronic acid, elastin and menthol with no treatment. Massage with the ointment was associated with less women developing stretch marks (OR 0.26, 95% CI 0.08 to 0.84).

AUTHORS' CONCLUSIONS: Trofolastin cream appears to help prevent the development of stretch marks in pregnancy in some women. Verum ointment may be helpful but the trial had no placebo and may show the benefit of massage alone.

☺ **INTERVENTIONS FOR LEG CRAMPS IN PREGNANCY:** leg cramps may be relieved by magnesium lactate or citrate. (Young GL, Jewell D) CD000121

BACKGROUND: Many women experience leg cramps in pregnancy. They become more common as pregnancy progresses and are especially troublesome at night.

OBJECTIVES: To assess methods of preventing and treating leg cramps in pregnancy.

METHODS: Standard PCG methods (see page xvii). Search date: October 2001.

MAIN RESULTS: Five trials involving 352 women were included. The trials were of moderate quality. The only placebo-controlled trial of calcium treatment showed no evidence of benefit. Trials comparing sodium chloride with placebo (odds ratio 0.54, 95% confidence interval 0.23 to 1.29) and calcium with sodium chloride (odds ratio 1.23, 95% confidence interval 0.47 to 3.27) showed no evidence of benefit. Placebo controlled trials of multivitamin with mineral supplements (odds ratio 0.23, 95% confidence interval 0.05 to 1.01) and magnesium (odds ratio 0.18, 95% confidence interval 0.05 to 0.60) provided some suggestion of benefit.

AUTHORS' CONCLUSIONS: The evidence that calcium reduces cramp is weak and seems to depend on placebo effect. The evidence for sodium chloride is stronger but the results of the sodium chloride trial may no longer be relevant because of dietary changes which include an increased sodium intake in the general population. It is not possible to recommend multivitamins with mineral supplementation, as it is not clear which ingredient, if any, is helping. If a woman finds cramp troublesome in pregnancy, the best evidence is for magnesium lactate or citrate taken as 5 mmol in the morning and 10 mmol in the evening.

> **INTERVENTIONS FOR PREVENTING AND TREATING PELVIC AND BACK PAIN IN PREGNANCY:** water gymnastics, acupuncture and a specially shaped pillow may possibly be of benefit. (Pennick VE, Young G) CD001139

BACKGROUND: More than two-thirds of pregnant women experience back pain and almost one-fifth experience pelvic pain. The pain increases with advancing pregnancy and interferes with work, daily activities and sleep.

OBJECTIVES: To assess the effects of interventions for preventing and treating back and pelvic pain in pregnancy.

METHODS: Standard PCG methods (see page xvii). Search date: February 2006.

DATA COLLECTION AND ANALYSIS: Two authors independently assessed trial quality and extracted data.

MAIN RESULTS: We found no studies dealing specifically with prevention of back or pelvic pain. We included eight studies (1305 participants) that examined the effects of adding various pregnancy-specific exercises, physiotherapy, acupuncture and pillows to usual prenatal care.

For women with low-back pain, participating in strengthening exercises, sitting pelvic tilt exercises (standardised mean difference (SMD) −5.34; 95% confidence interval (CI) −6.40 to −4.27) and water gymnastics reduced pain intensity and back pain-related sick leave (relative risk (RR) 0.40; 95% CI 0.17 to 0.92) better than usual prenatal care alone.

The specially-designed Ozzlo pillow was more effective than a regular one in relieving back pain (RR 1.84; 95% CI 1.32 to 2.55), but is no longer commercially available. Both acupuncture and stabilising exercises relieved pelvic pain more than usual prenatal care. Acupuncture gave more relief from evening pain than exercises. For women with both pelvic and back pain, in one study, acupuncture was more effective than physiotherapy in reducing the intensity of their pain; stretching exercises resulted in more total pain relief (60%) than usual care (11%); and 60% of those who received acupuncture reported less intense pain, compared to 14% of those receiving usual prenatal care. Women who received usual prenatal care reported more use of analgesics, physical modalities and sacroiliac belts.

AUTHORS' CONCLUSIONS: All but one study had moderate to high potential for bias, so results must be viewed cautiously. Adding pregnancy-specific exercises, physiotherapy or acupuncture to usual prenatal care appears to relieve back or pelvic pain more than usual prenatal care alone, although the effects are small. We do not know if they actually prevent pain from starting in the first place. Water gymnastics appear to help women stay at work. Acupuncture shows better results compared to physiotherapy.

INTERVENTIONS FOR TREATING CONSTIPATION IN PREGNANCY: fibre supplements were effective; stimulant laxatives were more effective than bulk-forming laxatives, but with more side-effects. (Jewell DJ, Young G) CD001142

BACKGROUND: Constipation is a common problem in late pregnancy. Circulating progesterone may be the cause of slower gastrointestinal movement in mid and late pregnancy.

OBJECTIVES: The objective of this review was to assess the effects of different methods for treating constipation in pregnancy.

METHODS: Standard PCG methods (see page xvii). Search date: January 2001.

MAIN RESULTS: Two suitable trials were identified. Fibre supplements increase the frequency of defaecation (odds ratio 0.18, 95% confidence interval 0.05 to 0.67), and lead to softer stools. Stimulant laxatives are more effective than bulk-forming laxatives (odds ratio 0.30, 95% confidence interval 0.14 to 0.61), but may cause more side-effects.

AUTHORS' CONCLUSIONS: Dietary supplements of fibre in the form of bran or wheat fibre are likely to help women experiencing constipation in pregnancy. If the problem fails to resolve, stimulant laxatives are likely to prove more effective.

> **INTERVENTIONS FOR VARICOSE VEINS AND LEG OEDEMA IN PREGNANCY:** rutoside was effective in relieving symptoms of leg oedema and varicosity; immersion in water at 32 °C reduced proxy measures; there was not enough evidence on external pneumatic compression. (Bamigboye AA, Smyth R) CD001066

BACKGROUND: Pregnancy is presumed to be a major contributory factor in the increased incidence of varicose veins in women, which can in turn lead to venous insufficiency and leg oedema. The most common symptom of varicose veins and oedema is the substantial pain experienced, as well as night cramps, numbness, tingling and the legs may feel heavy, achy and possibly be unsightly. Treatments of varicose veins are usually divided into three main groups: surgery, pharmacological and non-pharmacological treatments. Treatments of leg oedema comprise mostly of symptom reduction rather than cure and use pharmacological and non-pharmacological approaches.

OBJECTIVES: To assess any form of intervention used to relieve the symptoms associated with varicose veins and leg oedema in pregnancy.

METHODS: Standard PCG methods (see page xvii). Search date: October 2006.

MAIN RESULTS: Three trials, involving 159 women, were included.

Varicose veins
One trial, involving 69 women, reported that rutoside significantly reduced the symptoms associated with varicose veins (relative risk (RR) 1.89, 95% confidence interval (CI) 1.11 to 3.22). There were no significant differences in side-effects (RR 0.86, 95% CI 0.13 to 5.79) or incidence of deep vein thrombosis (RR 0.17, 95% CI 0.01 to 3.49).

Oedema

One trial, involving 35 women, reported no significant difference in lower leg volume when compression stockings were compared against rest (weighted mean difference −258.80, 95% CI −566.91 to 49.31). Another trial, involving 55 women, compared reflexology with rest. Reflexology significantly reduced the symptoms associated with oedema (reduction in symptoms: RR 9.09, 95% CI 1.41 to 58.54). There was no evidence of significant difference in the women's satisfaction and acceptability with either intervention (RR 6.00, 95% CI 0.92 to 39.11).

AUTHORS' CONCLUSIONS: Rutosides appear to help relieve the symptoms of varicose veins in late pregnancy. However, this finding is based on one small study (69 women) and there are not enough data presented in the study to assess its safety in pregnancy. It therefore cannot be routinely recommended. Reflexology appears to help improve symptoms for women with leg oedema, but again this is based on one small study (43 women). External compression stockings do not appear to have any advantages in reducing oedema.

2.7 Use of medicines during pregnancy

With the exception of large molecules such as heparin, and topical applications which are not absorbed, most medicines given to pregnant or breastfeeding women may reach their baby. While some medicines and vaccines have well-defined dangers and are contra-indicated, knowledge about risks to the baby of many medicines is sketchy. Decisions about the use of medicines during pregnancy need to balance the benefits to the mother with the known and potential risks to the baby, in relation to the stage of pregnancy. 'Tried and tested' remedies tend to be favoured because of the greater likelihood that unexpected harms would have surfaced over time.

The litany of physical and mental ill-health in the offspring of women treated with diethylstilboestrol for two decades after it was known to be ineffective underscores the importance of avoiding medicines or other interventions in pregnancy which have not been shown to be effective (see 'Oestrogen supplementation, mainly diethylstilbestrol, for preventing miscarriages and other adverse pregnancy outcomes', page 45) Effective medicines have a chance of doing more good than harm. Ineffective medicines do not.

MODIFICATIONS OF MATERNAL CAFFEINE INTAKE FOR IMPROVING PREGNANCY OUTCOME: (Jahanfar S, Sharifah H) Protocol [*see* page xviii] CD006965

ABRIDGED BACKGROUND: Studies investigating antenatal caffeine intake and pregnancy outcome have had mixed results. Animal studies suggest that caffeine is teratogenic when administered in large amounts. Excessive maternal caffeine consumption may lead to utero-placental vasoconstriction, fetal tachycardia and arrhythmias and, as a consequence, fetal hypoxia. Some authors have concluded that caffeine intake is harmful, causing stillbirth and fetal death; some that it has no effect; and others that it is beneficial in reducing the risk of gestational diabetes mellitus.

OBJECTIVES: To assess the effects of either avoidance of caffeine or caffeine supplementation used by mother on pregnancy outcome.

2.8   Miscarriage

Miscarriage is so common that it is accepted by professionals as part of the normal reproductive process. About 20% of recognised pregnancies miscarry, and for biochemically diagnosed pregnancies the rate may be as high as 50%. The great majority of miscarriages occur in the first trimester and are associated with sporadic chromosomal errors incompatible with life. Efforts to prolong such pregnancies would be misplaced.

A small proportion of miscarriages may be amenable to prediction, and prevention. In general, miscarriages are investigated if they differ from the common pattern of 'chromosomal' miscarriage (e.g. if they occur after the first trimester), or if they are 'recurrent' (three consecutive spontaneous miscarriages).

The clinical pattern of second trimester miscarriages differs according to the underlying cause. Impaired placental function may present with impaired growth of the baby, reduced amniotic fluid volume and death of the baby preceding miscarriage; the first intimation of cervical incompetence may be rupture of the amniotic sac, followed by relatively painless loss of a live or recently live baby.

Because miscarriage is so common, medical professionals may lose sight of the fact that, for women and their families, loss of a child through miscarriage may be a deeply felt loss. Professionals may cause unnecessary additional suffering by thoughtless actions such as use of the word 'abortion' (which in lay terms implies active termination of the pregnancy) and failing to support the grieving process.

Care of women with miscarriage requires considerable empathy and understanding. Most women will want to know at least three things, even if they do not verbalise the questions: 'what was the cause?'; 'was it my fault?'; and 'will it happen again?'

2.8.1 Prevention

Many strategies have been tried to prevent miscarriage in women with increased risk due to previous history of miscarriage or current complications such as vaginal bleeding.

ANTICOAGULANTS FOR THE TREATMENT OF RECURRENT PREGNANCY LOSS IN WOMEN WITHOUT ANTIPHOSPHOLIPID SYNDROME: not enough data to provide reliable evidence. (Di Nisio M, Peters LW, Middeldorp S) CD004734

BACKGROUND: Since hypercoagulability might result in recurrent pregnancy loss, anticoagulant agents could potentially increase the livebirth rate in subsequent pregnancies in women with either inherited thrombophilia or unexplained pregnancy loss.
OBJECTIVES: To evaluate the efficacy and safety of anticoagulant agents, such as aspirin and heparin, in women with a history of at least two spontaneous miscarriages or one later intrauterine fetal death without apparent causes other than inherited thrombophilias.
METHODS: Standard PCG methods (see page xvii). Search date: March 2004.
MAIN RESULTS: Two studies (242 participants) were included in the review and for both of them data were extracted for the subgroups of women fulfilling the inclusion criteria of the review. In one study,

54 pregnant women with recurrent spontaneous abortion without detectable anticardiolipin antibodies were randomised to low-dose aspirin or placebo. Similar live-birth rates were observed with aspirin and placebo (relative risk (RR) 1.00, 95% confidence interval (CI) 0.78 to 1.29). In another study, a subgroup of 20 women who had had a previous fetal loss after the 20th week and had a thrombophilic defect were randomised to enoxaparin or aspirin. Enoxaparin treatment resulted in an increased live-birth rate, as compared to low-dose aspirin (RR 10.00, 95% CI 1.56 to 64.20).

AUTHORS' CONCLUSIONS: The evidence on the efficacy and safety of thromboprophylaxis with aspirin and heparin in women with a history of at least two spontaneous miscarriages or one later intrauterine fetal death without apparent causes other than inherited thrombophilias is too limited to recommend the use of anticoagulants in this setting. Large, randomised, placebo-controlled trials are urgently needed.

> **BED REST DURING PREGNANCY FOR PREVENTING MISCARRIAGE:** not enough data to provide reliable evidence. (Aleman A, Althabe F, Belizán J, Bergel E) CD003576 (in RHL 11)

BACKGROUND: Miscarriage is pregnancy loss before 23 weeks of gestational age and it happens in 10% to 15% of pregnancies depending on maternal age and parity. It is associated with chromosomal defects in about a half or two thirds of cases. Many interventions have been used to prevent miscarriage but bed rest is probably the most commonly prescribed, especially in cases of threatened miscarriage and history of previous miscarriage. Since the aetiology of miscarriage in most of the cases is not related to an excess of activity, it is unlikely that bed rest could be an effective strategy to reduce spontaneous miscarriage.

OBJECTIVES: To evaluate the effect of prescription of bed rest during pregnancy to prevent miscarriage in women at high risk of miscarriage.

METHODS: Standard PCG methods (see page xvii). Search date: October 2007.

MAIN RESULTS: Only two studies including 84 women were identified. There was no statistically significant difference in the risk of miscarriage in the bed rest group versus the no bed rest group (placebo or other treatment) (relative risk (RR) 1.54, 95% confidence interval (CI)

0.92 to 2.58). Neither bed rest in hospital nor bed rest at home showed a significant difference in the prevention of miscarriage. There was a higher risk of miscarriage in those women in the bed rest group than in those in the human chorionic gonadotrophin therapy group with no bed rest (RR 2.50, 95% CI 1.22 to 5.11). It seems that the small number of participants included in these studies is a main factor to make this analysis inconclusive.

AUTHORS' CONCLUSIONS: There is insufficient evidence of high quality that supports a policy of bed rest in order to prevent miscarriage in women with confirmed fetal viability and vaginal bleeding in the first half of pregnancy.

IMMUNOTHERAPY FOR RECURRENT MISCARRIAGE: was not shown to be effective for improving the live birth rate. (Porter TF, LaCoursiere Y, Scott JR) CD000112

BACKGROUND: Because immunological aberrations might be the cause of miscarriage in some women, several immunotherapies have been used to treat women with otherwise unexplained recurrent pregnancy loss.

OBJECTIVES: To assess the effects of any immunotherapy, including paternal leukocyte immunization and intravenous immune globulin on the live birth rate in women with previous unexplained recurrent miscarriages.

METHODS: Standard PCG methods (see page xvii). Search date: December 2005.

MAIN RESULTS: 20 trials of high quality were included. The various forms of immunotherapy did not show significant differences between treatment and control groups in terms of subsequent live births: paternal cell immunization (12 trials, 641 women), Peto odds ratio (Peto OR) 1.23, 95% confidence interval (CI) 0.89 to 1.70; third party donor cell immunization (three trials, 156 women), Peto OR 1.39, 95% CI 0.68 to 2.82; trophoblast membrane infusion (one trial, 37 women), Peto OR 0.40, 95% CI 0.11 to 1.45; intravenous immune globulin, Peto OR 0.98, 95% CI 0.61 to 1.58.

AUTHORS' CONCLUSIONS: Paternal cell immunization, third party donor leukocytes, trophoblast membranes, and intravenous immune

globulin provide no significant beneficial effect over placebo in improving the live birth rate.

⊗ **OESTROGEN SUPPLEMENTATION, MAINLY DIETHYLSTILBES-TROL, FOR PREVENTING MISCARRIAGES AND OTHER ADVERSE PREGNANCY OUTCOMES:** was ineffective, with multiple long-term complications for the offspring. (Bamigboye AA, Morris J) CD004353

BACKGROUND: Laboratory evidence in the 1940s demonstrated a positive role of placental hormones in the continuation of pregnancy. It was suggested that diethylstilbestrol was the oestrogen of choice for prevention of miscarriages. Observational studies were carried out with apparently positive results, on which clinical practice was based. This led to a worldwide usage of diethylstilbestrol despite controlled studies with contrary findings.

OBJECTIVES: To determine the effects of antenatal administration of oestrogens, mainly diethylstilbestrol, on high risk and unselected pregnancy as regards miscarriages and other outcomes.

METHODS: Standard PCG methods (see page xvii). Search date: November 2002.

MAIN RESULTS: Miscarriage, preterm labour, low birthweight and stillbirth or neonatal death were not positively influenced by the intervention (diethylstilbestrol) as compared to the control group. Diethylstilbestrol in utero exposure led to increased rate of miscarriage and preterm birth. There was also an increase in the numbers of babies weighing less than 2500 grams. The maternal outcome in terms of pre-eclampsia was not influenced. Exposed female offspring have a non-significant trend towards more cancer of the genital tract and cancer other than of the genital tract. Primary infertility, adenosis of the vagina/cervix in female offspring and testicular abnormality in male offspring were significantly higher in those exposed to diethylstilbestrol before birth.

AUTHORS' CONCLUSIONS: There was no benefit with the use of diethylstilbestrol in preventing miscarriages. Both short and long-term adverse outcomes in exposed offspring were demonstration of the harm that this intervention caused women and their offspring during its usage.

PREVENTION OF RECURRENT MISCARRIAGE FOR WOMEN WITH ANTIPHOSPHOLIPID ANTIBODY OR LUPUS ANTICOAGULANT:

heparin reduced the risk of miscarriage; there was no reduced risk of miscarriage with aspirin, prednisone nor intravenous immunoglobulin. (Empson M, Lassere M, Craig J, Scott J) CD002859 (in RHL 11)

BACKGROUND: A range of treatments have been proposed to improve pregnancy outcome in recurrent pregnancy loss associated with antiphospholipid antibody (APL). Small studies have not resolved uncertainty about benefits and risks.

OBJECTIVES: To examine outcomes of all treatments given to maintain pregnancy in women with prior miscarriage and APL.

METHODS: Standard PCG methods (see page xvii). Search date: May 2004.

MAIN RESULTS: 13 studies were found (849 participants). The quality was not high; 50% had clear evidence of allocation concealment. Participant characteristics varied between trials.

Unfractionated heparin combined with aspirin (two trials; n = 140) significantly reduced pregnancy loss compared to aspirin alone (relative risk (RR) 0.46, 95% confidence interval (CI) 0.29 to 0.71). Low molecular weight heparin (LMWH) combined with aspirin compared to aspirin (one trial; n = 98) did not significantly reduce pregnancy loss (RR 0.78, 95% CI 0.39 to 1.57). There was no advantage in high-dose, over low-dose, unfractionated heparin (one trial; n = 50). Three trials of aspirin alone (n = 135) showed no significant reduction in pregnancy loss (RR 1.05, 95% CI 0.66 to 1.68). Prednisone and aspirin (three trials; n = 286) resulted in a significant increase in prematurity when compared to placebo, aspirin, and heparin combined with aspirin, and an increase in gestational diabetes, but no significant benefit. Intravenous immunoglobulin +/− unfractionated heparin and aspirin (two trials; n = 58) was associated with an increased risk of pregnancy loss or premature birth when compared to unfractionated heparin or LMWH combined with aspirin (RR 2.51, 95% CI 1.27 to 4.95). When compared to prednisone and aspirin, intravenous immunoglobulin (one trial; n = 82) was not significantly different in outcomes.

AUTHORS' CONCLUSIONS: Combined unfractionated heparin and aspirin may reduce pregnancy loss by 54%. Large, randomised

controlled trials with adequate allocation concealment are needed to explore potential differences between unfractionated heparin and LMWH.

> **PROGESTOGEN FOR PREVENTING MISCARRIAGE:** appeared to reduce the risk of miscarriage only in the subgroup of women with recurrent miscarriage. (Oates-Whitehead RM, Haas DM, Carrier JAK) CD003511 (in RHL 11)

BACKGROUND: Progesterone, a female sex hormone, is known to induce secretory changes in the lining of the uterus essential for successful implantation of a fertilized egg. It has been suggested that a causative factor in many cases of miscarriage may be inadequate secretion of progestogens. Therefore, progestational agents have been used, beginning in the first trimester of pregnancy, in an attempt to prevent spontaneous miscarriage.

OBJECTIVES: To determine the efficacy and safety of progestogens as a preventative therapy against miscarriage.

METHODS: Standard PCG methods (see page xvii). Search date: April 2003.

MAIN RESULTS: 14 trials (1988 women) met the inclusion criteria. The meta-analysis of all women, regardless of gravidity and number of previous miscarriages, showed no statistically significant difference in the risk of miscarriage between progestogen and placebo or no treatment groups (odds ratio (OR) 1.05, 95% confidence interval (CI) 0.83 to 1.34) and no statistically significant difference in the incidence of adverse effect in either mother or baby.

In a subgroup analysis of three trials involving women who had recurrent miscarriages (three or more consecutive miscarriages), progestogen treatment showed a statistically significant decrease in miscarriage rate compared to placebo or no treatment (OR 0.39, 95% CI 0.17 to 0.91). No statistically significant differences were found between the route of administration of progestogen (oral, intramuscular, vaginal) versus placebo or no treatment.

AUTHORS' CONCLUSIONS: There is no evidence to support the routine use of progestogen to prevent miscarriage in early to mid pregnancy. However, further trials in women with a history of recurrent miscarriage may be warranted, given the trend for improved live birth rates

in these women and the finding of no statistically significant difference between treatment and control groups in rates of adverse effects suffered by either mother or baby in the available evidence.

> **VITAMIN SUPPLEMENTATION FOR PREVENTING MISCARRIAGE:** was found not to be effective; multiple pregnancy was increased; pre-eclampsia was reduced. (Rumbold A, Middleton P, Crowther CA) CD004073

BACKGROUND: Miscarriage is a common complication of pregnancy that can be caused by a wide range of factors. Poor dietary intake of vitamins has been associated with an increased risk of miscarriage, therefore supplementing women with vitamins either prior to or in early pregnancy may help prevent miscarriage.

OBJECTIVES: To determine the effectiveness and safety of any vitamin supplementation, on the risk of spontaneous miscarriage, maternal adverse outcomes and fetal and infant adverse outcomes.

METHODS: Standard PCG methods (see page xvii). Search date: September 2004.

MAIN RESULTS: We identified 17 trials assessing supplementation with any vitamin(s) starting prior to 20 weeks' gestation and reporting at least one primary outcome that were eligible for the review. Overall, the included trials involved 35 812 women and 37 353 pregnancies. Two trials were cluster randomised and contributed data for 20 758 women and 22 299 pregnancies in total. No difference was seen between women taking any vitamins compared with controls for total fetal loss (relative risk (RR) 1.05, 95% confidence interval (CI) 0.95 to 1.15), early or late miscarriage (RR 1.08, 95% CI 0.95 to 1.24) or stillbirth (RR 0.85, 95% CI 0.63 to 1.14) and most of the other primary outcomes, using fixed-effect models. For the other primary outcomes, women given any type of vitamin(s) compared with controls were less likely to develop pre-eclampsia (RR 0.68, 95% CI 0.54 to 0.85, four trials, 5580 women) and more likely to have a multiple pregnancy (RR 1.38, 95% CI 1.12 to 1.70, three trials, 20 986 women).

AUTHORS' CONCLUSIONS: Taking vitamin supplements, alone or in combination with other vitamins, prior to pregnancy or in early pregnancy does not prevent women experiencing miscarriage or stillbirth. However, women taking vitamin supplements may be less likely to develop pre-eclampsia and more likely to have a multiple pregnancy.

2.8.2 Treatment of threatened miscarriage

Bleeding from the uterus in early pregnancy may cause considerable anxiety. Parents may be anxious for 'something to be done', despite the lack of evidence of effectives.

> **PROGESTOGEN FOR TREATING THREATENED MISCARRIAGE:** not enough data to provide reliable evidence. (Wahabi HA, Abed Althagafi NF, Elawad M) CD005943

BACKGROUND: Miscarriage is a common complication encountered during pregnancy. The role of progesterone in preparing the uterus for the implantation of the embryo and its role in maintaining the pregnancy have been known for a long time. Inadequate secretion of progesterone in early pregnancy has been linked to the aetiology of miscarriage and progesterone supplementation has been used as a treatment for threatened miscarriage to prevent spontaneous pregnancy loss.

OBJECTIVES: To determine the efficacy and the safety of progestogens in the treatment of threatened miscarriage.

METHODS: Standard PCG methods (see page xvii). Search date: December 2006.

MAIN RESULTS: Two studies (84 participants) were included in the meta-analysis. In one study, all the participants met the inclusion criteria, and in the other study, only the subgroup of participants who met the inclusion criteria was included in the meta-analysis. There was no evidence of effectiveness with the use of vaginal progesterone compared to placebo in reducing the risk of miscarriage (relative risk 0.47; 95% confidence interval (CI) 0.17 to 1.30).

AUTHORS' CONCLUSIONS: Based on scarce data from two methodologically poor trials, there is no evidence to support the routine use of progestogens for the treatment of threatened miscarriage. Information about potential harms to the mother or child, or both, with the use of progestogens is lacking. Further, larger, randomized controlled trials on the effect of progestogens on the treatment of threatened miscarriage, which investigate potential harms as well as benefits, are needed.

> **UTERINE MUSCLE RELAXANT DRUGS FOR THREATENED MISCARRIAGE:** not enough data to provided reliable evidence. (Lede R, Duley L) CD002857

BACKGROUND: Miscarriage is the spontaneous loss of a pregnancy before the fetus is viable. Uterine muscle relaxant drugs have been used for women at risk of miscarriage in the belief that they relax uterine muscle, and hence reduce the risk of miscarriage.

OBJECTIVES: To assess the effects for the woman and her baby of uterine muscle relaxant drugs when used for threatened miscarriage.

METHODS: Standard PCG methods (see page xvii). Search date: May 2004.

MAIN RESULTS: One poor quality trial (170 women) was included. This compared a beta-agonist with placebo. There was a lower risk of intrauterine death associated with the use of a beta-agonist (relative risk (RR) 0.25, 95% confidence interval (CI) 0.12 to 0.51). Preterm birth was the only other outcome reported (RR 1.67, 95% CI 0.63 to 4.38).

AUTHORS' CONCLUSIONS: There is insufficient evidence to support the use of uterine muscle relaxant drugs for women with threatened miscarriage. Any such use should be restricted to the context of randomised trials.

2.8.3   Treatment of miscarriage

Traditionally, miscarriage has been treated by surgically evacuating the uterus. The options of medical or expectant management are receiving increasing attention.

> ☺ **EXPECTANT CARE VERSUS SURGICAL TREATMENT FOR MIS-CARRIAGE:** was associated with more days of bleeding; more incomplete miscarriages; more unplanned surgery; less infection. (Nanda K, Peloggia A, Grimes D, Lopez L, Nanda G) CD003518 (in RHL 11)

BACKGROUND: Miscarriage is a common complication of early pregnancy that can have both medical and psychological consequences like depression and anxiety. The need for routine surgical evacuation with miscarriage has been questioned because of potential complications such as cervical trauma, uterine perforation, hemorrhage, or infection.

OBJECTIVES: To compare the safety and effectiveness of expectant management versus surgical treatment for early pregnancy loss.

METHODS: Standard PCG methods (see page xvii). Search date: December 2005.

MAIN RESULTS: Five trials were included in this review with 689 total participants. The expectant-care group was more likely to have an incomplete miscarriage (RR 5.37; 95% CI 2.57 to 11.22). However, the time frames for declaring the process incomplete varied across the studies. The need for unplanned surgical treatment (such as vacuum aspiration or D&C) was greater for the expectant-care group (RR 4.78; 95% CI 1.99 to 11.48). The expectant-care group had more days of bleeding (WMD 1.59; 95% CI 0.74 to 2.45) and a greater amount of bleeding (WMD 1.00; 95% CI 0.60 to 1.40). Post-procedure diagnosis of infection was lower in the expectant-care group (RR 0.29; 95% CI 0.09 to 0.87). Information on psychological outcomes and pregnancy was too limited to draw conclusions.

AUTHORS' CONCLUSIONS: Expectant management led to a higher risk of incomplete miscarriage, need for surgical emptying of the uterus, and bleeding. None of these were serious. In contrast, surgical evacuation was associated with a significantly higher risk of infection. Given the lack of clear superiority of either approach, the woman's preference should play a dominant role in decision making. Medical management has added choices for women and their clinicians, but these were not reviewed here.

> **MEDICAL TREATMENT FOR EARLY FETAL DEATH (LESS THAN 24 WEEKS):** vaginal misoprostol reduced the need for surgical curettage; was more effective than dinoprostone, oral misoprostol or lower dose misoprostol and similar to gemeprost; sublingual misoprostone had more side-effects; moistened vaginal misopostol, adding methotrexate and adding laminaria tents were not effective; mifepristone results were conflicting. (Neilson JP, Hickey M, Vazquez J) CD002253 (in RHL 11)

BACKGROUND: In most pregnancies that miscarry, arrest of embryonic or fetal development occurs some time (often weeks) before the miscarriage occurs. Ultrasound examination can reveal abnormal findings during this phase by demonstrating anembryonic pregnancies or embryonic or fetal death. Treatment before 14 weeks has traditionally been surgical but medical treatments may be effective, safe and acceptable, as may be waiting for spontaneous miscarriage.

OBJECTIVES: To assess the effectiveness, safety and acceptability of any medical treatment for early pregnancy failure (anembryonic pregnancies or embryonic and fetal deaths before 24 weeks).

METHODS: Standard PCG methods (see page xvii). Search date: November 2005.

MAIN RESULTS: 24 studies (1888 women) were included.

Vaginal misoprostol hastens miscarriage (complete or incomplete) when compared with placebo: e.g. miscarriage less than 24 hours (two trials, 138 women, relative risk (RR) 4.73, 95% confidence interval (CI) 2.70 to 8.28), with less need for uterine curettage (two trials, 104 women, RR 0.40, 95% CI 0.26 to 0.60) and no significant increase in nausea or diarrhoea. Lower-dose regimens of vaginal misoprostol tend to be less effective in producing miscarriage (three trials, 247 women, RR 0.85, 95% CI 0.72 to 1.00), with similar incidence of nausea. There seems no clear advantage to administering a 'wet' preparation of vaginal misoprostol or of adding methotrexate, or of using laminaria tents after 14 weeks. Vaginal misoprostol is more effective than vaginal prostaglandin E in avoiding surgical evacuation. Oral misoprostol was less effective than vaginal misoprostol in producing complete miscarriage (two trials, 218 women, RR 0.90, 95% CI 0.82 to 0.99). Sublingual misoprostol had equivalent efficacy to vaginal misoprostol in inducing complete miscarriage but was associated with more frequent diarrhoea. The two trials of mifepristone treatment generated conflicting results. There was no statistically significant difference between vaginal misoprostol and gemeprost in the induction of miscarriage for fetal death after 13 weeks.

AUTHORS' CONCLUSIONS: Available evidence from randomised trials supports the use of vaginal misoprostol as a medical treatment to terminate non-viable pregnancies before 24 weeks. Further research is required to assess effectiveness and safety, optimal route of administration and dose. Conflicting findings about the value of mifepristone need to be resolved by additional study.

☺ **SURGICAL PROCEDURES TO EVACUATE INCOMPLETE ABORTION:** manual vacuum aspiration was preferable to traditional dilatation and curettage in several respects. (Forna F, Gülmezoglu AM) CD001993 (in RHL 11)

BACKGROUND: Incomplete abortion is a major problem that should be effectively managed with safe and appropriate procedures. Surgical evacuation of the uterus for management of incomplete abortion usually involves vacuum aspiration or sharp curettage.

OBJECTIVES: To compare the safety and effectiveness of surgical uterine evacuation methods for management of incomplete abortion.

METHODS: Standard PCG methods (see page xvii). Search date: December 2002.

MAIN RESULTS: Two trials were included. Vacuum aspiration was associated with statistically significantly decreased blood loss (−17 ml weighted mean difference, 95% confidence interval (CI) −24 to −10 ml), less pain (relative risk (RR): 0.74, 95% CI 0.61–0.90), and shorter duration of procedure (−1.2 minutes weighted mean difference, 95% CI −1.5 to −0.87 minutes) than sharp curettage, in the single study that evaluated these outcomes. Serious complications such as uterine perforation and other morbidity were rare and the sample sizes of the trials were not large enough to evaluate small or moderate differences.

AUTHORS' CONCLUSIONS: Vacuum aspiration is safe, quick to perform, and less painful than sharp curettage, and should be recommended for use in the management of incomplete abortion. Analgesia and sedation should be provided as necessary for the procedure.

COMBINATION CHEMOTHERAPY FOR HIGH-RISK GESTATIONAL TROPHOBLASTIC TUMOUR: not enough data to provide reliable evidence. (Xue Y, Zhang J, Wu TX, An RF) CD005196 (Gynaecological Cancer Group)

BACKGROUND: Gestational trophoblastic disease (GTD) includes gestational trophoblastic tumour (GTT) and hydatidiform mole. Many women of reproductive age are affected by this disease although its incidence differs by geographical location. A number of chemotherapy regimens are used for treating the disease, such as methotrexate, actinomycin D and cyclophosphamide (MAC), methotrexate, actinomycin D, cyclophosphamide, doxorubicin, melphalan, hydroxyurea and vincristine (CHAMOC), etoposide, methotrexate and actinomycin (EMA) plus cyclophosphamide and vincristine (CO) (EMA-CO), and etoposide, methotrexate and actinomycin (EMA) plus etoposide and cisplatin (EP) (EMA-EP). The efficacy of these drugs has not been systematically reviewed.

OBJECTIVES: To determine the efficacy and safety of combination chemotherapy in treating high-risk GTT.

SEARCH STRATEGY: Electronic searches of MEDLINE, EMB, Cochrane Central Register of Controlled Trials (CENTRAL) and CBM were carried out. Four journals were handsearched and other searching methods were used for identifying more studies.

SELECTION CRITERIA: The review included randomized controlled trials (RCTs) or quasi-RCTs of combination chemotherapy for treating high-risk GTT. Patients with placental-site trophoblastic tumour (PSTT), who had received chemotherapy in the previous two weeks, or patients with chemotherapy intolerance were excluded.

DATA COLLECTION AND ANALYSIS: Two investigators independently collected data using a data extraction form. Meta-analysis was not performed and the review was conducted as a narrative review

MAIN RESULTS: One study with 42 participants was included in this review. It indicated that a MAC regimen was better than a CHAMOCA regimen for high-risk GTT because of lower toxicity. The quality of the study was unclear.

AUTHORS' CONCLUSIONS: The methodological limitations of the included study prevent any firm conclusions about the best combination chemotherapy regimen for high-risk GTT. High quality studies are required.

Chapter 3: Medical Problems During Pregnancy

3.1 Hypertension during pregnancy

In 1969 Carey wrote: 'The concept of a circulating toxin as the cause of raised blood pressure and albuminuria in pregnancy has now been discarded and it is to be hoped that the term "toxaemia" will suffer a similar fate' (HM Carey in Donald I, *Practical Obstetric Problems*, 4th ed., 1969; 239). We have come full circle in the light of evidence of endotheliotoxic substances originating in the placenta.

This section includes evidence on the prevention, detection and care of women with hypertensive disorders of pregnancy

3.1.1 Preventing hypertensive disorders

> **INTERVENTIONS FOR PREVENTING PRE-ECLAMPSIA AND ITS CONSEQUENCES: GENERIC PROTOCOL.** (Meher S, Duley L, on behalf of the Prevention of Pre-eclampsia Cochrane Review authors) Protocol CD005301

ABRIDGED BACKGROUND: Hypertension (high blood pressure) is common during pregnancy. For women who have hypertension alone, pregnancy outcome is similar to that for women with normal blood pressure. Outcome deteriorates once proteinuria develops. Women with mild pre-eclampsia generally have no symptoms. Women with severe pre-eclampsia or very high blood pressure may feel unwell with symptoms such as headache, upper abdominal pain or visual disturbances. Rare but serious complications include eclampsia (seizures in a woman with pre-eclampsia), stroke, HELLP syndrome (haemolysis, elevated liver enzymes and low platelets) and disseminated intravascular coagulation.

A Cochrane Pocketbook: Pregnancy and Childbirth   G.J. Hofmeyr et al.
Copyright © 2008, Z. Alfiervic, C. A. Crowther, L. Duley, A. M. Gulmezoglu, G. ML. Gyte , E. D. Hodnett, G. J. Hofmeyr, J. P. Neilson

These complications are associated with an increased risk of maternal death. The placenta is also involved in pre-eclampsia, and so risks for the baby are increased. The most common problems are those related to poor growth and premature birth.

Four main categories of hypertensive disorders of pregnancy are now widely agreed.

(1) *Gestational hypertension or pregnancy-induced hypertension*
    This is hypertension detected for the first time during the second half of pregnancy (after 20 weeks gestation) in the absence of proteinuria. It resolves within three months of birth.
(2) *Pre-eclampsia/eclampsia*
    Pre-eclampsia is defined as hypertension and proteinuria detected for the first time in the second half of pregnancy (after 20 weeks gestation). Eclampsia is the occurrence of seizures in a woman with pre-eclampsia.
(3) *Chronic hypertension*
    This is hypertension known to be present before pregnancy, or detected before 20 weeks gestation.
(4) *Pre-eclampsia superimposed on chronic hypertension*
    Women with chronic hypertension may develop pre-eclampsia.

Despite a growing understanding of the pathophysiology of pre-eclampsia, the underlying cause of the syndrome remains unclear. Factors that appear to have a role include the placenta, maternal immune response, genetic predisposition, maternal vascular disease, and diet.

Current thinking is that inadequate blood supply to the placenta leads to the release of unknown factors or materials into the maternal circulation which activate or injure the endothelial cells, resulting in endothelial dysfunction (abnormal functioning of cells lining blood vessels). Endothelial dysfunction results in a series of changes including reduced production of vasodilators and anticoagulants (such as prostacyclin and nitric oxide), increased production of vasoconstrictors and platelet aggregators (such as thromboxane A2 and endothelin), increased responsiveness of endothelium to the vasopressor Angiotensin II, and an elevation in the proteins of the coagulation cascade (such as von Willebrand factor). These changes result in widespread vasoconstriction and activation of platelets and the coagulation system. Injured endothelial cells allow leakage of fluid out of the blood vessels and into surrounding tissues, causing oedema and a reduction in the circulating blood volume. There is then inadequate blood flow to many of the woman's organs, especially the kidneys, liver and brain. It is the vasoconstriction, micro clots and reduced circulating blood volume that result in the clinical manifestations of pre-eclampsia.

Routine screening for pre-eclampsia is based on measurement of blood pressure and urinalysis for proteinuria.

As the cause of pre-eclampsia is not completely understood, and screening tests remain unreliable, it is difficult to develop rational strategies for prevention of pre-eclampsia. Current strategies for prevention focus on antenatal surveillance, modification of lifestyle, nutritional supplementation and pharmacological therapy.

OBJECTIVES: To determine the effectiveness and safety of interventions for prevention of pre-eclampsia and its complications.

⊗ **DIURETICS FOR PREVENTING PRE-ECLAMPSIA:** No clear benefits found; significant adverse effects. More data needed. (D Churchill, C Rhodes, G Beevers) CD004451

BACKGROUND: Diuretics are used to reduce blood pressure and oedema in non-pregnant individuals. Formerly, they were used in pregnancy with the aim of preventing or delaying the development of pre-eclampsia. This practice became controversial when concerns were raised that diuretics may further reduce plasma volume in women with pre-eclampsia, thereby increasing the risk of adverse effects on the mother and baby, particularly fetal growth.

OBJECTIVES: To assess the effects of diuretics on prevention of pre-eclampsia and its complications.

METHODS: Standard methods (see page xvii). Search date: April 2005.

MAIN RESULTS: Five studies (1836 women) were included. All were of uncertain quality. The studies compared thiazide diuretics with either placebo or no intervention. There were no clear differences between the diuretic and control groups for any reported pregnancy outcomes including pre-eclampsia (four trials, 1391 women; relative risk (RR) 0.68, 95% confidence interval (CI) 0.45 to 1.03), perinatal death (five trials, 1836 women; RR 0.72, 95% CI 0.40 to 1.27), and preterm birth (two trials, 465 women; RR 0.67, 95% CI 0.32 to 1.41). There were no small-for-gestational age babies in the one trial that reported this outcome, and there was insufficient evidence to demonstrate any clear differences between the two groups for birthweight (one trial, 20 women; weighted mean difference 139 grams, 95% CI -484.40 to 762.40).

Thiazide diuretics were associated with an increased risk of nausea and vomiting (two trials, 1217 women; RR 5.81, 95% CI 1.04 to 32.46), and women allocated diuretics were more likely to stop treatment due to side-effects compared to those allocated placebo (two trials, 1217 women; RR 1.85, 95% CI 0.81 to 4.22).

AUTHORS' CONCLUSIONS: There is insufficient evidence to draw reliable conclusions about the effects of diuretics on prevention of pre-eclampsia and its complications. However, from this review, no clear benefits have been found from the use of diuretics to prevent pre-eclampsia. Taken together with the level of adverse effects found, the use of diuretics for the prevention of pre-eclampsia and its complications cannot be recommended.

REST DURING PREGNANCY FOR PREVENTING PRE-ECLAMPSIA AND ITS COMPLICATIONS IN WOMEN WITH NORMAL BLOOD PRESSURE: not enough data to provide reliable evidence. (Meher S, Duley L) CD005939

BACKGROUND: Women at risk of pre-eclampsia or gestational hypertension are sometimes advised to rest. Whether this does more good than harm overall is unclear.

OBJECTIVES: To assess the effects of rest or advice to reduce physical activity during pregnancy for preventing pre-eclampsia and its complications in women with normal blood pressure.

METHODS: Standard PCG methods (see page xvii). Search: December 2005.

MAIN RESULTS: Two small trials (106 women) of uncertain quality were included. Both recruited women with a singleton pregnancy at moderate risk of pre-eclampsia from 28 to 32 weeks' gestation. There was a statistically significant reduction in the relative risk of pre-eclampsia with four to six hours rest per day (one trial, 32 women; relative risk (RR) 0.05, 95% confidence interval (CI) 0.00 to 0.83), but not of gestational hypertension (RR 0.25, 95% CI 0.03 to 2.00), compared to normal activity. Rest of 30 minutes per day plus nutritional supplementation was associated with a reduction in the risk of pre-eclampsia (one trial, 74 women; RR 0.13, 95% CI 0.03 to 0.51) and also of gestational hypertension (RR 0.15, 95% CI 0.04 to 0.63). The effect on caesarean section was unclear (RR 0.82, 95% CI 0.48 to 1.41). No other outcomes were reported.

AUTHORS' CONCLUSIONS: **Daily rest, with or without nutrient supplementation, may reduce the risk of pre-eclampsia for women with normal blood pressure, although the reported effect may reflect bias and/or random error rather than a true effect. There is no information about outcomes such as perinatal mortality and morbidity, maternal morbidity, women's views, adverse effects, and costs. Current evidence is insufficient to support recommending rest or reduced activity to women for preventing pre-eclampsia and its complications. Whether women rest during pregnancy should therefore be a matter of personal choice.**

> ## EXERCISE OR OTHER PHYSICAL ACTIVITY FOR PREVENTING PRE-ECLAMPSIA AND ITS COMPLICATIONS: not enough data to provide reliable evidence. (Meher S, Duley L) CD005942

BACKGROUND: The association between an increase in regular physical activity and a reduction in the risk of hypertension is well documented for non-pregnant people. It has been suggested that exercise may help prevent pre-eclampsia and its complications. Possible adverse effects of increased physical activity during pregnancy, particularly on the risk of preterm birth and fetal growth restriction, are unclear. It is, therefore, important to assess whether exercise reduces the risk of pre-eclampsia and its complications and, if so, whether these benefits outweigh the risks.

OBJECTIVES: To assess the effects of exercise, or increased physical activity, on prevention of pre-eclampsia and its complications.

METHODS: Standard PCG methods (see page xvii). Search date: December 2005.

MAIN RESULTS: Two small, good quality trials (45 women) were included. Both compared moderate intensity regular aerobic exercise with maintenance of normal physical activity during pregnancy. The confidence intervals were wide and crossed the line of no effect for all reported outcomes including pre-eclampsia (relative risk 0.31, 95% confidence interval 0.01 to 7.09).

AUTHORS' CONCLUSIONS: There is insufficient evidence for reliable conclusions about the effects of exercise on prevention of pre-eclampsia and its complications.

> **GARLIC FOR PREVENTING PRE-ECLAMPSIA AND ITS COMPLI-CATIONS:** not enough data to provide reliable evidence. (Meher S, Duley L) CD006065

BACKGROUND: The suggestion that garlic may lower blood pressure, inhibit platelet aggregation and reduce oxidative stress has led to the hypothesis that it may have a role in preventing pre-eclampsia and its complications.

OBJECTIVES: To assess the effects of garlic on prevention of pre-eclampsia and its complications.

METHODS: Standard PCG methods (see page xvii). Search date: October 2007.

MAIN RESULTS: One trial (100 women) of uncertain quality compared garlic with placebo. Another study was excluded as 29% of women were lost to follow up. There was no clear difference between the garlic and control groups in the risk of developing gestational hypertension (relative risk (RR) 0.50, 95% confidence interval (CI) 0.25 to 1.00) or pre-eclampsia (RR 0.78, 95% CI 0.31 to 1.93). Women allocated garlic were more likely to report odour than those allocated placebo (RR 8.50, 95% CI 2.07 to 34.88), but there were no significant differences in other reported side-effects. The only other outcomes reported were caesarean section (RR 1.35, 95% CI 0.93 to 1.95) and perinatal mortality. There were no perinatal deaths in the study.

AUTHORS' CONCLUSIONS: There is insufficient evidence to recommend increased garlic intake for preventing pre-eclampsia and its complications. Although garlic is associated with odour, other more serious side-effects have not been reported. Further large randomised trials evaluating the effects of garlic are needed before any recommendations can be made to guide clinical practice.

> **ALTERED DIETARY SALT FOR PREVENTING PRE-ECLAMPSIA, AND ITS COMPLICATIONS:** was not found to be effective but there were not enough data to assess this intervention properly. (Duley L, Henderson-Smart D, Meher S) CD005548

BACKGROUND: In the past, women have been advised that lowering their salt intake might reduce their risk of developing pre-eclampsia. Although this practice has largely ceased, it remains important to assess the evidence about possible effects of altered dietary salt intake during pregnancy.

OBJECTIVES: To assess the effects of altered dietary salt during pregnancy on the risk of developing pre-eclampsia and its complications.

METHODS: Standard PCG methods (see page xvii). Search date: April 2005.

MAIN RESULTS: Two trials were included, with 603 women. Both compared advice to reduce dietary salt intake with advice to continue a normal diet. The confidence intervals were wide and crossed the no-effect line for all the reported outcomes, including pre-eclampsia (relative risk 1.11, 95% confidence interval 0.46 to 2.66). In other words, there was insufficient evidence for reliable conclusions about the effects of advice to reduce dietary salt.

AUTHORS' CONCLUSIONS: In the absence of evidence that advice to alter salt intake during pregnancy has any beneficial effect for prevention of pre-eclampsia or any other outcome, salt consumption during pregnancy should remain a matter of personal preference.

> **REDUCED SALT INTAKE COMPARED TO NORMAL DIETARY SALT, OR HIGH INTAKE, IN PREGNANCY:** not enough data to provide reliable evidence. (Duley L, Henderson-Smart D) CD001687

BACKGROUND: In the past women have been advised that lowering their salt intake might reduce their risk of pre-eclampsia. Although this practice has largely ceased, it remains important to assess the evidence about possible effects of advice to alter dietary salt intake during pregnancy.

OBJECTIVES: The objective of this review was to assess the effects of dietary advice to alter salt intake, compared to continuing a normal diet, on the risk of pre-eclampsia and its consequences.

METHODS: Standard PCG methods (see page xvii). Search date: October 1998.

MAIN RESULTS: Two trials were included, with 603 women. They compared advice about a low salt diet with no dietary advice. The confidence intervals for all of the outcomes reported were wide, and cross the no effect line. This includes pre-eclampsia (relative risk 1.11, 95% confidence interval 0.46 to 2.66). Even when taken together, these trials are insufficient to provide reliable information about the effects of advice on salt restriction during normal pregnancy. None of the trials included women with pre-eclampsia, so this review provides no reliable information about changes in salt intake for treatment of pre-eclampsia.

AUTHORS' CONCLUSIONS: Salt consumption during pregnancy should remain a matter of personal preference.

☺ **CALCIUM SUPPLEMENTATION DURING PREGNANCY FOR PREVENTING HYPERTENSIVE DISORDERS AND RELATED PROBLEMS:** reduced the incidence of pre-eclampsia and severe morbidity, particularly for women with low dietary calcium intake (Hofmeyr GJ, Atallah AN, Duley L) CD001059 (in RHL 11)

BACKGROUND: Pre-eclampsia and eclampsia are common causes of serious morbidity and death. Calcium supplementation may reduce the risk of pre-eclampsia through a number of mechanisms, and may help to prevent preterm labour.

OBJECTIVES: To assess the effects of calcium supplementation during pregnancy on hypertensive disorders of pregnancy and related maternal and child outcomes.

METHODS: Standard PCG methods (see page xvii). Search date: February 2006.

MAIN RESULTS: 12 studies of good quality were included. The risk of high blood pressure was reduced with calcium supplementation rather than placebo (11 trials, 14 946 women: relative risk (RR) 0.70, 95% confidence interval (CI) 0.57 to 0.86). There was also a reduction in the risk of pre-eclampsia associated with calcium supplementation (12 trials, 15 206 women: RR 0.48, 95% CI 0.33 to 0.69). The effect was greatest for high-risk women (five trials, 587 women: RR 0.22, 95% CI 0.12 to 0.42), and those with low baseline calcium intake (seven trials, 10 154 women: RR 0.36, 95% CI 0.18 to 0.70).

The composite outcome of maternal death or serious morbidity was reduced (four trials, 9732 women; RR 0.80, 0.65 to 0.97). Almost all the women in these trials were low risk and had a low calcium diet. Maternal deaths were reported in only one trial. One death occurred in the calcium group and six in the placebo group, a difference which was not statistically significant (RR 0.17, 95% CI 0.02 to 1.39).

There was no overall effect on the risk of preterm birth (10 trials, 14 751 women: RR 0.81, 95% CI 0.64 to 1.03), or stillbirth or death before discharge from hospital (10 trials 15 141 babies; RR 0.89, 95% CI 0.73 to 1.09).

Blood pressure in childhood has been assessed in one study: childhood systolic blood pressure greater than 95th percentile was reduced (514 children: RR 0.59, 95% CI 0.39 to 0.91).

AUTHORS' CONCLUSIONS: Calcium supplementation appears to almost halve the risk of pre-eclampsia, and to reduce the rare occurrence of the composite outcome 'death or serious morbidity'. There were no other clear benefits, or harms.

MARINE OIL, AND OTHER PROSTAGLANDIN PRECURSOR, SUPPLEMENTATION FOR PREGNANCY UNCOMPLICATED BY PRE-ECLAMPSIA OR INTRAUTERINE GROWTH RESTRICTION: decreased risk for birth before 34 weeks but there were not enough data to support routine use. (Makrides M, Duley L, Olsen SF) CD003402

BACKGROUND: Population studies have shown that higher intakes of marine foods during pregnancy are associated with longer gestations, higher infant birthweights and a low incidence of pre-eclampsia. It is suggested that the fatty acids of marine foods may be the underlying cause of these associations.

OBJECTIVES: To estimate the effects of marine oil, and other prostaglandin precursor, supplementation during pregnancy on the risk of pre-eclampsia, preterm birth, low birthweight and small-for-gestational age.

METHODS: Standard PCG methods (see page xvii). Search date: December 2005.

MAIN RESULTS: Six trials, involving 2783 women, are included in this review. Three of these were rated as high quality, including the largest trial with 1477 women. Women allocated a marine oil supplement had a mean gestation that was 2.6 days longer than women allocated to placebo or no treatment (weighted mean difference (WMD), 2.55 days, 95% confidence interval (CI) 1.03 to 4.07 days; three trials, 1621 women). This was not reflected in a clear difference between the two groups in the relative risk (RR) of birth before 37 completed weeks, although women allocated marine oil did have a lower risk of giving birth before 34 completed weeks' gestation (RR 0.69, 95% CI 0.49 to 0.99; two trials, 860 women). Birthweight was slightly greater in infants born to women in the marine oil group compared with control (WMD 47 g, 95% CI 1 g to 93 g; three trials, 2440 women). However, there were no overall differences between the groups in the proportion of low birthweight or small-for-gestational-age babies. There was no clear difference in the relative risk of pre-eclampsia between the two groups.

AUTHORS' CONCLUSIONS: There is not enough evidence to support the routine use of marine oil, or other prostaglandin precursor, supplements during pregnancy to reduce the risk of pre-eclampsia, preterm birth, low birthweight or small-for-gestational age.

⊗ **ANTIOXIDANTS FOR PREVENTING PRE-ECLAMPSIA:** vitamins C and E showed promise in earlier, poor quality studies. No benefit was found in more recent trials. (Rumbold A, Duley L, Crowther C, Haslam R) CD004227 (in RHL 11)

BACKGROUND: Oxidative stress has been proposed as a key factor involved in the development of pre-eclampsia. Supplementing women with antioxidants during pregnancy may help to counteract oxidative stress and thereby prevent or delay the onset of pre-eclampsia.

OBJECTIVES: To determine the effectiveness and safety of any antioxidant supplementation during pregnancy and the risk of developing pre-eclampsia and its related complications.

METHODS: Standard PCG methods (see page xvii). Search date: May 2007

MAIN RESULTS: Ten trials, involving 6533 women, were included in this review; five trials were rated high quality. For the majority of trials, the antioxidant assessed was combined vitamin C and E therapy. There was no significant difference between antioxidant and control groups for the relative risk (RR) of pre-eclampsia (RR 0.73, 95% confidence interval (CI) 0.51 to 1.06; nine trials, 5446 women) or any other primary outcome: severe pre-eclampsia (RR 1.25, 95% CI 0.89 to 1.76; two trials, 2495 women), preterm birth (before 37 weeks) (RR 1.10, 95% CI 0.99 to 1.22; five trials, 5198 women), small-for-gestational-age infants (RR 0.83, 95% CI 0.62 to 1.11; five trials,

5271 babies) or any baby death (RR 1.12, 95% CI 0.81 to 1.53; four trials, 5144 babies). Women allocated antioxidants were more likely to self-report abdominal pain late in pregnancy (RR 1.61, 95% CI 1.11 to 2.34; one trial, 1745 women), require antihypertensive therapy (RR 1.77, 95% CI 1.22 to 2.57; two trials, 4272 women) and require an antenatal hospital admission for hypertension (RR 1.54, 95% CI 1.00 to 2.39; one trial, 1877 women). However, for the latter two outcomes, this was not clearly reflected in an increase in any other hypertensive complications.

AUTHORS' CONCLUSIONS: Evidence from this review does not support routine antioxidant supplementation during pregnancy to reduce the risk of pre-eclampsia and other serious complications in pregnancy.

☺ **ANTIPLATELET AGENTS FOR PREVENTING PRE-ECLAMPSIA AND ITS COMPLICATIONS:** antiplatelet agents (largely low-dose aspirin) showed small to moderate benefit. (Duley L, Henderson-Smart DJ, Meher S, King JF) CD004659 (in RHL 11)

BACKGROUND: Pre-eclampsia is associated with deficient intravascular production of prostacyclin, a vasodilator, and excessive production of thromboxane, a vasoconstrictor and stimulant of platelet aggregation. These observations led to the hypotheses that antiplatelet agents, low-dose aspirin in particular, might prevent or delay development of pre-eclampsia.

OBJECTIVES: To assess the effectiveness and safety of antiplatelet agents for women at risk of developing pre-eclampsia.

METHODS: Standard PCG methods (see page xvii). Search date: July 2006.

MAIN RESULTS: 59 trials (37560 women) are included. There is a 17% reduction in the risk of pre-eclampsia associated with the use of antiplatelet agents ((46 trials, 32891 women, relative risk (RR) 0.83, 95% confidence interval (CI) 0.77 to 0.89), number needed to treat (NNT) 72 (52, 119)). Although there is no statistical difference in RR based on maternal risk, there is a significant increase in the absolute risk reduction of pre-eclampsia for high risk (risk difference (RD) −5.2% (−7.5, −2.9), NNT 19 (13, 34)) compared with moderate risk women (RD −0.84 (−1.37, −0.3), NNT 119 (73, 333)).

Antiplatelets were associated with an 8% reduction in the relative risk of preterm birth (29 trials, 31 151 women, RR 0.92, 95% CI 0.88 to 0.97); NNT 72 (52, 119)), a 14% reduction in fetal or neonatal deaths (40 trials, 33 098 women, RR 0.86, 95% CI 0.76 to 0.98)); NNT 243 (131, 1666) and a 10% reduction in small-for-gestational age babies (36 trials, 23 638 women, RR 0.90, 95% CI 0.83 to 0.98). There were no statistically significant differences between treatment and control groups for any other outcomes.

AUTHORS' CONCLUSIONS: Antiplatelet agents, largely low-dose aspirin, have moderate benefits when used for prevention of pre-eclampsia and its consequences. Further information is required to assess which women are most likely to benefit, when treatment is best started and at what dose.

NITRIC OXIDE FOR PREVENTING PRE-ECLAMPSIA AND ITS COMPLICATIONS: not enough data to provide reliable evidence. (Meher S, Duley L) CD006490

BACKGROUND: Pre-eclampsia, a multisystem disorder of pregnancy characterised by high blood pressure and protein in the urine, is associated with endothelial dysfunction. Nitric oxide mediates many functions of the endothelium, including vasodilatation and inhibition of platelet aggregation. Pre-eclampsia may be associated with nitric oxide deficiency, but the evidence to support this suggestion is contradictory. Nevertheless, it has been hypothesised that agents which increase nitric oxide may prevent pre-eclampsia.

OBJECTIVES: To assess the effectiveness and safety of nitric oxide donors and precursors for preventing pre-eclampsia and its complications.

METHODS: Standard PCG methods (see page xvii). Search date: November 2006.

SELECTION CRITERIA: Studies were included if they were randomised trials evaluating nitric oxide donors or precursors for preventing pre-eclampsia and its complications.

DATA COLLECTION AND ANALYSIS: Both review authors independently assessed studies for inclusion. Data were extracted and double checked for accuracy.

MAIN RESULTS: Six trials (310 women) were included. Four were of good quality and two were of uncertain quality. Four trials

(170 women) compared nitric oxide donors (glyceryl trinitrate) or precursors (L-arginine) with either placebo or no intervention. There are insufficient data for reliable conclusions about the effects on pre-eclampsia (four trials, 170 women; relative risk (RR) 0.83, 95% confidence interval (CI) 0.49 to 1.41) or its complications. One trial (36 women) compared a nitric oxide donor with nifedipine, and another (76 women) compared it with antiplatelet agents. Both were too small for reliable conclusions about possible differential effects.

Glyceryl trinitrate was associated with an increased risk of headache (two trials, 56 women; RR 6.85, 95% CI 1.42 to 33.04) and of stopping treatment (two trials, 56 women; RR 4.02, 95% CI 1.15 to 14.09) compared to placebo. However, the increase for both outcomes was due to an extreme result in one small trial (7/7 versus 0/9 for both outcomes).

AUTHORS' CONCLUSIONS: There is insufficient evidence to draw reliable conclusions about whether nitric oxide donors and precursors prevent pre-eclampsia or its complications.

PROGESTERONE FOR PREVENTING PRE-ECLAMPSIA AND ITS COMPLICATIONS: not enough data to provide reliable evidence (Meher S, Duley L) CD006175

BACKGROUND: In the past, progesterone has been advocated for prevention of pre-eclampsia and its complications. Although progestogens are not used for this purpose in current clinical practice, it remains relevant to assess the evidence on their possible benefits and harms.
OBJECTIVES: To assess the effects of progesterone during pregnancy on the risk of developing pre-eclampsia and its complications.
METHODS: Standard PCG methods (see page xvii). Search date: April 2006.
MAIN RESULTS: Two trials of uncertain quality were included (296 women). These trials compared progesterone injections with no progesterone. There was insufficient evidence to demonstrate any clear differences between the two groups on the risk of pre-eclampsia (one trial, 128 women; relative risk (RR) 0.21, 95% confidence interval (CI) 0.03 to 1.77), death of the baby (two trials, 296 women; RR 0.72, 95% CI 0.21 to 2.51), preterm birth (one trial, 168 women; RR 1.10, 95% CI 0.33 to 3.66), small-for-gestational-age babies (one trial, 168 women;

RR 0.83, 95% CI 0.19 to 3.57) or major congenital defects (one trial, 168 women; RR 1.65, 95% CI 0.28 to 9.62). There were no reported cases of masculinisation of female babies (one trial, 128 women).

Long-term follow up for the children has been reported in one trial, but the data are excluded from the review as 54% were lost to follow up at one year and 80% at 16 years.

AUTHORS' CONCLUSIONS: There is insufficient evidence for reliable conclusions about the effects of progesterone for preventing pre-eclampsia and its complications. Therefore, progesterone should not be used for this purpose in clinical practice at present. Unless new and plausible hypotheses emerge for the role of progesterone in the development of pre-eclampsia, further trials of progesterone are unlikely to be a priority.

ANTIBIOTICS FOR PREVENTING HYPERTENSIVE DISEASES IN PREGNANCY: (Mathew D, Khan K, Thornton JG, Todros T) Protocol [see page xviii] CD006841

ABRIDGED BACKGROUND: A number of authors have suggested that infective agents may be responsible for hypertensive disease in pregnancy including pre-eclampsia. A case-control study comparing primiparous women with pre-eclampsia and controls found a five-times increased risk of urinary tract infection during pregnancy among cases. A historical comparison of ten days' antibiotic treatment for women at high risk of pre-eclampsia suggested that the incidence fell from 8.0% to 3.8%.

OBJECTIVES: To test the hypotheses:

(1) that antibiotics prescribed in the first half of pregnancy (before 20 weeks) reduce the risk of hypertensive disease in general, and on pre-eclampsia specifically;

(2) that antibiotics prescribed in the first half of pregnancy (before 20 weeks) increase the risk of hypertensive disease in general, and on pre-eclampsia specifically;

(3) to explore the effects of different types of antibiotics on the risk of hypertensive disease in general, and on pre-eclampsia specifically.

> **ANTITHROMBOTIC THERAPY FOR IMPROVING MATERNAL OR INFANT HEALTH OUTCOMES IN WOMEN CONSIDERED AT RISK OF PLACENTAL DYSFUNCTION:** (Dodd JM, Kingdom J, McLeod A, Windrim RC) Protocol [*see* page xviii] CD006780

ABRIDGED BACKGROUND: Pregnancy complications such as pre-eclampsia and eclampsia, intrauterine growth restriction and placental abruption are thought to have a common origin related to abnormalities in the development and function of the placenta. Pathological examination of the placenta after birth, which has occurred secondary to pre-eclampsia or intrauterine growth restriction occurring in early pregnancy, has identified the presence of ischaemic thrombotic lesions, including infarction (or damage to the placental tissue due to clots forming in the placental blood vessels). While there may be benefits in the use of antenatal antithrombotic therapy for women considered to be at risk of complications related to placental dysfunction, in terms of improved maternal and infant health outcomes, there may also be harms related to the potential side effects of medication.

OBJECTIVES: To compare, using the best available evidence, the benefits and harms of antenatal antithrombotic therapy to improve maternal or infant health outcomes in women considered at risk of placental dysfunction, when compared with other treatments, placebo or no treatment.

3.1.2 Detection of hypertensive disorders

> **AMBULATORY VERSUS CONVENTIONAL METHODS FOR MONITORING BLOOD PRESSURE DURING PREGNANCY:** there were no randomised trials to provide reliable evidence. (Bergel E, Carroli G, Althabe F) CD001231

BACKGROUND: Hypertensive disorders are among the most common medical complications of pregnancy and a leading cause of maternal and perinatal morbidity and mortality world-wide. Blood pressure measurement plays a central role in the screening and management of hypertension during pregnancy. In recent years the validity of conventional (clinic) blood pressure measurement has been questioned and efforts have been made to improve the technique with ambulatory automated devices that provide a large number of measurements over a period of time, usually a 24-hour period.

OBJECTIVES: To assess whether the use of ambulatory blood pressure monitoring during pregnancy improves subsequent maternal and feto-neonatal outcomes, women–newborn quality of life or use of health service resources, compared with conventional (clinic) blood pressure measurements. These effects will be assessed for the following sub-groups: (1) Women at low or average risk of hypertensive disorders of pregnancy (unselected). (2) Women defined as high risk of hypertensive disorders of pregnancy. (3) Women with hypertension without other signs of pre-eclampsia. (4) Women with established pre-eclampsia.

METHODS: Standard PCG methods (see page xvii). Search date: January 2005.

MAIN RESULTS: No trials included.

AUTHORS' CONCLUSIONS: There is no randomised controlled trial evidence to support the use of ambulatory blood pressure monitoring during pregnancy. Randomised trials with adequate design and sample sizes are needed to evaluate the possible advantages and risks of ambulatory blood pressure monitoring during pregnancy, in particular in hypertensive pregnant women. These trials should evaluate not only clinical outcomes, but also use of health care resources and women's views.

3.1.3   Treatment of mild/moderate hypertension

The extent to which the blood pressure of hypertensive pregnant women is lowered represents a trade-off between protecting the mother from complications of severe hypertension such as intracranial haemorrhage, and the concern that lowered blood pressure may reduce maternal blood flow to the placenta.

ANTIHYPERTENSIVE DRUG THERAPY FOR MILD TO MODERATE HYPERTENSION DURING PREGNANCY: reduced severe hypertension; but not pre-eclampsia or substantive outcomes. (Abalos E, Duley L, Steyn DW, Henderson-Smart DJ) CD002252 (in RHL 11)

BACKGROUND: Mild to moderate hypertension during pregnancy is common. Antihypertensive drugs are often used in the belief that lowering blood pressure will prevent progression to more severe disease, and thereby improve outcome.

OBJECTIVES: To assess the effects of antihypertensive drug treatments for women with mild to moderate hypertension during pregnancy.

METHODS: Standard PCG methods (see page xvii). Search date: March 2006.

MAIN RESULTS: Forty-six trials (4282 women) were included. Twenty-eight trials compared an antihypertensive drug with placebo/no antihypertensive drug (3200 women). There is a halving in the risk of developing severe hypertension associated with the use of antihypertensive drug(s) (19 trials, 2409 women; relative risk (RR) 0.50; 95% confidence interval (CI) 0.41 to 0.61; risk difference (RD) −0.10 (−0.12 to −0.07); number needed to treat (NNT) 10 (8 to 13)) but little evidence of a difference in the risk of pre-eclampsia (22 trials, 2702 women; RR 0.97; 95% CI 0.83 to 1.13). Similarly, there is no clear effect on the risk of the baby dying (26 trials, 3081 women; RR 0.73; 95% CI 0.50 to 1.08), preterm birth (14 trials, 1992 women; RR 1.02; 95 % CI 0.89 to 1.16) or small-for-gestational-age babies (19 trials, 2437 women; RR 1.04; 95 % CI 0.84 to 1.27). There were no clear differences in any other outcomes.

Nineteen trials (1282 women) compared one antihypertensive drug with another. Beta blockers seem better than methyldopa for reducing the risk of severe hypertension (10 trials, 539 women, RR 0.75 (95 % CI 0.59 to 0.94); RD −0.08 (−0.14 to 0.02); NNT 12 (6 to 275)). There is no clear difference between any of the alternative drugs in the risk of developing proteinuria/pre-eclampsia. Other outcomes were only reported by a small proportion of studies, and there were no clear differences.

AUTHORS' CONCLUSIONS: It remains unclear whether antihypertensive drug therapy for mild to moderate hypertension during pregnancy is worthwhile.

TIGHT VERSUS VERY TIGHT CONTROL OF MILD–MODERATE PRE-EXISTING OR NON-PROTEINURIC GESTATIONAL HYPERTENSION FOR IMPROVING OUTCOMES: (Nabhan AF, Adel A) Protocol [see page xviii] CD006907

ABRIDGED BACKGROUND: There is a lack of consensus on when and how women with mild and moderate pre-existing or non-proteinuric gestational hypertension should be treated. In general, antihypertensive treatment is used to reduce cardiovascular disease risk and thus morbidity and mortality rates. On the other hand, there has been speculation that aggressive blood pressure lowering may decrease placental perfusion and jeopardize fetal well-being and might lead to fetal growth restriction while providing no extra benefit to the mother.

OBJECTIVES: To compare tight versus very tight control of mild–moderate pre-existing or non-proteinuric gestational hypertension for improving outcomes.

BED REST WITH OR WITHOUT HOSPITALISATION FOR HYPERTENSION DURING PREGNANCY: reduced the risk of severe hypertension and preterm birth but there was insufficient evidence to recommend its routine use. (Meher S, Abalos E, Carroli G) CD003514 (in RHL 11)

BACKGROUND: Bed rest or restriction of activity, with or without hospitalisation, have been advocated for women with hypertension during pregnancy to improve pregnancy outcome. However, benefits need to be demonstrated before such interventions can be recommended since restricted activity may be disruptive to women's lives, expensive and increase the risk of thromboembolism.

OBJECTIVES: To assess the effects on the mother and the baby of different degrees of bed rest, compared with each other, and with routine activity, in hospital or at home, for primary treatment of hypertension during pregnancy.

METHODS: Standard PCG methods (see page xvii). Search date: October 2007.

MAIN RESULTS: Four small trials (449 women) were included. Three were of good quality. Two trials (145 women) compared strict bed rest with some rest, in hospital, for women with proteinuric hypertension. There was insufficient evidence to demonstrate any differences between the groups for reported outcomes. Two trials (304 women) compared some bed rest in hospital with routine activity at home for non-proteinuric hypertension. There was reduced risk of severe hypertension (one trial, 218 women; RR 0.58, 95% CI 0.38 to 0.89) and a borderline reduction in risk of preterm birth (one trial, 218 women; RR 0.53, CI 0.29 to 0.99) with some rest compared to normal activity. More women in the bed rest group opted not to have the same management in future pregnancies, if the choice were given (one trial, 86 women; RR 3.00,

95% CI 1.43 to 6.31). There were no significant differences for any other outcomes.

AUTHORS' CONCLUSIONS: Few randomised trials have evaluated rest for women with hypertension during pregnancy, and important information on side-effects and cost implication is missing from available trials. Although one small trial suggests that some bed rest may be associated with reduced risk of severe hypertension and preterm birth, these findings need to be confirmed in larger trials. At present, there is insufficient evidence to provide clear guidance for clinical practice. Therefore, bed rest should not be recommended routinely for hypertension in pregnancy, especially since more women appear to prefer unrestricted activity, if the choice were given.

ORAL BETA-BLOCKERS FOR MILD TO MODERATE HYPERTENSION DURING PREGNANCY: reduced severe hypertension; increased growth impairment of the baby; did not improve substantive outcomes. (Magee LA, Duley L) CD002863

BACKGROUND: Antihypertensives, such as beta-blockers, are used for pregnancy hypertension in the belief that these will improve outcome for mother and baby.

OBJECTIVES: To assess whether oral beta-blockers are better than placebo, or no beta-blocker, and have advantages over other antihypertensives, for women with mild to moderate pregnancy hypertension.

METHODS: Standard PCG methods (see page xvii). Search date: January 2004.

MAIN RESULTS: 29 trials (approximately 2500 women) are included. 13 trials (1480 women) compared beta-blockers with placebo/no beta-blocker. Oral beta-blockers decrease the risk of severe hypertension (relative risk (RR) 0.37, 95% confidence interval (CI) 0.26 to 0.53; 11 trials, N = 1128 women) and the need for additional antihypertensives (RR 0.44, 95% CI 0.31 to 0.62; seven trials, N = 856 women). There are insufficient data for conclusions about the effect on perinatal mortality or preterm birth. Beta-blockers seem to be associated with an increase in small-for-gestational-age (SGA) infants (RR 1.36, 95% CI 1.02 to 1.82; 12 trials; N = 1346 women). Maternal hospital admission may be decreased, neonatal bradycardia increased and respiratory distress syndrome decreased, but these outcomes are reported in only a small proportion of trials. In 13 trials (854 women), beta-blockers were compared with methyldopa. Beta-blockers appear to be no more effective and probably equally as safe. Single small trials have compared beta-blockers with hydralazine, nicardipine or isradipine. It is unusual for women to change drugs due to side effects.

AUTHORS' CONCLUSIONS: Improvement in control of maternal blood pressure with use of beta-blockers would be worthwhile only if it were reflected in substantive benefits for mother and/or baby, and none have been clearly demonstrated. The effect of beta-blockers on perinatal outcome is uncertain; the worrying trend to an increase in SGA infants is partly dependent on one small outlying trial. Large randomised trials are needed to determine whether antihypertensive therapy in general (rather than beta-blocker therapy specifically) results in greater benefit than risk, for treatment of mild–moderate pregnancy hypertension. If so, then it would be appropriate to consider which antihypertensive is best, and beta-blockers should be evaluated.

CHINESE HERBAL MEDICINE FOR THE TREATMENT OF PRE-ECLAMPSIA: no randomised trials to provide reliable evidence. (Zhang J, Wu TX, Liu GJ) CD005126

BACKGROUND: Pre-eclampsia is a common disorder of pregnancy with uncertain aetiology. In Chinese herbal medicines, a number of herbs are used for treating pre-eclampsia. Traditional Chinese medicine considers that, when a woman is pregnant, most of the blood of the mother is directed to the placenta to provide the baby with the required nutrition; other maternal organs may in consequence be vulnerable to damage. These organs include the liver, the spleen and the kidneys. The general effects of Chinese herbal medicines that can protect these organs may be valuable in pre-eclampsia by encouraging vasodilatation, increasing blood flow and decreasing platelet aggregation. The use of Chinese herbal medicine is often based on the individual and presence of traditional Chinese medicine symptoms.

OBJECTIVES: To assess the effect of Chinese herbal medicine for treating pre-eclampsia and compare it with that of placebo, no treatment or Western medicine.

METHODS: Standard PCG methods (see page xvii). Search date: March 2005, including handsearching several main journals published in China.
MAIN RESULTS: No trials were suitable for inclusion in this review.

AUTHORS' CONCLUSIONS: The effect of Chinese herbal medicine for treating pre-eclampsia remains unclear. There are currently no randomised controlled trials to address the efficacy and safety of Chinese herbal medicine for the treatment of pre-eclampsia. Well conducted randomised controlled trials are required.

PREVENTION AND TREATMENT OF POSTPARTUM HYPERTEN-SION: not enough data to provide reliable evidence. (Magee L, Sadeghi S) CD004351

BACKGROUND: Postpartum blood pressure (BP) is highest three to six days after birth when most women have been discharged home. A significant rise in BP may be dangerous (e.g., lead to stroke), but there is little information about how to prevent or treat postpartum hypertension.
OBJECTIVES: To assess the relative benefits and risks of interventions to:

(1) prevent postpartum hypertension, by assessing whether 'routine' postpartum administration of oral antihypertensive therapy is better than placebo/no treatment; and
(2) treat postpartum hypertension, by assessing whether (i) oral anti-hypertensive therapy is better than placebo/no therapy for mild–moderate postpartum hypertension; and (ii) one antihypertensive agent offers advantages over another for mild–moderate or severe postpartum hypertension.

METHODS: Standard PCG methods (see page xvii). Search date March 2004.
MAIN RESULTS: Six trials are included.
Prevention: Three trials (315 women; six comparisons) compared furo-semide or nifedipine capsules with placebo/no therapy. There are insufficient data for conclusions about possible benefits and risks of these management strategies. Most outcomes included data from only one trial. No trial reported severe maternal hypertension or breastfeeding.

Treatment: In two trials (106 women; three comparisons), oral timolol or hydralazine was compared with oral methyldopa for treatment of mild to moderate postpartum hypertension. In one trial (38 women; one comparison), oral hydralazine plus sublingual nifedipine was compared with sublingual nifedipine for treatment of severe postpartum hypertension. The need for additional antihypertensive therapy did not differ between groups (relative risk 4.24, 95% confidence interval 0.96 to 18.84; three trials, N = 144 women), but three antihypertensive drugs were studied. All were well tolerated.

AUTHORS' CONCLUSIONS: There are no reliable data to guide management of women who are hypertensive postpartum or at increased risk of becoming so. If a clinician feels that hypertension is severe enough to treat, the agent used should be based on his/her familiarity with the drug. Future studies of prevention or treatment of postpartum hypertension should include information about use of postpartum analgesics and outcomes of severe maternal hypertension, breastfeeding, hospital length of stay and maternal satisfaction with care.

See also reviews of: Antenatal day care units versus hospital admission for women with complicated pregnancy (page 9), Patterns of routine antenatal care for low-risk pregnancy (page 7), energy and protein intake in pregnancy (page 23), Magnesium supplementation in pregnancy (page 26), Pyridoxine (vitamin B6) supplementation in pregnancy (page 27), Vitamin C supplementation in pregnancy (page 29), Vitamin E supplementation in pregnancy (page 31), Abdominal decompression in normal pregnancy (page 140), Abdominal decompression for suspected fetal compromise/pre-eclampsia (page 140), Vitamin supplementation for preventing miscarriage (page 48), Oestrogen supplementation, mainly diethylstilbestrol, for preventing miscarriages and other adverse pregnancy outcomes (page 45) and Multiple-micronutrient supplementation for women during pregnancy (page 32).

3.1.4 *Treatment of severe pre-eclampsia/eclampsia*

'In NO cases have I detected albumin, except in those in which there have been convulsions, or in which symptoms have presented themselves, and which are readily recognised as the precursors of puerperal fits.' Lever

JCW, Cases of puerperal convulsions, with remarks. *Guys Hospital Record* 1843; 2: 495–517.

Because of the potential for progression and serious complications, severe pre-eclampsia is usually managed in hospital. When severe pre-eclampsia develops before term, the interests of the mother and those of the baby are generally opposed. For the mother, expediting the birth is the safest option, while expectant care may benefit the baby by allowing more time to mature. When the benefits of delaying birth to the baby are considered to outweigh the risks to the mother, the condition of both is kept under close surveillance and delivery undertaken as soon as the balance shifts, for example because of deteriorating condition of the mother or baby, or relative maturity of the baby.

Very little empirical research has addressed the question of the optimal timing or method of giving birth for women with severe pre-eclampsia/eclampsia. Caesarean section offers the most rapid route for the birth, but carries significant risks for women whose clinical condition is already compromised. Rapid labour induction is sometimes considered a safer option.

Some of these clinical dilemmas are addressed in the following reviews.

In 1995, the only mention of magnesium sulphate in a major obstetric textbook was the following: 'Intravenous diazepam is the agent of choice to stop convulsions, but is inappropriate for longer-term prevention of fits. For the latter purpose phenytoin has been used, although in the USA parenteral magnesium sulphate is preferred.' G. Chamberlain, Editor, *Turnbull's Obstetrics* (second ed.), Churchill Livingstone, Edinburgh (1995). The Collaborative Eclampsia Trial which dominates some of the reviews below has overturned entrenched doctrines.

INTERVENTIONIST VERSUS EXPECTANT CARE FOR SEVERE PRE-ECLAMPSIA BEFORE TERM: larger studies are needed to confirm the benefits to the baby of expectant care. (Churchill D, Duley L) CD003106 (in RHL 11)

BACKGROUND: Severe pre-eclampsia can cause significant mortality and morbidity for both mother and child, particularly when it occurs well before term. The only known cure for this disease is delivery.

Some obstetricians advocate early delivery to prevent the development of serious maternal complications, such as eclampsia (fits) and kidney failure. Others prefer a more expectant approach in an attempt to delay delivery and, hopefully, reduce the mortality and morbidity for the child associated with being born too early.

OBJECTIVES: To compare the effects of a policy of interventionist care and early delivery with a policy of expectant care and delayed delivery for women with early onset severe pre-eclampsia.

METHODS: Standard PCG methods (see page xvii). Search date: April 2006.

MAIN RESULTS: Two trials (133 women) are included in this review. There are insufficient data for reliable conclusions about the comparative effects on outcome for the mother. For the baby, there is insufficient evidence for reliable conclusions about the effects on stillbirth or death after delivery (relative risk (RR) 1.50, 95% confidence interval (CI) 0.42 to 5.41). Babies whose mothers had been allocated to the interventionist group had more hyaline membrane disease (RR 2.30, 95% CI 1.39 to 3.81), more necrotising enterocolitis (RR 5.54, 95% CI 1.04 to 29.56) and were more likely to need admission to neonatal intensive care (RR 1.32, 95% CI 1.13 to 1.55) than those allocated an expectant policy. Nevertheless, babies allocated to the interventionist policy were less likely to be small-for-gestational age (RR 0.36, 95% CI 0.14 to 0.90). There were no statistically significant differences between the two strategies for any other outcomes.

AUTHORS' CONCLUSIONS: There are insufficient data for any reliable recommendation about which policy of care should be used for women with severe early onset pre-eclampsia. Further large trials are needed.

PLASMA VOLUME EXPANSION FOR TREATMENT OF PRE-ECLAMPSIA: not enough data to provide reliable evidence. (Duley L, Williams J, Henderson-Smart DJ) CD001805

BACKGROUND: Plasma volume is reduced amongst women with pre-eclampsia. This association has led to the suggestion that expanding the plasma volume might improve maternal and uteroplacental circulation, and so potentially improve outcome for both the woman and her baby.

OBJECTIVES: The aim of this review was to assess the effects of plasma volume expansion for the treatment of women with pre-eclampsia.
METHODS: Standard PCG methods (see page xvii). Search date: December 2000.
Women who were postpartum at trial entry were excluded.
MAIN RESULTS: Three trials involving 61 women were included in this review. All compared a colloid solution with no plasma volume expansion. For every outcome reported, the confidence intervals are very wide and cross the no effect line.

AUTHORS' CONCLUSIONS: There is insufficient evidence for any reliable estimates of the effects of plasma volume expansion for women with pre-eclampsia.

CORTICOSTEROIDS FOR HELLP SYNDROME IN PREGNANCY: showed some benefits in terms of laboratory tests; the evidence was insufficient to recommend routine use. (Matchaba P, Moodley J) CD002076

BACKGROUND: Hemolysis, elevated liver enzymes and low platelets (HELLP) syndrome is a severe form of pre-eclampsia. Pre-eclampsia is a multi-system disease of pregnancy associated with an increase in blood pressure and increased perinatal and maternal morbidity and mortality. 80% of women with HELLP syndrome present before term. There are suggestions from observational studies that steroid treatment in HELLP syndrome may improve disordered maternal hematological and biochemical features and perhaps perinatal mortality and morbidity.
OBJECTIVES: To summarize the evidence on the effects of corticosteroids on maternal and neonatal mortality and morbidity in women with HELLP syndrome.
METHODS: Standard PCG methods (see page xvii). Search date: October 2003.
MAIN RESULTS: Of the five studies reviewed (n = 170), three were conducted antepartum and two postpartum. Four of the studies randomized participants to standard therapy or dexamethasone. One study compared dexamethasone with betamethasone.
Dexamethasone versus control: There were no significant differences in the primary outcomes of maternal mortality and morbidity due to placental abruption, pulmonary edema and liver hematoma or rupture. Of the secondary maternal outcomes, there was a tendency to a greater

platelet count increase over 48 hours, statistically significantly less mean number of hospital stay days (weighted mean difference (WMD) −4.50, 95% confidence interval (CI) −7.13 to −1.87), and mean interval (hours) to delivery (41 ± 15) versus (15 ± 4.5) (p = 0.0068) in favour of women allocated to dexamethasone.

There were no significant differences in perinatal mortality or morbidity due to respiratory distress syndrome, need for ventilatory support, intracerebral hemorrhage, necrotizing enterocolitis and a five minute Apgar less than seven. The mean birthweight was significantly greater in the group allocated to dexamethasone (WMD 247.00, 95% CI 65.41 to 428.59).

Dexamethasone versus betamethasone: There were no significant differences in all the maternal and perinatal mortality and in primary morbidity outcomes. Women randomized to dexamethasone fared significantly better for: oliguria, mean arterial pressure, mean increase in platelet count, mean increase in urinary output and liver enzyme elevations.

AUTHORS' CONCLUSIONS: There is insufficient evidence to determine whether adjunctive steroid use in HELLP syndrome decreases maternal and perinatal mortality, and major maternal and perinatal morbidity.

DRUGS FOR TREATMENT OF VERY HIGH BLOOD PRESSURE DURING PREGNANCY: the best drug is not known, but calcium channel blockers or labetalol appear to be better alternatives than diazoxide, ketanserin, nimodipine and magnesium sulphate. (Duley L, Henderson-Smart DJ, Meher S) CD001449 (in RHL 11)

BACKGROUND: Very high blood pressure during pregnancy poses a serious threat to women and their babies. Antihypertensive drugs lower blood pressure. Their comparative effects on other substantive outcomes, however, are uncertain.

OBJECTIVES: To compare different antihypertensive drugs for very high blood pressure during pregnancy.

METHODS: Standard PCG methods (see page xvii). Search date: February 2006.

MAIN RESULTS: 24 trials (2949 women) with 12 comparisons were included. Women allocated to calcium channel blockers rather than hydralazine were less likely to have persistent high blood pressure (five trials, 263 women; 6% versus 18%; relative risk (RR) 0.33, 95% confidence interval (CI) 0.15 to 0.70). Ketanserin was associated with more persistent high blood pressure than hydralazine (four trials, 200 women; 27% versus 6%; RR 4.79, 95% CI 1.95 to 11.73), but fewer side-effects (three trials, 120 women; RR 0.32, 95% CI 0.19 to 0.53) and a lower risk of HELLP (Haemolysis, Elevated Liver enzymes and Lowered Platelets) syndrome (one trial, 44 women, RR 0.20, 95% CI 0.05 to 0.81).

Labetalol was associated with a lower risk of hypotension (one trial 90 women; RR 0.06, 95% CI 0.00 to 0.99) and caesarean section (RR 0.43, 95% CI 0.18 to 1.02) than diazoxide. Data were insufficient for reliable conclusions about other outcomes.

The risk of persistent high blood pressure was greater for nimodipine compared to magnesium sulphate (two trials 1683 women; 47% versus 65%; RR 0.84, 95% CI 0.76 to 0.93). Nimodipine was also associated with a higher risk of eclampsia (RR 2.24, 95% CI 1.06 to 4.73) and respiratory difficulties (RR 0.28, 95% CI 0.08 to 0.99), but fewer side-effects (RR 0.68, 95% CI 0.54 to 0.86) and less postpartum haemorrhage (RR 0.41, 95% CI 0.18 to 0.92) than magnesium sulphate. Stillbirths and neonatal deaths were not reported.

There are insufficient data for reliable conclusions about the comparative effects of any other drugs.

AUTHORS' CONCLUSIONS: Until better evidence is available, the choice of antihypertensive should depend on the clinician's experience and familiarity with a particular drug and what is known about adverse effects. Exceptions are diazoxide, ketanserin, nimodipine and magnesium sulphate, which are probably best avoided.

MAGNESIUM SULPHATE AND OTHER ANTICONVULSANTS FOR WOMEN WITH PRE-ECLAMPSIA: magnesium sulphate greatly reduced the risk of eclampsia and possibly maternal death though it has side effects. (Duley L, Gülmezoglu AM, Henderson-Smart DJ) CD000025 (in RHL 11)

BACKGROUND: Pre-eclampsia is a relatively common complication of pregnancy. Eclampsia, the occurrence of one or more convulsions (fits) in association with the syndrome of pre-eclampsia, is a rare but serious complication. Anticonvulsants are used in the belief that they help prevent eclamptic fits and so improve outcome.

OBJECTIVES: The objective was to assess the effects of anticonvulsants for pre-eclampsia on the women and their children.

METHODS: Standard PCG methods (see page xvii). Search date: November 2002.

MAIN RESULTS: Six trials (11 444 women) compared magnesium sulphate with placebo or no anticonvulsant. There was more than a halving in the risk of eclampsia associated with magnesium sulphate (relative risk (RR) 0.41, 95% confidence interval (CI) 0.29 to 0.58; number needed to treat (NNT) 100, 95% CI 50 to 100). The risk of dying was non-significantly reduced by 46% for women allocated magnesium sulphate (RR 0.54, 95% CI 0.26 to 1.10). For serious maternal morbidity RR 1.08, 95% CI 0.89 to 1.32. Side effects were more common with magnesium sulphate (24% versus 5%; RR 5.26, 95% CI 4.59 to 6.03; NNT for harm 6, 95% CI 6 to 5). The main side effect was flushing. Risk of placental abruption was reduced for women allocated magnesium sulphate (RR 0.64, 95% CI 0.50 to 0.83; NNT 100, 95% CI 50 to 1000). Women allocated magnesium sulphate had a small increase (5%) in the risk of caesarean section (95% CI 1% to 10%). There was no overall difference in the risk of stillbirth or neonatal death (RR 1.04, 95% CI 0.93 to 1.15).

Magnesium sulphate was better than phenytoin for reducing the risk of eclampsia (two trials, 2241 women; RR 0.05, 95% CI 0.00 to 0.84), but with an increased risk of caesarean section (RR 1.21, 95% CI 1.05 to 1.41). It was also better than nimodipine (one trial, 1650 women; RR 0.33, 95% CI 0.14 to 0.77).

AUTHORS' CONCLUSIONS: Magnesium sulphate more than halves the risk of eclampsia, and probably reduces the risk of maternal death. It does not improve outcome for the baby, in the short term. A quarter of women have side effects, particularly flushing.

☺ **MAGNESIUM SULPHATE VERSUS DIAZEPAM FOR ECLAMPSIA:** reduced maternal deaths and substantially reduced recurrent convulsions and other morbidity. (Duley L, Henderson-Smart D) CD000127 (in RHL 11)

BACKGROUND: Eclampsia, the occurrence of a convulsion in association with pre-eclampsia, remains a rare but serious complication of pregnancy. A number of different anticonvulsants are used to control eclamptic fits and to prevent further fits.

OBJECTIVES: The objective of this review was to assess the effects of magnesium sulphate compared with diazepam when used for the care of women with eclampsia. Magnesium sulphate is compared with phenytoin and with lytic cocktail in other Cochrane reviews.

METHODS: Standard PCG methods (see page xvii). Search date: November 2002.

MAIN RESULTS: Seven trials involving 1441 women are included. Most of the data are from trials of good quality. Magnesium sulphate is associated with a reduction in maternal death when compared to diazepam (six trials 1336 women; relative risk (RR) 0.59, 95% confidence interval (CI) 0.37 to 0.94). There is also a substantial reduction in the risk of recurrence of further fits (seven trials 1441 women; RR 0.44, 95% CI 0.34 to 0.57). There were few differences in any other measures of outcome, except for fewer Apgar scores less than seven at five minutes (two trials 597 babies; RR 0.72, 95% CI 0.55 to 0.94) and fewer babies with a length of stay in special care baby unit more than seven days (three trials 631 babies; RR 0.66, 95% CI 0.46 to 0.95) associated with magnesium sulphate.

AUTHORS' CONCLUSIONS: Magnesium sulphate appears to be substantially more effective than diazepam for treatment of eclampsia.

☺ **MAGNESIUM SULPHATE VERSUS LYTIC COCKTAIL FOR ECLAMPSIA:** substantially reduced recurrent convulsions and other morbidity. (Duley L, Gulmezoglu AM) CD002960 (in RHL 11)

BACKGROUND: Eclampsia, the occurrence of a seizure in association with pre-eclampsia, is a rare but serious complication of pregnancy. A number of different anticonvulsants are used to control eclamptic fits and to prevent further seizures.

OBJECTIVES: To compare the effects of magnesium sulphate with those of lytic cocktail when used for the care of women with eclampsia.

METHODS: Standard PCG methods (see page xvii). Search date: April 2000.

MAIN RESULTS: Two trials with 199 women were included in the review. These were both small and of average quality. Magnesium sulphate was better than lytic cocktail at preventing further fits (relative risk (RR) 0.09, 95% confidence interval (CI) 0.03–0.24; risk difference (RD) 0.43, 95% CI −0.53, −0.34; number needed to treat (NNT) 3,

95% CI 2–3) and was associated with less respiratory depression (RR 0.12, 95% CI 0.02–0.91). Magnesium sulphate was also associated with fewer maternal deaths than lytic cocktail, but the difference was not statistically significant (RR 0.25, 95% CI 0.04–1.43).

AUTHORS' CONCLUSIONS: Magnesium sulphate is the anticonvulsant of choice for women with eclampsia. Lytic cocktail should be abandoned.

© **MAGNESIUM SULPHATE VERSUS PHENYTOIN FOR ECLAMPSIA:** substantially reduced recurrent convulsions and other morbidity. (Duley L, Henderson-Smart D) CD000128 (in RHL 11)

BACKGROUND: Eclampsia, the occurrence of a convulsion (fit) in association with pre-eclampsia, remains a rare but serious complication of pregnancy. A number of different anticonvulsants are used to control eclamptic fits and to prevent further convulsions.

OBJECTIVES: To assess the effects of magnesium sulphate compared with phenytoin when used for the care of women with eclampsia. Magnesium sulphate is compared with diazepam and with lytic cocktail in other Cochrane reviews.

METHODS: Standard PCG methods (see page xvii). Search date: November 2002.

MAIN RESULTS: Six trials involving 897 women are included. Most of the data are from trials of good quality. Magnesium sulphate is associated with a substantial reduction in the recurrence of convulsions, when compared to phenytoin (five trials, 895 women; relative risk (RR) 0.31, 95% confidence interval (CI) 0.20 to 0.47). The trend in maternal mortality favours magnesium sulphate, but this difference is not statistically significant (two trials, 797 women; RR 0.50, 95% CI 0.24 to 1.05). There are also reductions in the risk of pneumonia (RR 0.44, 95% CI 0.24 to 0.79), ventilation (RR 0.66, 95% CI 0.49 to 0.90) and admission to an intensive care unit (RR 0.67, 95% CI 0.50 to 0.89) associated with the use of magnesium sulphate. For the baby, magnesium sulphate was associated with fewer admissions to a special care baby unit (SCBU) (one trial, 518 babies; RR 0.73, 95% CI 0.58 to 0.91) and fewer babies who died or were in SCBU for more than seven days (one trial, 665 babies; RR 0.77, 95% CI 0.63 to 0.95).

AUTHORS' CONCLUSIONS: Magnesium sulphate appears to be substantially more effective than phenytoin for treatment of eclampsia.

> **LOW-DOSE DOPAMINE FOR WOMEN WITH SEVERE PRE-ECLAMPSIA:** not enough data to provide reliable evidence. (Steyn DW, Steyn P) CD003515

BACKGROUND: Hypertensive disorders during pregnancy are important causes of maternal mortality and morbidity worldwide. The long-term outcome of surviving mothers will depend largely on whether intracranial haemorrhage or renal failure developed. Low-dose dopamine is used for the prevention and treatment of acute renal failure, but its role in the management of pregnant women with severe pre-eclampsia is unclear.

OBJECTIVES: To assess the effects of low-dose dopamine used for oliguria in severe pre-eclampsia on mothers and their children.

METHODS: Standard PCG methods (see page xvii). Search date: June 2006.

MAIN RESULTS: Only one randomised placebo controlled trial of six hours' duration, including 40 postpartum women, was found. This study showed a significant increase in urinary output over six hours in women receiving dopamine. It is unclear if this was of any benefit to the women.

AUTHORS' CONCLUSIONS: It is unclear whether low-dose dopamine therapy for pre-eclamptic women with oliguria is worthwhile. It should not be used other than in prospective trials.

3.2   Anaemia during pregnancy

> Her face, which...was distinguished by rosiness of cheeks and redness of lips, is some how as if exsanguinated, sadly paled, the heart trembles with every movement of her body, and the arteries of her temples pulsate, & she is seized with dyspnoea in dancing or climbing the stairs. Lange J. Medicinalium Epistolarum Miscellanea. *Basel: J. Oporinus* 1554; 74.

Lower haemoglobin levels are common during pregnancy, mainly because of the diluting effect of increased plasma volume. Modestly reduced haemoglobin levels are generally regarded as physiological, but severe anaemia is a major health problem in pregnant women, particularly in poor communities and those exposed to malaria. The commonest cause is dietary iron deficiency. The additional iron requirements in pregnancy are about 1000 mg, and dietary iron is preferentially diverted to the baby. Other causes of anaemia include folate deficiency and rarely vitamin B12 deficiency, haemoglobinopathies and chronic blood loss. In evaluating preventive and treatment strategies, it is important to distinguish between laboratory evidence of an effect on haemoglobin levels, and clinical evidence of improved health.

3.2.1 Prevention of anaemia

Iron supplementation may be used routinely in communities at risk of iron deficiency, or selectively in women with iron deficiency anaemia or reduced iron stores. A public health risk of routine iron supplementation during pregnancy is childhood iron poisoning, because of the tablets (which may look like sweets) being accessible to children in the community. Fortification of staple foods such as wheat flour with elemental iron or maize flour with sodium iron edetic acid may reduce iron deficiency at a population level.

EFFECTS OF ROUTINE ORAL IRON SUPPLEMENTATION WITH OR WITHOUT FOLIC ACID FOR WOMEN DURING PREGNANCY: daily or weekly dosage regimens increased haemoglobin levels; but there was insufficient evidence regarding substantive health outcomes. (Pena-Rosas JP, Viteri FE) CD004736 (in RHL 11)

BACKGROUND: It has been suggested that routine intake of supplements containing iron or a combination of iron and folic acid during pregnancy improves maternal health and pregnancy outcomes.

OBJECTIVES: To assess the efficacy, effectiveness and safety of routine antenatal daily or intermittent iron supplementation with or without folic acid during pregnancy on the health of mothers and newborns.

METHODS: Standard PCG methods (see page xvii). Search date: June 2005.

MAIN RESULTS: 40 trials, involving 12 706 women, were included in the review. Overall, the results showed significant heterogeneity across most prespecified outcomes. Heterogeneity could not be explained by standard sensitivity analyses including quality assessment; therefore, all results were analysed assuming random-effects. Very limited information related to clinical maternal and infant outcomes was available in the included trials.

The data suggest that daily antenatal iron supplementation increases haemoglobin levels in maternal blood both antenatally and postnatally. It is difficult to quantify this increase due to significant heterogeneity between the studies. Women who receive daily antenatal iron supplementation are less likely to have iron deficiency and iron-deficiency anaemia at term as defined by current cut-off values. Side-effects and haemoconcentration are more common in women who receive daily iron supplementation. No differences were evident between daily and weekly supplementation with regards to gestational anaemia; haemoconcentration during pregnancy appears less frequent with the weekly regimen. The clinical significance of haemoconcentration, defined as haemoglobin greater than 130 g/l remains uncertain.

AUTHORS' CONCLUSIONS: Further studies are needed to assess the effects of routine antenatal supplementation with iron or a combination of iron and folic acid on clinically important maternal and infant outcomes.

3.2.2 Treatment of anaemia

> **TREATMENTS FOR IRON-DEFICIENCY ANAEMIA IN PREGNANCY:** oral iron reduced anaemia; intramuscular and intravenous iron showed potential for adverse effects; there was insufficient evidence on clinical health outcomes or other methods of treatment. (Reveiz L, Gyte GML, Cuervo LG) CD003094 (in RHL 11)

BACKGROUND: Iron deficiency, the most common cause of anaemia in pregnancy worldwide, can be mild, moderate or severe. Severe anaemia can have very serious consequences for mothers and babies, but there is controversy about whether treating mild or moderate anaemia provides more benefit than harm.

OBJECTIVES: To assess the effects of different treatments for iron-deficiency anaemia in pregnancy (defined as haemoglobin less than 11 g/dl) on maternal and neonatal morbidity and mortality.

METHODS: Standard PCG methods (see page xvii). Search date: January 2007.

MAIN RESULTS: The trials were small and generally methodologically poor. They covered a very wide range of differing drugs, doses and routes of administration, making it difficult to pool data. Oral iron in pregnancy showed a reduction in the incidence of anaemia (one trial, 125 women; relative risk 0.38; 95% confidence interval 0.26 to 0.55). It was not possible to assess the effects of treatment by severity of anaemia. A trend was found between dose and reported adverse effects. We found that most trials had no assessments on relevant clinical outcomes and a paucity of data on adverse effects, including some that are known to be associated with iron administration. Although the intramuscular and intravenous routes produced better haematological indices in women than the oral route, no clinical outcomes were assessed and there were insufficient data on adverse effects, for example, on venous thrombosis and severe allergic reactions.

AUTHORS' CONCLUSIONS: Despite the high incidence and burden of disease associated with this condition, there is a paucity of good quality trials assessing clinical maternal and neonatal effects of iron administration in women with anaemia. Daily oral iron treatment improves haematological indices but causes frequent gastrointestinal adverse effects. Parenteral (intramuscular and intravenous) iron enhances haematological response, compared with oral iron, but there are concerns about possible important adverse effects. Large, good quality trials assessing clinical outcomes (including adverse effects) are required.

TREATMENT FOR WOMEN WITH POSTPARTUM IRON DEFICIENCY ANAEMIA: haemopoietin reduced anaemia; there was inadequate evidence regarding substantive outcomes and other methods of treatment. (Dodd J, Dare MR, Middleton P) CD004222 (in RHL 11)

BACKGROUND: Postpartum anaemia is associated with breathlessness, tiredness, palpitations and maternal infections. Blood transfusions or iron supplementation have been used in the treatment of iron deficiency anaemia. Recently other anaemia treatments, in particular erythropoietin therapy, have also been used.

OBJECTIVES: To assess the clinical effects of treatments for postpartum anaemia, including oral, intravenous or subcutaneous iron/folate supplementation and erythropoietin administration, and blood transfusion.

METHODS: Standard PCG methods (see page xvii). Search date: May 2004.

MAIN RESULTS: Six included RCTs involving 411 women described treatment with erythropoietin or iron as their primary interventions. No RCTs were identified that assessed treatment with blood transfusion. Few outcomes relating to clinical maternal and neonatal factors were reported: studies focused largely on surrogate outcomes such as haematological indices. Overall, the methodological quality of the included RCTs was reasonable; however, their usefulness in this review is restricted by the interventions and outcomes reported. When compared with iron therapy only, erythropoietin increased the likelihood of lactation at discharge from hospital (one RCT, n = 40; relative risk (RR) 1.90, 95% confidence interval (CI) 1.21 to 2.98). No apparent effect on need for blood transfusions was found when erythropoietin plus iron was compared to treatment with iron only (two RCTs, n = 100; RR 0.20, 95% CI 0.01 to 3.92), although the RCTs may have been of insufficient size to rule out important clinical differences. Haematological indices (haemoglobin and haemocrit) showed some increases when erythropoietin was compared to iron only, iron and folate, but not when compared with placebo.

AUTHORS' CONCLUSIONS: There is some limited evidence of favourable outcomes for treatment of postpartum anaemia with erythropoietin. However, most of the available literature focuses on laboratory haematological indices, rather than clinical outcomes. Further high-quality trials assessing the treatment of postpartum anaemia with iron supplementation and blood transfusions are required. Future trials may also examine the significance of the severity of anaemia in relation to treatment, and an iron-rich diet as an intervention.

3.3   Diabetes mellitus

'Those labouring with this Disease, piss a great deal more than they drink....The Urine in all .... Was wonderfully sweet as if it were imbued with Honey or Sugar.' Willis T. The Diabetes or Pissing Evil. In: *Pharmaceuticae Rationalis Sive Diatriba de Medicamentorum Operationibus in Humano Corpore*. London: R Scott, 1672: 252.

During pregnancy hormonal changes, including secretion of human placental lactogen from the placenta, modify glucose metabolism. This promotes glucose transfer to the baby, but places the mother at risk for hyperglycaemia. Some healthy women become diabetic (gestational diabetes), while pre-existing diabetes may be aggravated. Diabetes is usually defined as a fasting plasma glucose level of 7.0 mmol/l or more; or 11.1 mmol/l or more 2 hours after a 75 gram glucose load. Levels of 6.1 to 7 or 7.8 to 11.1 mmol/l respectively are referred to as impaired glucose tolerance.

Hyperglycaemia has adverse effects on the baby: congenital anomalies; macrosomia (large baby) with the risk of obstructed labour and birth injuries; polyhydramnios; intrauterine death; neonatal hypoglycaemia; polycythaemia; hyperbilirubinaemia; and respiratory distress syndrome. Diabetic women with microvascular disease may develop impaired fetal growth.

The pillars of treatment have been diet and insulin, though in type II diabetics with high body mass index recent evidence has favoured the use of oral hypoglycaemic agents.

Because of the unpredictability of late intrauterine death in diabetic women, curtailment of pregnancy at 38 weeks has been suggested. During labour, sugar levels may be controlled with simultaneous infusion of glucose and insulin. After delivery of the placenta, insulin requirements are greatly reduced.

> **EXERCISE FOR DIABETIC PREGNANT WOMEN:** not enough data to provide reliable evidence. (Ceysens G, Rouiller D, Boulvain M) CD004225

BACKGROUND: Diabetes in pregnancy may result in unfavourable maternal and neonatal outcomes. Exercise was proposed as an additional strategy to improve glycaemic control. The effect of exercise during pregnancies complicated by diabetes needs to be assessed.
OBJECTIVES: To evaluate the effect of exercise programmes, alone or in conjunction with other therapies, compared to no specific program or to other therapies, in pregnant women with diabetes on perinatal and maternal morbidity and on the frequency of prescription of insulin to control glycaemia. To compare the effectiveness of different types of exercise programmes on perinatal and maternal morbidity.

METHODS: Standard PCG methods (see page xvii). Search date: December 2005

MAIN RESULTS: Four trials, involving 114 pregnant women with gestational diabetes, were included in the review. None included pregnant women with type 1 or type 2 diabetes. Women were recruited during the third trimester and the intervention was performed for about six weeks. The programmes generally consisted in exercising three times a week for 20 to 45 minutes. We found no significant difference between exercise and the other regimen in all the outcomes evaluated.

AUTHORS' CONCLUSIONS: There is insufficient evidence to recommend, or advise against, diabetic pregnant women to enrol in exercise programmes. Further trials, with larger sample size, involving women with gestational diabetes, and possibly type 1 and 2 diabetes, are needed to evaluate this intervention.

DIETARY ADVICE IN PREGNANCY FOR PREVENTING GESTATIONAL DIABETES MELLITUS: (Tieu J, Crowther CA., Middleton P) Protocol [see page xviii] CD006674

ABRIDGED BACKGROUND: Gestational diabetes mellitus (GDM) is defined as 'glucose intolerance that begins or is first detected during pregnancy'. Gestational glucose intolerance usually resolves after birth. However, the risk of perinatal complications such as macrosomia is elevated even at low levels of glucose intolerance. Placental hormones secreted in pregnancy, including oestrogen, progesterone, cortisol, placental lactogen, prolactin and growth hormone, create an insulin resistant state to direct sufficient nutrition to the fetus. More severe insulin resistance accompanied by insufficient compensatory insulin release in GDM limits glucose transport into cells, increasing maternal glucose concentration. This results in hyperglycaemia in the developing fetus, stimulating insulin production. Insulin allows greater glucose and amino acid entry into cells, increasing metabolism and, ultimately, fetal growth. Neonatal hypoglycaemia can result from hyperinsulinaemia when linked to the mother's excess glucose. Excess fetal growth also poses problems for delivery, increasing non-traditional modes of birth and complications such as shoulder dystocia. Stillbirths and perinatal mortality are also linked to GDM.

Where GDM is undetected or poorly controlled, polyuria (increased urinary frequency), polydipsia (excessive thirst), fatigue, macrosomia (birthweight greater than 4000 g), polyhydramnios (excess amniotic fluid volume) and blurred vision may arise. GDM is identified by diagnostic oral glucose tolerance test, indicated for by positive screening from an oral glucose challenge test, 'high risk' based on the risk factors stated above or presence of symptoms such as polydipsia and polyuria.

Treatment aims to reduce glucose levels to lessen excessive fetal growth and other associated adverse outcomes. Less invasive treatments include dietary therapy and exercise. If these interventions alone cannot limit maternal hyperglycaemia, insulin therapy may be necessary. Additionally, oral hypoglycaemics such as glyburide have been demonstrated to be as efficient as insulin therapy in controlling hyperglycaemia and perinatal outcomes.

OBJECTIVES: To assess the effect of dietary advice in preventing gestational diabetes in pregnant women.

TREATMENTS FOR GESTATIONAL DIABETES AND IMPAIRED GLUCOSE TOLERANCE IN PREGNANCY: not enough data to provide reliable evidence. (Tuffnell DJ, West J, Walkinshaw SA) CD003395

BACKGROUND: Gestational diabetes and impaired glucose tolerance (IGT) in pregnancy affect between 3 and 6% of all pregnancies and both have been associated with pregnancy complications. A lack of conclusive evidence has led clinicians to equate the risk of adverse perinatal outcome with pre-existing diabetes. Consequently, women are often intensively managed with increased obstetric monitoring, dietary regulation and in some cases insulin therapy. However, there has been no sound evidence base to support intensive treatment. The key issue for clinicians and consumers is whether treatment of gestational diabetes and IGT will improve perinatal outcome.

OBJECTIVES: To compare alternative policies of care for women with gestational diabetes and IGT in pregnancy.

METHODS: Standard PCG methods (see page xvii). Search date: September 2002.

MAIN RESULTS: Three studies with a total of 223 women were included. All three included studies involved women with IGT. No trials reporting treatments for gestational diabetes met the criteria. There are insufficient data for any reliable conclusions about the effect of treatments for IGT on perinatal outcome. The difference in abdominal operative delivery rates is not statistically significant (relative risk (RR) 0.86, 95% confidence interval 0.51 to 1.45) and the effect on special care baby unit admission is also not significant (RR 0.49, 95% confidence interval (CI) 0.19 to 1.24). Reduction in birthweight greater than 90th centile (RR 0.55, 95% CI 0.19 to 1.61) was not found to be significant. This review suggests that an interventionist policy of treatment may be associated with a reduced risk of neonatal hypoglycaemia (RR 0.25, 95% CI 0.07 to 0.86). No other statistically significant differences were detected. A number of outcomes are only reported by one study resulting in a small sample and wide confidence intervals.

AUTHORS' CONCLUSIONS: There are insufficient data for any reliable conclusions about the effects of treatments for impaired glucose tolerance on perinatal outcome.

CONTINUOUS SUBCUTANEOUS INSULIN INFUSION VERSUS MULTIPLE DAILY INJECTIONS OF INSULIN FOR PREGNANT WOMEN WITH DIABETES: not enough data to provide reliable evidence. (Farrar D, Tuffnell DJ, West J) CD005542

BACKGROUND: Diabetes causes a rise in blood glucose above normal physiological levels, causing damage to many systems including the cardiovascular and renal systems. Pregnancy causes a physiological reduction in insulin action; for those women who have pre-gestational diabetes, this results in an increasing insulin requirement. There are several methods of administering insulin. Conventionally, insulin has been administered subcutaneously, formally referred to as intensive conventional treatment, but now more usually referred to as multiple daily injections (MDI). An alternative insulin administration method is the continuous subcutaneous insulin infusion pump (CSII).

OBJECTIVE: To compare continuous subcutaneous insulin infusion with MDI of insulin for pregnant women with diabetes.

METHODS: Standard PCG methods (see page xvii). Search date: November 2006.

MAIN RESULTS: Two studies (60 women with 61 pregnancies) were included. There was a significant increase in mean birthweight associated with CSII as opposed to MDI (weighted mean difference 220.56, 95% confidence interval (CI) −2.09 to 443.20; two trials, 61 participants).

However, taking into consideration the lack of significant difference in rate of macrosomia (birthweight greater than 4000 g) (relative risk (RR) 3.20, 95% CI 0.14 to 72.62; two trials, 61 participants), this is not viewed by the authors as clinically significant. No significant differences were found in any other outcomes measured, which may reflect the small number of trials suitable for meta-analysis and the small number of participants in the included studies. No significant differences were found in perinatal mortality (RR 2.00, 95% CI 0.20 to 19.91), fetal anomaly (RR 1.07, 95% CI 0.07 to 15.54), maternal hypoglycaemia (RR 3.00, 95% CI 0.35 to 25.87) or maternal hyperglycaemia (RR 7.00, 95% CI 0.39 to 125.44).

AUTHORS' CONCLUSIONS: There is a dearth of robust evidence to support the use of one particular form of insulin administration over another for pregnant women with diabetes. The data are limited because of the small number of trials appropriate for meta-analysis, small study sample size and questionable generalisability of the trial population. Conclusions cannot be made from the data available and therefore a robust randomised trial is needed. The trial should be adequately powered to assess the efficacy of continuous subcutaneous insulin infusion versus multiple daily injections in terms of appropriate outcomes for women with diabetes.

3.4 Thrombocytopenia

Thrombocytopenia is when there are low platelet concentrations in the blood, platelets being required for normal blood clotting. In autoimmune ('idiopathic') thrombocytopenic purpura, antiplatelet antibodies may affect both the mother's and the baby's platelets. Treatments used for the mother include steroids, immunoglobulin and splenectomy. Babies with very low platelet counts are at risk of intracranial haemorrhage during labour or after birth. Because the levels of the baby's platelets correlate poorly with those of the mother, strategies used include cordocentesis, taking fetal scalp blood platelet counts in early labour or empirical caesarean section if the mother's platelet count is below 50000 /μl.

Secondary thrombocytopenia may be due to pre-eclampsia, placental abruption, septicaemia, systemic lupus erythematosis, antiphospholipid syndrome, severe obstetric haemorrhage, megaloblastic anaemia, HIV infection or bone marrow depression due to infection, drugs, alcoholism or neoplastic infiltration.

Alloimmune thrombocytopenia is due to fetomaternal incompatibility for the human platelet antigen. Screening is not routinely performed, so the condition is usually identified after one baby has been affected. Treatments used include weekly fetal transfusions of compatible platelets, or weekly maternal infusions of IgG.

Despite considerable uncertainty concerning the optimal management of these conditions, there is a dearth of information from randomised trials, and no Cochrane systematic reviews of the topic.

3.5 Inherited coagulation defects

These may be suspected in women with a family history or with easy bruising or bleeding, or unexplained postpartum haemorrhage.

There are no Cochrane reviews of this topic.

3.6 Thrombophilias

Susceptibility to thrombosis is increased in women with thrombophilias. Women with a personal or family history of thromboembolism or a history of recurrent miscarriage are generally offered coagulation screening.

> **HEPARIN FOR PREGNANT WOMEN WITH ACQUIRED OR INHERITED THROMBOPHILIAS:** no randomised trials to provide reliable evidence. (Walker MC, Ferguson SE, Allen VM) CD003580

BACKGROUND: Thrombophilias, which are associated with a predisposition to thrombotic events, have been implicated in adverse obstetrical outcomes such as intrauterine growth restriction, stillbirth, severe early onset pre-eclampsia and placental abruption. Heparin administration in pregnancy may reduce the risk of these events.
OBJECTIVES: To assess the effects of heparin on pregnancy outcomes for women with a thrombophilia.
METHODS: Standard PCG methods (see page xvii). Search date: July 2002.
MAIN RESULTS: No studies were included.

AUTHORS' CONCLUSIONS: There are no completed trials to determine the effects of heparin on pregnancy outcomes for women with a thrombophilia.

PROPHYLAXIS FOR VENOUS THROMBOEMBOLIC DISEASE IN PREGNANCY AND THE EARLY POSTNATAL PERIOD: not enough data to provide reliable evidence. (Gates S, Brocklehurst P, Davis LJ) CD001689

BACKGROUND: Venous thromboembolic disease (TED), although very rare, is a major cause of maternal mortality and morbidity; hence methods of prophylaxis are often used for women at risk. This may include women delivered by caesarean section, those with a personal or family history of TED and women with inherited or acquired thrombophilias (conditions that predispose people to thrombosis). Many methods of prophylaxis carry a risk of side effects, and as the risk of thromboembolic disease is low, it is possible that the benefits of thromboprophylaxis may be outweighed by harm. Current guidelines for clinical practice are based on expert opinion only, rather than high quality evidence from randomised trials.

OBJECTIVES: To determine the effects of thromboprophylaxis in association with pregnancy in women who are pregnant or have recently delivered on the incidence of venous thromboembolic disease and side effects.

METHODS: Standard PCG methods (see page xvii). Search date: January 2002.

MAIN RESULTS: Eight trials involving 649 women were included. Four of them compared methods of antenatal prophylaxis: low molecular weight versus unfractionated heparin (two studies), aspirin plus heparin versus aspirin alone (one study) and unfractionated heparin versus no treatment (one study). Four studies assessed postnatal prophylaxis after caesarean section; one compared hydroxyethyl starch with unfractionated heparin, two compared heparin with placebo (one low molecular weight heparin, one unfractionated heparin) and the other compared unfractionated heparin with low molecular weight heparin. It was not possible to assess the effects of any of these interventions on most outcomes, especially rare outcomes such as death, thromboembolic disease and osteoporosis, because of small sample sizes and the small number of trials making the same comparisons.

AUTHORS' CONCLUSIONS: There is insufficient evidence on which to base recommendations for thromboprophylaxis during pregnancy and the early postnatal period. Large scale randomised trials of currently-used interventions should be conducted.

3.7 Haemoglobinopathies

> **INTERVENTIONS FOR TREATING PAINFUL SICKLE CELL CRISIS DURING PREGNANCY:** (Martí-Carvajal A, Peña-Martí G, Comunitn G, Martí-Peña). Protocol [see page xviii] CD006786

ABRIDGED BACKGROUND: Sickle cell disease (SCD) is a group of genetic haemoglobin disorders – abnormal structure of the haemoglobin – which have their origins in sub-Saharan Africa and the Indian sub-continent. The term SCD includes sickle cell anemia (Hb SS); haemoglobin S combined with haemoglobin C (Hb SC); haemoglobin S associated with βThalassemia (Sβ0 Thal and Sβ+ Thal) and other double heterozygous conditions which cause clinical disease. Haemoglobin S combined with normal haemoglobin (A), known as sickle trait (AS), is asymptomatic and therefore not part of this review.

Although SCD is primarily a defect of red blood cells (a haematological defect), changes in the red blood cells result in chronic vasculopathy (damage to blood vessels). The most frequent complication of SCD is vaso-occlusive or painful crises; this is a process of vascular obstruction in very small and, sometimes, large vessels that is initiated by sickle erythrocytes. The remarkable symptom is severe or moderate bone pain, which indicates a haematological emergency. Vaso-oclusive sickle cell crisis tends to occur more frequently during pregnancy and is the most common maternal complication in pregnancy associated with sickle haemoglobinopathies.

OBJECTIVES: To assess the effectiveness and safety of different regimens of packed red cell transfusion, oxygen therapy, fluid replacement therapy, analgesic drugs and steroids for the treatment of painful sickle cell crisis during pregnancy.

3.8 Thromboembolic disease

'...the wealthier patients who remained in bed and formed large clots in their legs and pelvises suffered the major consequences of large pulmonary emboli.' Dock W. In Weisse AB, *Conversations in Medicine: The Story of Twentieth-Century American Medicine in the Words of Those Who Created It*. New York: New York University Press, 1984: 28.

The risk of thromboembolism is increased during pregnancy because of a physiological hypercoagulable state and venous stasis, as well as complications such as vessel wall damage from pre-eclampsia. Clinical signs of deep vein thrombosis may not be prominent. There needs to be a high index of suspicion to diagnose both deep vein thrombosis and pulmonary embolism. The cornerstones of prevention and treatment are anticoagulation and physical measures such as mobilisation and elastic stockings.

There are no Cochrane reviews of this topic.

3.9   Myasthenia gravis

Pregnant women with myasthenia gravis usually continue with anti-cholinesterase medication. Magnesium sulphate is generally avoided, and these women may need assistance in the second stage of labour. There are no Cochrane reviews of this topic.

3.10   Cardiac disease

Trophoblast invasion causes widening of the spiral arterioles supplying the placenta. This large volume, low resistance circulation, together with other physiological changes of pregnancy, reduces peripheral resistance and increases cardiac output considerably. The additional demands of pregnancy and particularly labour on the heart may aggravate the effects of pre-existing heart disease. Previously healthy women may present with heart failure, particularly during the puerperium, due to peripartum cardiomyopathy (a disorder of the heart muscle).

Generally accepted principles for the care of women with heart disease who are pregnant or intend to become pregnant include:

- pre-conceptual counselling and modification of treatment. Women with high-risk conditions such as right-to-left shunt with pulmonary hypertension may be advised to avoid pregnancy.

- screening of pregnant women for silent heart disease, particularly mitral stenosis.
- functional assessment according to the New York Heart Association grading.
- antibiotic prophylaxis for women at risk for recurrent rheumatic valvular disease.
- anticoagulation for women at risk of thrombo-embolism.
- antibiotic prophylaxis during procedures or labour for women at risk for subacute bacterial endocarditis.
- preference for spontaneous labour and vaginal birth, with assisted second stage if necessary.
- careful fluid management during labour.
- prophylactic diuretic at delivery for women with significant functional impairment.
- vigilance for heart failure during the early postpartum period.

There has been relatively little systematic research to evaluate the effectiveness of these strategies.

There are no Cochrane reviews of this topic.

3.11   Renal disease

Women with serious renal disease are usually counselled about the possibility of complications during pregnancy. If not diagnosed before pregnancy, renal disease with proteinuria and hypertension may be mistaken for pre-eclampsia. Urinary tract infections are particularly common during pregnancy (see page 207)

There are no Cochrane reviews of this topic.

3.12   Epilepsy

Preconceptually, women with epilepsy are often counselled about the risk of congenital anomalies related to their medication. If women with epilepsy have been free of convulsions for some years, stopping medication may be considered. The risks of congenital anomalies with single drug treatment are less than with multiple drugs. In most cases, continuing medication is advised because the risks of convulsions appear greater than the risks of medication. Folate is given periconceptually.

During pregnancy, serum drug levels are monitored and dosages increased as necessary to maintain therapeutic levels.

> **COMMON ANTIEPILEPTIC DRUGS IN PREGNANCY IN WOMEN WITH EPILEPSY:** monotherapy appeared safer than multiple drug therapy; more research is needed. (Adab N, Tudur Smith C, Vinten J, Williamson PR, Winterbottom JB) CD004848 (Epilepsy Group)

BACKGROUND: The potential adverse effects of antiepileptic drug (AED) exposure in pregnancy have been well recognised but the relative risks of specific antiepileptic drug exposures remain poorly understood.

OBJECTIVES: To assess the adverse effects of commonly used antiepileptic drugs on maternal and fetal outcomes in pregnancy in women with epilepsy. Comparison of outcomes following specific antiepileptic drug exposures in utero to unexposed pregnancies in the general population or women with epilepsy is described. The current manuscript reports the first phase of this review which focuses upon neurodevelopmental outcomes in children exposed to antiepileptic drugs in utero.

SEARCH STRATEGY: We searched MEDLINE, Pharmline, EMBASE, Reprotox and TERIS from 1966 to December 2003. Review articles and conference abstracts were also hand searched.

SELECTION CRITERIA: All randomised controlled trials, prospective cohorts of children of pregnant women with and without epilepsy and case control studies (cases: developmental delay or impaired cognitive outcome, control: normal development) were included.

DATA COLLECTION AND ANALYSIS: Methodological quality was assessed using an adapted version of the Newcastle-Ottawa Scale. The wide variety of outcome measures and methodological approaches made meta-analysis difficult and a descriptive analysis of the results is presented.

MAIN RESULTS: *PART A 1b – Developmental outcomes*
The majority of studies were of limited quality. There was little evidence about which specific drugs carry more risk than others to the development of children exposed in utero. The results between studies are conflicting and while most failed to find a significant detrimental outcome with in utero exposure to monotherapy with carbamazepine, phenytoin or phenobarbitone, this should be interpreted cautiously. There were very few studies of exposure to sodium valproate. Polytherapy exposure in utero was more commonly associated with poorer outcomes,

as was exposure to any AEDs when analysis did not take into account the type of AED. The latter may reflect the large proportion of children included in these studies who were in fact exposed to polytherapy.

AUTHORS' CONCLUSIONS: *PART A 1b – Developmental outcomes* **Based on the best current available evidence it would seem advisable for women to continue medication during pregnancy using monotherapy at the lowest dose required to achieve seizure control. Polytherapy would seem best avoided where possible. More population based studies adequately powered to examine the effects of in utero exposure to specific monotherapies which are used in everyday practice are required.**

3.13   Human immunodeficiency virus infection (HIV)

In countries with high infection rates, deaths from HIV may outstrip all other causes of maternal mortality. Highly active antiretroviral treatment (HAART) for immunodeficient women has the potential to reverse this mortality trend, but implementation in resource-poor countries is difficult.

Mother to child transmission of HIV is in theory almost entirely preventable, but achieving this goal in resource-poor environments has been elusive. For women not receiving triple antiretroviral therapy, several low-cost interventions to reduce mother to child transmission of HIV infection during and after pregnancy have emerged.

Infant feeding is a particularly fraught issue in low-income populations, where the risks of HIV infection need to be weighed against the increased mortality from other causes in non-breastfed infants.

The Cochrane HIV/AIDS Group and the Child Health Field are in the process of completing an umbrella review on Interventions for preventing mother-to-child transmission of HIV.

☺ **ANTIRETROVIRALS FOR REDUCING THE RISK OF MOTHER-TO-CHILD TRANSMISSION OF HIV INFECTION:** are effective in various regimens including short courses. (Volmink J, Siegfried NL, van der Merwe L, Brocklehurst P) CD003510 (HIV/AIDS Group) (in RHL 11)

BACKGROUND: Antiretroviral drugs (ARV) reduce viral replication and can reduce mother-to-child transmission of HIV either by lower plasma viral load in pregnant women or through post-exposure prophylaxis in their newborns. In rich countries, highly active antiretroviral therapy (HAART) has reduced the vertical transmission rates to around 1–2%, but HAART is not yet widely available in low and middle income countries. In these countries, various simpler and less costly antiretroviral regimens have been offered to pregnant women or to their newborn babies, or to both.

OBJECTIVES: To determine whether, and to what extent, antiretroviral regimens aimed at decreasing the risk of mother-to-child transmission of HIV infection achieve a clinically useful decrease in transmission risk, and what effect these interventions have on maternal and infant mortality and morbidity.

SEARCH STRATEGY: We sought to identify all relevant studies regardless of language or publication status by searching the Cochrane HIV/AIDS Review Group Trials Register, The Cochrane Library, Medline, EMBASE and AIDSearch and relevant conference abstracts. We also contacted research organisations and experts in the field for unpublished and ongoing studies. The original review search strategy was updated in 2006.

SELECTION CRITERIA: Randomised controlled trials of any antiretroviral regimen aimed at decreasing the risk of mother-to-child transmission of HIV infection compared with placebo or no treatment.

DATA COLLECTION AND ANALYSIS: Two authors independently selected relevant studies, extracted data and assessed trial quality. For the primary outcomes, we used survival analysis to estimate the probability of infants being infected with HIV (the observed proportion) at various specific time-points and calculated efficacy at a specific time as the relative reduction in the proportion infected. Efficacy, at a specific time, is defined as the preventive fraction in the exposed group compared to the reference group, which is the relative reduction in the proportion infected: $1-(Re/Rf)$. For those studies where efficacy and hence confidence intervals were not calculated, we calculated the approximate confidence intervals for the efficacy using recommended methods. For analysis of results that are not based on survival analyses we present the relative risk for each trial outcome based on the number randomised. No meta-analysis was conducted as no trial assessed the identical drug regimens.

MAIN RESULTS: Eighteen trials including 14398 participants conducted in 16 countries were eligible for inclusion in the review. The first trial began in April 1991 and assessed zidovudine (ZDV) versus placebo and since then the type, dosage and duration of drugs to be compared have been modified in each subsequent trial.

Antiretrovirals versus placebo: In breastfeeding populations, three trials found that:

ZDV given to mothers from 36 to 38 weeks' gestation, during labour and for seven days after delivery significantly reduced HIV infection at four to eight weeks (Efficacy 32.00%; 95% CI 0.64 to 63.36), three to four months (Efficacy 34.00%; 95% CI 6.56 to 61.44), six months (Efficacy 35.00%; 95% CI 9.52 to 60.48), 12 months (Efficacy 34.00%; 95% CI 8.52 to 59.48) and 18 months (Efficacy 30.00%; 95% CI 2.56 to 57.44).

ZDV given to mothers from 36 weeks' gestation and during labour significantly reduced HIV infection at four to eight weeks (Efficacy 44.00%; 95% CI 8.72 to 79.28) and three to four months (Efficacy 37.00%; 95% CI 3.68 to 70.32) but not at birth.

ZDV plus lamivudine (3TC) given to mothers from 36 weeks gestation, during labour and for seven days after delivery and to babies for the first seven days of life (PETRA 'regimen A') significantly reduced HIV infection (Efficacy 63.00%; 95% CI 41.44 to 84.56) and a combined endpoint of HIV infection or death (Efficacy 61.00%; 95% CI 41.40 to 80.60) at four to eight weeks but these effects were not sustained at 18 months.

ZDV plus 3TC given to mothers from the start of labour until seven days after delivery and to babies for the first seven days of life (PETRA 'regimen B') significantly reduced HIV infection (Efficacy 42.00%; 95% CI 12.60 to 71.40) and HIV infection or death at four to eight weeks (Efficacy 36.00%; 95% CI 8.56 to 63.44) but the effects were not sustained at 18 months.

ZDV plus 3TC given to mothers during labour only (PETRA 'regimen C') with no treatment to babies did not reduce the risk of HIV infection at either four to eight weeks or 18 months.

In non-breastfeeding populations, three trials found that:

ZDV given to mothers from 14 to 34 weeks' gestation and during labour and to babies for the first six weeks of life significantly reduced HIV infection in babies at 18 months (Efficacy 66.00%; 95% CI 34.64 to 97.36).

ZDV given to mothers from 36 weeks' gestation and during labour with no treatment to babies ('Thai-CDC regimen') significantly reduced HIV infection at four to eight weeks (Efficacy 50.00%; 95% CI 12.76 to 87.24) but not at birth.

ZDV given to mothers from 38 weeks' gestation and during labour with no treatment to babies did not influence HIV transmission at six months.

Longer versus shorter regimens using the same antiretrovirals: One trial in a breastfeeding population found that:

ZDV given to mothers during labour and to their babies for the first three days of life compared with ZDV given to mothers from 36 weeks and during labour (similar to 'Thai-CDC') resulted in HIV infection rates that were not significantly different at birth, four to eight weeks, three to four months, six months and 12 months.

Three trials in non-breastfeeding populations found that:

ZDV given to mothers from 28 weeks' gestation during labour and to infants for the first three days after birth compared with ZDV given to mothers from 35 weeks' gestation through labour and to infants from birth to six weeks significantly reduced HIV infection rate at six months (Efficacy 45.00%; 95% CI 1.88 to 88.12) but compared with the same regimen ZDV given to mothers from 28 weeks' gestation through labour and to infants from birth to six weeks did not result in a statistically significant difference in HIV infection at six months. ZDV given to mothers from 35 weeks' gestation during labour and to infants for the first three days after birth was considered ineffective for reducing transmission rates and this regimen was discontinued.

An antenatal/intrapartum course of ZDV used for a median of 76 days compared with an antenatal/intrapartum ZDV regimen used for a median 28 days with no treatment to babies in either group did not result in HIV infection rates that were significantly different at birth or at three to four months.

In a programme where mothers were routinely receiving ZDV in the third trimester of pregnancy and babies were receiving one week of ZDV therapy, a single dose of nevirapine (NVP) given to mothers in labour and to their babies soon after birth compared with a single dose of NVP given to mothers only resulted in HIV infection rates that were not significantly different at birth or six months. However the reduction in risk of HIV infection or death at six months was marginally significant (Efficacy 45.00%; 95% CI −4.00 to 94.00).

Antiretroviral regimens using different drugs and durations of treatment: In breastfeeding populations, three trials found that:

A single dose of NVP given to mothers at the onset of labour plus a single dose of NVP given to their babies immediately after birth ('HIVNET 012 regimen') compared with ZDV given to mothers during labour and to their babies for a week after birth resulted in lower HIV infection rates at 4–8 weeks (Efficacy 41.00%; 95% CI 11.60 to 70.40), three to four months (Efficacy 39.00%; 95% CI 11.56 to 66.44), 12 months (Efficacy 36.00%; 95% CI 8.56 to 63.44) and 18 months (Efficacy 39.00%; 95% CI 13.52 to 64.48). In addition, the NVP regimen significantly reduced the risk of HIV infection or death at four to eight weeks (Efficacy 42.00%; 95% CI 14.56 to 69.44), three to four months (Efficacy 40.00%; 95% CI 14.52 to 65.48), 12 months (Efficacy 32.00%; 95% CI 8.48 to 55.52) and 18 months (Efficacy 33.00%; 95% CI 9.48 to 56.52).

The 'HIVNET 012 regimen' plus ZDV given to babies for 1 week after birth compared with the 'HIVNET 012 regimen' alone did not result in a statistically significant difference in HIV infection at four to eight weeks.

A single dose of NVP given to babies immediately after birth plus ZDV given to babies for one week after birth compared with a single dose of NVP given to babies only significantly reduced the HIV infection rate at four to eight weeks (Efficacy 37.00%; 95% CI 3.68 to 70.32).

Five trials in non-breastfeeding populations found that:

In a population in which mothers were receiving 'standard' ARV for HIV infection a single dose of NVP given to mothers in labour plus a single dose of NVP given to babies immediately after birth ('HIVNET 012 regimen') compared with placebo did not result in a statistically significant difference in HIV infection rates at birth or at four to eight weeks.

The 'Thai CDC regimen' compared with the 'HIVNET 012 regimen' did not result in a significant difference in HIV infection at four to eight weeks.

A single dose of NVP given to babies immediately after birth compared to ZDV given to babies for the first six weeks of life did not result in a significant difference in HIV infection rates at four to eight weeks or three to four months.

ZDV plus 3TC given to mothers in labour and for a week after delivery and to their infants for a week after birth (similar to 'PETRA regimen B') compared with NVP given to mothers in labour and immediately after delivery plus a single dose of NVP to their babies immediately after birth (similar to 'HIVNET 012 regimen') did not result in a significant difference in the HIV infection rate at four to eight weeks.

An evaluation of various ARV drugs given to mothers from 34 to 36 weeks and during labour with the same drugs given to their babies for six weeks after birth – stavudine (d4T) versus ZDV, didanosine (ddI) versus ZDV and d4T plus ddI versus ZDV – did not result in statistically important differences in HIV infection rates at birth, four to eight weeks, three to four months or six months.

Adverse effects:

The incidence of serious or life threatening events was not significantly different in any of the trials included in this review.

AUTHORS' CONCLUSIONS: Short courses of antiretroviral drugs are effective for reducing mother-to-child transmission of HIV and are not associated with any safety concerns in the short term. A combination of ZDV and 3TC given to mothers in the antenatal, intrapartum and postpartum periods and to babies for a week after delivery or a single dose of NVP given to mothers in labour and babies immediately after birth may be most effective. Where HIV- infected women present late for delivery, post-exposure prophylaxis with a single dose of NVP immediately after birth plus ZDV for the first 6 weeks of life is beneficial. The long-term implications of the emergence of resistant mutations following the use of these regimens require further study.

EFFICACY AND SAFETY OF CESAREAN DELIVERY FOR PREVENTION OF MOTHER-TO-CHILD TRANSMISSION OF HIV-1: is effective for women not receiving highly active antiretroviral therapy. (Read JS, Newell ML) CD005479 (HIV/AIDS Group) (in RHL 11)

BACKGROUND: Cesarean section before labor and before ruptured membranes ("elective cesarean section", or ECS) has been introduced as an intervention for the prevention of mother-to-child transmission

(MTCT) of HIV-1. The role of mode of delivery in the management of HIV-1-infected women should be assessed in light of risks as well as benefits, since HIV-1-infected pregnant women must be provided with available information with which to make informed decisions regarding cesarean section and other options to prevent transmission of infection to their children.

OBJECTIVES: Our objectives were to assess the efficacy (for prevention of MTCT of HIV-1) and the safety of ECS among HIV-1-infected women.

SEARCH STRATEGY: Electronic searches were undertaken using MEDLINE and other databases. Hand searches of reference lists of pertinent reviews and studies, as well as abstracts from relevant conferences, were also conducted. Experts in the field were contacted to locate any other studies. The search strategy was iterative.

SELECTION CRITERIA: Randomized clinical trials assessing the efficacy and safety of ECS for prevention of MTCT of HIV-1 were included in the analysis, as were observational studies with relevant data.

DATA COLLECTION AND ANALYSIS: Data regarding HIV-1 infection status of infants born to HIV-1-infected women according to mode of delivery were extracted from the reports of the studies. Similarly, data regarding postpartum morbidity (PPM) (including minor (e.g. febrile morbidity, urinary tract infection) and major (e.g. endometritis, thromboembolism) morbidity) of the HIV-1-infected women, and infant morbidity, according to mode of delivery were extracted.

MAIN RESULTS: One randomized clinical trial of the efficacy of ECS for prevention of MTCT of HIV-1 was identified. No data regarding infant morbidity according to the HIV-1-infected mother's mode of delivery were available. Data regarding PPM according to mode of delivery were available from this clinical trial as well as from five observational studies. Among HIV-1-infected women not taking antiretrovirals (ARVs) during pregnancy or taking only zidovudine, ECS was found to be efficacious for prevention of MTCT of HIV-1. PPM is generally higher among HIV-1-infected women who undergo cesarean as compared to vaginal delivery, with the risk with ECS being intermediate between that of vaginal delivery and NECS (including emergency procedures). Other factors associated with the risk of PPM among HIV-1-infected women include HIV-1 disease stage (more advanced disease, as manifested by lower CD4 counts and higher viral loads, being associated with a greater risk of PPM) and co-morbid conditions (e.g., diabetes).

AUTHORS' CONCLUSIONS: ECS is an efficacious intervention for the prevention of MTCT among HIV-1-infected women not taking ARVs or taking only zidovudine. The risk of PPM with ECS is higher than that associated with vaginal delivery, yet lower than with NECS. Among HIV-1-infected women, more advanced maternal HIV-1 disease stage and concomitant medical conditions (e.g. diabetes) are independent risk factors for PPM. The risk of MTCT of HIV-1 according to mode of delivery among HIV-1-infected women with low viral loads (low either because the woman's HIV-1 disease is not advanced, or because her HIV-1 disease is well-controlled with ARVs) is unclear. Therefore, an important issue to be addressed in one or more large studies (individual studies or an individual patient data meta-analysis combining data from more than one study) is assessment of the effectiveness of ECS for prevention of MTCT of HIV-1 among HIV-1-infected women with undetectable viral loads (with or without receipt of highly active ARV therapy (HAART)).

☺ **INTERVENTIONS FOR REDUCING THE RISK OF MOTHER-TO-CHILD TRANSMISSION OF HIV INFECTION:** zidovudine, nevirapine and delivery by elective caesarean section are effective (Brocklehurst P) CD000102 (HIV/AIDS Group)

BACKGROUND: At the end of 1998 over 33 million people were infected with the human immunodeficiency virus (HIV) and over one million children had been infected from their mothers.

OBJECTIVES: The objective of this review was to assess what interventions may be effective in decreasing the risk of mother-to-child transmission of HIV infection as well as their effect on neonatal and maternal mortality and morbidity.

SEARCH STRATEGY: The Cochrane Pregnancy and Childbirth Group trials register and the Cochrane Controlled Trials Register were searched.

SELECTION CRITERIA: Randomised trials comparing any intervention aimed at decreasing the risk of mother-to-child transmission of HIV infection compared with placebo or no treatment, or any two or more interventions aimed at decreasing the risk of mother-to-child transmission of HIV infection.

DATA COLLECTION AND ANALYSIS: Trial quality assessments and data extraction were undertaken by the reviewer.

MAIN RESULTS: Zidovudine: Four trials comparing zidovudine with placebo involving 1585 participants were included. Compared with placebo, there was a significant reduction in the risk of mother-to-child transmission with any zidovudine (relative risk (RR) 0.54, 95% confidence interval (CI) 0.42–0.69). There is no evidence that 'long course therapy' is superior to 'short course therapy'.

Nevirapine: One trial compared intrapartum and postnatal nevirapine with intrapartum and postnatal zidovudine in 626 women, the majority of whom breast fed their infants. Compared with zidovudine, there was a significant reduction in the risk of mother-to-child transmission of HIV with nevirapine (RR 0.58, 95% CI 0.40–0.83). No trials are available comparing nevirapine with placebo.

Caesarean section: One trial comparing elective caesarean section with anticipation of vaginal delivery involving 436 participants was included. Compared with vaginal delivery, there was a significant reduction in the risk of mother-to-child transmission of HIV infection with caesarean section (RR 0.17, 95% CI 0.05–0.55).

Immunoglobulin: One trial comparing hyperimmune immunoglobulin plus zidovudine with non-specific immunoglobulin plus zidovudine involving 501 participants was included. The addition of hyperimmune immunoglobulin to zidovudine does not appear to have any additional effect on the risk of mother-to-child transmission (RR 0.67, 95% CI 0.29–1.55).

AUTHOR'S CONCLUSIONS: Zidovudine, nevirapine and delivery by elective caesarean section appear to be very effective in decreasing the risk of mother-to-child transmission of HIV infection.

VAGINAL DISINFECTION FOR PREVENTING MOTHER-TO-CHILD TRANSMISSION OF HIV INFECTION: not enough data to provide reliable evidence. (Wiysonge CS, Shey MS, Shang JD, Sterne JAC, Brocklehurst P) CD003651 (HIV/AIDS Group) (in RHL 11)

BACKGROUND: Mother-to-child transmission (MTCT) of HIV infection is one of the most tragic consequences of the HIV epidemic, especially in resource-limited countries, resulting in about 650 000 new paediatric HIV infections each year worldwide. The paediatric HIV epidemic threatens to seriously undermine decade-old child survival programmes.

OBJECTIVES: To estimate the effect of vaginal disinfection on the risk of MTCT of HIV and infant and maternal mortality and morbidity, as well as tolerability of vaginal disinfection in HIV-infected women.

SEARCH STRATEGY: We searched the Cochrane Controlled Trials Register, Cochrane Pregnancy and Childbirth Register, PubMed, EMBASE, AIDSLINE, LILACS, AIDSTRIALS and AIDSDRUGS, using standardised methodological filters for identifying trials. We also searched reference lists of identified articles, relevant editorials, expert opinions and letters to journal editors, and abstracts and proceedings of relevant conferences, and contacted subject experts and pharmaceutical companies. There were no language restrictions.

SELECTION CRITERIA: Randomised trials or clinical trials comparing vaginal disinfection during labour with placebo or no treatment, in known HIV-infected pregnant women. Trials had to include an estimate of the effect of vaginal disinfection on MTCT of HIV and/or infant and maternal mortality and morbidity.

DATA COLLECTION AND ANALYSIS: Three authors independently assessed trial eligibility and quality, and extracted data. Meta-analysis was performed using the Yusuf-Peto modification of Mantel-Haenszel's fixed effect method.

MAIN RESULTS: Only two trials that included 708 patients met the inclusion criteria. The effect of vaginal disinfection on the risk of MTCT of HIV (OR 0.93, 95% CI 0.65 to 1.33), neonatal death (OR 1.38, 95% CI 0.30 to 6.33) and death after the neonatal period (OR 1.45, 95% CI 0.47 to 4.45) is uncertain. There was no evidence that vaginal disinfection increased adverse effects in mothers (OR 1.15, 95% CI 0.41 to 3.22), and evidence from one trial showed that adverse effects decreased in neonates (OR 0.14, 95% CI 0.07 to 0.31).

AUTHORS' CONCLUSIONS: Currently, there is no evidence of an effect of vaginal disinfection on the risk of MTCT of HIV. Given its simplicity and low cost, there is need for a large well-designed and well-conducted randomised controlled trial to assess the additive

effect of vaginal disinfection on the risk of MTCT of HIV in antiretro-
viral-treated women.

**VITAMIN A SUPPLEMENTATION FOR REDUCING THE RISK OF
MOTHER-TO-CHILD TRANSMISSION OF HIV INFECTION:** was
not effective; further results awaited. (Wiysonge CS, Shey MS, Sterne
JAC, Brocklehurst P) CD003648 (HIV/AIDS Group) (in RHL 11)

BACKGROUND: Mother-to-child transmission (MTCT) of HIV is the
dominant mode of acquisition of HIV infection for children, currently
resulting in more than 2000 new paediatric HIV infections each day
worldwide.

OBJECTIVES: To assess the effects of antenatal and intrapartum vitamin
A supplementation on the risk of MTCT of HIV infection and infant and
maternal mortality and morbidity, and the tolerability of vitamin A supplementation.

SEARCH STRATEGY: We searched the Cochrane Central Register of Controlled Trials, PubMed, EMBASE, AIDSLINE, LILACS, AIDSTRIALS and
AIDSDRUGS, using standardised methodological filters for identifying
trials. We also searched reference lists of identified articles, relevant
editorials, expert opinions and letters to journal editors, and abstracts
or proceedings of relevant conferences; and contacted subject experts,
agencies, organisations, academic centres and pharmaceutical companies. There were no language restrictions.

SELECTION CRITERIA: Randomised trials comparing vitamin A supplementation with no vitamin A supplementation in known HIV-
infected pregnant women. Trials had to include an estimate of the
effect of vitamin A supplementation on MTCT of HIV and/or any
other adverse pregnancy outcome to be included.

DATA COLLECTION AND ANALYSIS: Two authors independently assessed trial eligibility and quality and extracted data. Effect measures
(odds ratio [OR] for binary variables and weighted mean difference
[WMD] for continuous variables) with their 95% confidence intervals
(CI) were estimated for each study and combined using the fixed effect (Mantel-Haenszel) method, by intention to treat. Heterogeneity
between studies was examined by graphical inspection of results followed by a chi-square test of homogeneity.

MAIN RESULTS: Four trials, which enrolled 3033 HIV-infected pregnant
women, are included in this review. There was no evidence of an effect

of vitamin A supplementation on MTCT of HIV infection (OR 1.14, 95% CI 0.93 to 1.38). There was evidence of heterogeneity between the three trials with information on MTCT of HIV (I^2 =75.7%, P=0.02). While the trials conducted in South Africa (OR 0.98, 95% CI 0.67 to 1.42 at three months) and Malawi (OR 0.78, 95% CI 0.53 to 1.15 at 24 months) did not find evidence that the effect of vitamin A supplementation was different from that of placebo, the trial in Tanzania did find evidence that vitamin A supplementation increased the risk of MTCT of HIV (OR 1.53, 95% CI 1.15 to 2.04 at 24 months). Vitamin A supplementation significantly improved birth weight (WMD 89.78, 95% CI 84.73 to 94.83), but there was no evidence of an effect of vitamin A supplementation on stillbirths (OR 0.99, 95% CI 0.67 to 1.46), preterm births (OR 0.89, 95% CI 0.71 to 1.11), death by 24 months among live births (OR 1.11, 95% CI 0.88 to 1.40), postpartum CD4 levels (WMD −4.00, 95% CI −51.06 to 43.06), or maternal death (OR 0.49, 95%CI 0.04 to 5.40).

AUTHORS' CONCLUSIONS: Implications for practice: Currently available evidence does not support the use of vitamin A supplementation of HIV-infected pregnant women to reduce MTCT of HIV, though there is an indication that vitamin A supplementation improves birth weight.

Implications for research: The awaited publication of data from a large trial involving 4495 HIV-infected pregnant women in Harare (Zimbabwe Vitamin A for Mothers and Babies Project) will further clarify the effect of vitamin A supplementation on MTCT of HIV. The current review will be updated as soon as the trial is published.

MICRONUTRIENT SUPPLEMENTATION IN CHILDREN AND ADULTS WITH HIV INFECTION: multivitamin supplementation for pregnant women and for those who are breastfeeding improved outcomes. More research is needed. (Irlam JH, Visser ME, Rollins N, Siegfried N) CD003650 (HIV/AIDS Group)

BACKGROUND: The scale and impact of the HIV/AIDS pandemic has made the search for simple, affordable, safe and effective public health interventions all the more urgent. Micronutrient supplements hold the promise of meeting these criteria, but their widespread use needs to be based on sound scientific evidence of effectiveness and safety.

OBJECTIVES: To assess whether micronutrient supplements are effective in reducing morbidity and mortality in adults and children with HIV infection.

SEARCH STRATEGY: The Cochrane Library (CENTRAL), EMBASE, MEDLINE, AIDSearch, CINAHL and conference proceedings were searched, and pharmaceutical manufacturers and researchers in the field were contacted to locate any ongoing or unpublished trials.

SELECTION CRITERIA: Randomised controlled trials comparing the effects of micronutrient supplements (vitamins, trace elements and combinations of these) with placebo or no treatment on mortality and morbidity in HIV-infected individuals.

DATA COLLECTION AND ANALYSIS: Two reviewers independently appraised trial quality and extracted data. Study authors were contacted for additional data where necessary. A meta-analysis was not deemed appropriate due to significant heterogeneity between trials.

MAIN RESULTS: 15 trials were included. Six trials comparing vitamin A/beta-carotene with placebo in adults failed to show any effects on mortality, morbidity, CD4 and CD8 counts, or on viral load. Four trials of other micronutrients in adults did not affect overall mortality, although there was a reduction in mortality in a low CD4 subgroup. In a large Tanzanian trial in pregnant and lactating women, daily multivitamin supplementation was associated with a number of benefits to both mothers and children: a reduction in maternal mortality from AIDS-related causes; a reduced risk of progression to stage four disease; fewer adverse pregnancy outcomes; less diarrhoeal morbidity; and a reduction in early-child mortality among immunologically- and nutritionally-compromised women. Vitamin A alone reduced all-cause mortality and improved growth in a small sub-group of HIV-infected children in one hospital-based trial, and reduced diarrhoea-associated morbidity in a small HIV-infected sub-group of infants in another trial.

AUTHORS' CONCLUSIONS: There is no conclusive evidence at present to show that micronutrient supplementation effectively reduces morbidity and mortality among HIV-infected adults. It is reasonable to support the current WHO recommendations to promote and support adequate dietary intake of micronutrients at RDA levels wherever possible. There is evidence of benefit of vitamin A supplementation in children. The long-term clinical benefits, adverse effects and optimal formulation of micronutrient supplements require further investigation.

3.14   Other viral infections

Primary rubella infection in early pregnancy may cause fetal anomaly, and can be prevented by vaccination of adolescent girls.

Primary cytomegalovirus infection during pregnancy may lead to congenital infection with serious morbidity and mortality.

Parvovirus B19 infection during pregnancy may cause haemolytic anaemia in the baby. Intrauterine transfusion may be needed in severe cases, but the infection is self-limiting.

Primary varicella infection during pregnancy may infect the baby. Between 11 and 19 weeks anomalies may occur, in which case calcification is almost always visible with ultrasound within five weeks. Birth of a recently-infected baby who has not had time to receive passive immunity may be fatal.

Active herpes simplex type II infections may cause serious neonatal infection during vaginal birth.

Human papilloma virus types 6 and 11 may rarely cause papillomas on the baby's vocal cords.

Measles is a serious illness in adults, and may cause pregnancy complications and congenital anomalies.

Influenza may be a serious infection in pregnant women. Data on effects on the baby are inconclusive.

There are no Cochrane reviews on these topics

3.15   Malaria

☺ **DRUGS FOR PREVENTING MALARIA IN PREGNANT WOMEN:** reduced parasitaemia, anaemia, low birthweight and possibly perinatal death. (Garner P, Gülmezoglu AM) CD000169 (Infectious Diseases Group) (in RHL 11)

BACKGROUND: Malaria contributes to maternal illness and anaemia in pregnancy, especially in first-time mothers, and can harm the mother and the baby. Drugs given routinely to prevent or mitigate the effects of malaria during pregnancy are often recommended.

OBJECTIVES: To assess drugs given to prevent malaria infection and its consequences in pregnant women living in malarial areas. This includes prophylaxis and intermittent preventive treatment (IPT).

SEARCH STRATEGY: We searched the Cochrane Infectious Diseases Group Specialized Register (March 2006) CENTRAL (*The Cochrane Library* 2006, Issue 1), MEDLINE (1966 to March 2006) EMBASE (1974 to March 2006), LILACS (1982 to March 2006), and reference lists. We also contacted researchers working in the field.

SELECTION CRITERIA: Randomized and quasi-randomized controlled trials comparing antimalarial drugs given regularly with no antimalarial drugs for preventing malaria in pregnant women living in malaria-endemic areas.

DATA COLLECTION AND ANALYSIS: Both authors extracted data and assessed methodological quality. Dichotomous variables were combined using relative risks (RR) and weighted mean differences (WMD) for mean values, both with 95% confidence intervals (CI).

MAIN RESULTS: Sixteen trials (12 638 participants) met the inclusion criteria; two used adequate methods to conceal allocation. Antimalarials reduced antenatal parasitaemia when given to all pregnant women (RR 0.53, 95% CI 0.33 to 0.86; 328 participants, two trials), placental malaria (RR 0.34, 95% CI 0.26 to 0.45; 1236 participants, three trials), but no effect was detected with perinatal deaths (2890 participants, four trials). In women in their first or second pregnancy, antimalarial drugs reduced severe antenatal anaemia (RR 0.62, 95% CI 0.50 to 0.78; 2809 participants, one prophylaxis and two IPT trials), antenatal parasitaemia (RR 0.27, 95% CI 0.17 to 0.44, random-effects model; 2906 participants, six trials) and perinatal deaths (RR 0.73, 95% CI 0.53 to 0.99; 1986 participants, two prophylaxis and one IPT trial); mean birthweight was higher (WMD 126.70 g, 95% CI 88.64 to 164.75 g; 2648 participants, eight trials) and low birthweight was less frequent (RR 0.57, 95% CI 0.46 to 0.72; 2350 participants, six trials).

Proguanil performed better than chloroquine in one trial of women of all parities in relation to maternal fever episodes. Sulfadoxine–pyrimethamine performed better than chloroquine in two trials of low-parity women.

AUTHORS' CONCLUSIONS: Chemoprophylaxis or IPT reduces antenatal parasite prevalence and placental malaria when given to women in all parity groups. They also have positive effects on birthweight and possibly on perinatal death in low-parity women.

DRUGS FOR TREATING UNCOMPLICATED MALARIA IN PREGNANT WOMEN: not enough data to provide reliable evidence. (Orton L, Garner P) CD004912 (Infectious Diseases Group)

BACKGROUND: Women are more vulnerable to malaria during pregnancy, and malaria infection may have adverse consequences for the fetus. Identifying safe and effective treatments is important.

OBJECTIVES: To compare the effects of drug regimens for treating uncomplicated falciparum malaria in pregnant women.

SEARCH STRATEGY: We searched the Cochrane Infectious Diseases Group Specialized Register (May 2005), Cochrane Central Register of Controlled Trials (*The Cochrane Library* Issue 2, 2005), MEDLINE (1966 to May 2005), EMBASE (1974 to May 2005), LILACS (May 2005), reference lists, and conference abstracts. We also contacted researchers in the field, organizations, and pharmaceutical companies.

SELECTION CRITERIA: Randomized and quasi-randomized controlled trials of antimalarial drugs for treating uncomplicated malaria in pregnant women.

DATA COLLECTION AND ANALYSIS: Both authors assessed trial eligibility and methodological quality, and extracted data. We performed a quantitative analysis only where we could combine the data. We combined dichotomous data using relative risk (RR) with 95% confidence intervals (CI).

MAIN RESULTS: Six trials (513 participants) met the inclusion criteria. Two were quasi-randomized, and none described allocation concealment. Data were scarce for the primary outcome, treatment failure. One trial compared artesunate plus mefloquine with quinine and reported fewer treatment failures at day 63 with the combination (RR 0.09, 95% CI 0.02 to 0.38; 106 participants).

AUTHORS' CONCLUSIONS: There is insufficient reliable research on malaria treatment options in pregnancy.

☺ **INSECTICIDE-TREATED NETS FOR PREVENTING MALARIA IN PREGNANCY:** reduced placental malaria, low birthweight and fetal loss in Africa; anaemia and fetal loss in Thailand. (Gamble C, Ekwaru JP, ter Kuile FO) CD003755 (Infectious Diseases Group) (in RHL 11)

BACKGROUND: Malaria in pregnancy is associated with adverse consequences for mother and fetus. Protection with insecticide-treated nets (ITNs) during pregnancy is widely advocated, but evidence of their benefit has been inconsistent.

OBJECTIVES: To compare the impact of ITNs with no nets or untreated nets on preventing malaria in pregnancy.

SEARCH STRATEGY: We searched the Cochrane Infectious Diseases Group Specialized Register (January 2006), CENTRAL (*The Cochrane Library* 2005, Issue 4), MEDLINE (1966 to January 2006), EMBASE (1974 to January 2006), LILACS (1982 to January 2006) and reference lists. We also contacted researchers working in the field.

SELECTION CRITERIA: Individual and cluster randomised controlled trials of ITNs in pregnant women.

DATA COLLECTION AND ANALYSIS: Three authors independently assessed trials for methodological quality and extracted data. Data were combined using the generic inverse variance method.

MAIN RESULTS: Six randomised controlled trials were identified, five of which met the inclusion criteria: four trials from sub-Saharan Africa compared ITNs with no nets, and one trial from Asia compared ITNs with untreated nets. Two trials randomised individual women and three trials randomised communities. In Africa, ITNs, compared with no nets, reduced placental malaria in all pregnancies (relative risk (RR) 0.79, 95% confidence interval (CI) 0.63 to 0.98). They also reduced low birthweight (RR 0.77, 95% CI 0.61 to 0.98) and fetal loss in the first to fourth pregnancy (RR 0.67, 95% CI 0.47 to 0.97), but not in women with more than four previous pregnancies. For anaemia and clinical malaria, results tended to favour ITNs, but the effects were not significant. In Thailand, one trial randomised individuals to ITNs or untreated nets showed a significant reduction in anaemia and fetal loss in all pregnancies but not for clinical malaria or low birthweight.

AUTHORS' CONCLUSIONS: ITNs have a beneficial impact on pregnancy outcome in malaria-endemic regions of Africa when used by

communities or by individual women. No further trials of ITNs in pregnancy are required in sub-Saharan Africa. Further evaluation of the potential impact of ITNs is required in areas with less intense and *Plasmodium vivax* transmission in Asia and Latin America.

3.16   Other infections

Gonorrhoea (a sexually transmitted disease) may cause various complications of pregnancy, and eye infection in the newborn baby. For this reason, silver nitrate or antibiotic eye drops or ointment may be given routinely to newborn babies.

Bacterial vaginosis has been linked to preterm labour, ruptured membranes and chorioamnionitis, and is susceptible to antibiotics such as metronidazole (see Preterm labour, p 157).

Group B beta-haemolytic streptococcus is commonly present in women's genital tracts without causing symptoms, and may cause complications of pregnancy and fatal infection in the newborn baby. Preventive strategies have included routine screening, and treatment of infected pregnant women or treatment on the basis of risk factors for infection.

Syphilis (a sexually transmitted disease) is an important cause of pregnancy loss, impaired fetal growth, preterm birth and congenital infection. Universal serological screening and treatment are recommended.

Toxoplasmosis infection acquired from cats, uncooked meat or soil causes pregnancy loss and anomalies. Routine screening is performed in some countries.

Vaginal trichomonas infection may be associated with the development of chorioamnionitis and preterm birth. Treatment may be based on routine screening or symptomatology.

Vulvovaginal candidiasis is a common infection in pregnancy, and may cause infection of the newborn bay.

There are no Cochrane reviews on these topics

3.17 Respiratory illness

Women with respiratory illness, for example, chronic lung disease, kyphoscoliosis (curvature of the spine) and severe asthma, may become progressively short of breath in late pregnancy. This may be due to both the increased oxygen demands of the pregnancy and splinting of the diaphragm by the uterus. Apart from appropriate medical care for the specific condition, early delivery may be needed to relieve the respiratory distress. Healthy women with multiple pregnancy or excessive amniotic fluid may also become progressively short of breath, requiring early delivery or repeated therapeutic amniocentesis.

There are no Cochrane reviews on this topic.

3.18 Liver disease

Liver disease during pregnancy may be specific to pregnancy (e.g. pre-eclampsia, intrahepatic cholestasis, acute fatty liver, complicated hyperemesis gravidarum) or incidental (e.g. viral hepatitis, gallstones, cirrhosis, drug-induced jaundice).

Acute fatty liver of pregnancy is potentially fatal for both mother and baby, and management includes expediting the birth and intensive supportive care for the mother.

> **INTERVENTIONS FOR TREATING CHOLESTASIS IN PREGNANCY:** not enough data to provide reliable evidence. (Burrows RF, Clavisi O, Burrows E) CD000493

BACKGROUND: Cholestasis of pregnancy has been linked to adverse maternal and fetal/neonatal outcomes. As the pathophysiology is poorly understood, therapies have been empiric.
OBJECTIVES: To evaluate the effectiveness and safety of therapeutic interventions in women with a clinical diagnosis of cholestasis of pregnancy.
METHODS: Standard PCG methods (see page xvii). Search date: March 2001.
MAIN RESULTS: Nine RCTs involving 227 women were included but adequate data for appropriate comparisons of effects of pruritus, bile

acids or liver enzymes were not consistently reported. S-adenosyl-methionine (SAMe) versus placebo (four trials, 82 women): only one trial showed significantly greater improvements in pruritus, bile salts and liver enzymes with SAMe. Ursodeoxycholic acid (UDCA) versus placebo (three trials, 56 women): in two trials a significant difference in pruritus relief was not detected. One trial observed greater reductions in bile salts and liver enzymes with UDCA. Preterm births were fewer with UDCA in one study while two studies reported no difference in fetal distress incidence. Guar gum versus placebo (one trial, 48 patients): no differences in pruritus, bile salts or fetal/neonatal outcomes were observed. Activated charcoal versus no treatment (one trial, 20 patients): the reduction in bile salts was greater with charcoal, but no difference in pruritus relief (relative risk (RR) 9.0, 95% confidence interval (CI) 0.6 – 148) or fetal/neonatal outcomes. UDCA versus SAMe (two trials, 36 patients): pruritus relief was better with UDCA in one study and with SAMe in the other. UDCA was better in reducing bile acids but not liver enzymes in one trial. UDCA + SAMe versus placebo, UDCA or SAMe (one study, eight patients/arm): UDCA + SAMe versus placebo or UDCA resulted in greater improvements in pruritus, bile salts and selected liver function assays; UDCA + SAMe versus SAMe resulted in greater improvements in bile salts and ALP only. No treatments were found to be unsafe.

AUTHORS' CONCLUSIONS: There is insufficient evidence to recommend guar gum, activated charcoal, SAMe and UDCA alone or in combination in treating women with cholestasis of pregnancy. Inconsistent and inadequate reporting of results precluded pooling the results of small studies.

3.19   Thyroid disease

Dietary iodine deficiency may be aggravated during pregnancy because iodine is diverted preferentially to the baby. Signs and symptoms of hypo-and hyperthyroidism are generally screened for as either may impair pregnancy outcomes. Thyroid hormone levels are corrected with replacement or antithyroid drugs, or occasionally surgery. Hyperthyroidism and hyperemesis gravidarum may co-exist, and both are linked to the effects of human chorionic gonadotrophin. Treatment of autoimmune thyrotoxicosis in the mother does not prevent the effects of persistent thyroid-stimulating antibody on the baby's thyroid. In poorly controlled thyrotoxicosis, labour may precipitate a thyroid crisis.

There are no Cochrane reviews on this topic.

3.20 Haemorrhoids

'Women during the state of pregnancy, and just after the menses have finally left them, are particularly subject to the piles.' Heberden W. *Commentaries on the History and Cure of Diseases*. London: T.Payne, Mews-Gate, 1802: 211.

> **CONSERVATIVE MANAGEMENT OF SYMPTOMATIC AND/OR COMPLICATED HAEMORRHOIDS IN PREGNANCY AND THE PUERPERIUM:** rutosides are effective; safety in pregnancy has not been confirmed. (Quijano CE, Abalos E) CD004077

BACKGROUND: Haemorrhoids (piles) are swollen veins at or near the anus, normally asymptomatic. They do not constitute a disease, unless they become symptomatic. Pregnancy and the puerperium predispose to symptomatic haemorrhoids, being the most common ano-rectal disease at these stages. Symptoms are usually mild and transient and include intermittent bleeding from the anus and pain. Depending on the degree of pain, quality of life could be affected, varying from mild discomfort to real difficulty in dealing with the activities of everyday life. Treatment during pregnancy is mainly directed to the relief of symptoms, especially pain control. The so-called conservative management includes dietary modifications, stimulants or depressants of the bowel transit, local treatment and phlebotonics (drugs that cause decreased capillary fragility, improving the micro-circulation in venous insufficiency). For many women, symptoms will resolve spontaneously soon after birth, and so any corrective treatment is usually deferred to some time after birth. Thus, the objective of this review is to evaluate the efficacy of conservative management of piles during pregnancy and the puerperium.
OBJECTIVES: To determine the possible benefits, risks and side-effects of the conservative management of symptomatic haemorrhoids during pregnancy and the puerperium.

METHODS: Standard PCG methods (see page xvii). Search date: June 2007. Randomised-controlled trials comparing any of the conservative treatments for symptomatic haemorrhoids during pregnancy and the puerperium (such as dietary modifications, stimulant/depressant of the bowel transit, local treatments, drugs that improve the microcirculation in venous insufficiency) with a placebo or no treatment.
MAIN RESULTS: From 10 potentially eligible studies, two were included in this review (150 women). Both compared oral rutosides against placebo. Rutosides seem to be effective in reducing the signs identified by the healthcare provider, and symptoms and signs reported by women, of haemorrhoidal disease. For the outcome no response to treatment: relative risk 0.07, 95% confidence interval 0.03 to 0.20. Regarding perinatal outcomes, one fetal death and one congenital malformation (possible not related to exposure) were reported in the control and treatment group respectively.

AUTHORS' CONCLUSIONS: Although the treatment with oral hydroxyethylrutosides looks promising for symptom relief in first and second degree haemorrhoids, its use cannot be recommended until new evidence reassures women and their clinicians about their safety. The most commonly used approaches, such as dietary modifications and local treatments, were not properly evaluated during pregnancy and the puerperium.

LAPAROSCOPIC SURGERY FOR PRESUMED BENIGN OVARIAN TUMOR DURING PREGNANCY: no randomized trials to provide reliable evidence. (Bunyavejchevin S, Phupong V) CD005459

BACKGROUND: The surgical management of ovarian tumors in pregnancy is similar to that of non-pregnant women. The procedures include resection of the tumor (enucleation), removal of an ovary or ovaries (oophorectomy), or surgical excision of the fallopian tube and ovary (salpingo-oophorectomy). The procedure can be done by open surgery (laparotomy) or keyhole surgery (laparoscopy) technique. The benefits of laparoscopic surgery include shorter hospital stay, earlier return to normal activity, and reduced postoperative pain. However, conventional laparoscopic surgery techniques required the infusion of carbon dioxide gas in the peritoneum to distend the abdomen and displace the bowel upward to create the room for surgical manipulation.

Serious complications such as abnormally high levels of carbon dioxide in the circulating blood (hypercarbia) and perforation of internal organs have also been reported. These serious complications may be harmful to the fetus.

OBJECTIVES: To compare the effects of using laparoscopic surgery for benign ovarian tumor during pregnancy on maternal and fetal health and the use of healthcare resources.

METHODS: Standard PCG methods (see page xvii). Search date June 2006.

MAIN RESULTS: There were no randomized controlled trials identified.

AUTHORS' CONCLUSIONS: The practice of laparoscopic surgery for benign ovarian tumour during pregnancy is associated with benefits and harms. However, the evidence for the magnitude of these benefits and harms is drawn from case series studies, associated with potential bias. The results and conclusions of these studies must therefore be interpreted with caution.

The available case series studies of laparoscopic surgery for benign ovarian tumour during pregnancy provide limited insight into the potential benefits and harms associated with this new surgical technique in pregnancy. Randomized controlled trials are required to provide the most reliable evidence regarding the benefits and harms of laparoscopic surgery for benign ovarian tumour during pregnancy.

3.21   Psychiatric disorders

Stress related to pregnancy may aggravate psychiatric disorders, as may hormonal changes, particularly after the birth. Cognitive behaviour therapy and antidepressants are used for mood disorders and anxiety disorders. During pregnancy lithium and tricyclic antidepressants are avoided because of teratogenicity.

Modern antipsychotic drugs are effective and have low side-effect profiles. Most psychotic women may be treated in the community, with family therapy and support.

> **PSYCHOSOCIAL AND PSYCHOLOGICAL INTERVENTIONS FOR TREATING ANTENATAL DEPRESSION:** not enough data to provide reliable evidence. (Dennis C-L, Ross LE, Grigoriadis S) CD006309

BACKGROUND: Although pregnancy was once thought of as a time of emotional wellbeing for many women, conferring 'protection' against psychiatric disorders, a recent meta-analysis of 21 studies suggests the mean prevalence rate for depression across the antenatal period is 10.7%, ranging from 7.4% in the first trimester to a high of 12.8% in the second trimester. Due to maternal treatment preferences and potential concerns about fetal and infant health outcomes, non-pharmacological treatment options are needed.

OBJECTIVES: The primary objective of this review is to assess the effects, on mothers and their families, of psychosocial and psychological interventions compared with usual antepartum care in the treatment of antenatal depression.

METHODS: Standard PCG methods (see page xvii). Search date: September 2006.

MAIN RESULTS: One US trial was included in this review, incorporating 38 outpatient antenatal women who met Diagnostic and Statistical Manual for Mental Disorders-IV criteria for major depression. Interpersonal psychotherapy, compared to a parenting education programme, was associated with a reduction in the risk of depressive symptomatology immediately post-treatment using the Clinical Global Impression Scale (one trial, n = 38; relative risk (RR) 0.46, 95% confidence interval (CI) 0.26 to 0.83) and the Hamilton Rating Scale for Depression (one trial, n = 38; RR 0.82, 95% CI 0.65 to 1.03).

AUTHORS' CONCLUSIONS: The evidence is inconclusive to allow us to make any recommendations for interpersonal psychotherapy for the treatment of antenatal depression. The one trial included was too small, with a non-generalisable sample, to make any recommendations.

INTERVENTIONS (OTHER THAN PHARMACOLOGICAL, PSYCHOSOCIAL OR PSYCHOLOGICAL) FOR TREATING ANTENATAL DEPRESSION: (Dennis C-L, Giavedoni K) Protocol [see page xviii] CD006795

ABRIDGED BACKGROUND: According to the World Health Organization, by the year 2020 depression will be second only to coronary heart disease in disability experienced worldwide. Major depression is a type of mood disturbance that lasts more than two weeks. Symptoms may include overwhelming feelings of sadness and grief, loss of interest or pleasure in activities usually enjoyed, and feelings of worthlessness or guilt. This type of depression may result in poor sleep, a change in appetite, severe fatigue and difficulty concentrating. Severe depression may increase the risk of suicide. Many people with depression also have symptoms of anxiety.

Although evidence exists that antidepressant medication may be safe for use antenatally, many depressed pregnant women fear teratogenic effects of medications and are thus reluctant to take antidepressants. Due to the limited amount of research evaluating the effectiveness of psychological and psychosocial interventions for the treatment of antenatal depression and the perceived risks of pharmacotherapy, alternative forms of treatment that have been evaluated for general depression (e.g., bright light therapy, massage therapy, acupuncture, or Omega-3 fatty acid supplementation) should be examined.

OBJECTIVES: The primary objective of this review is to assess the effects, on mothers and their families, of biological and other non-pharmacological/psychosocial/psychological interventions compared with usual antepartum care in the treatment of antenatal depression.

3.22   Skin diseases

Physiological skin changes during pregnancy may cause concern. Certain skin diseases are specific to pregnancy:

- pruritic urticarial papules and plaques of pregnancy/polymorphic eruption of pregnancy
- pemphigoid (herpes) gestationis, a rare auto-immune condition occurring in the second half of pregnancy and particularly the puerperium
- impetigo herpetiformis and
- papular eruptions of pregnancy – prurigo gestationis.

There are no Cochrane reviews on this topic.

Chapter 4: Disorders Affecting The Unborn Baby

4.1 Routine assessment of the baby during pregnancy

4.1.1 Can routine screening tests do harm?

We believe there is an ethical difference between everyday clinical practice and screening. If a patient asks a medical practitioner for help, the doctor does the best possible. The doctor is not responsible for defects in medical knowledge. If, however, the practitioner initiates screening procedures the doctor is in a very different situation. The doctor should, in our view, have conclusive evidence that screening can alter the natural history of disease in a significant proportion of those screened. Cochrane AL, Holland WW. Validation of screening procedures. *British Medical Bulletin* 1971; 27 (1): 3–8.

Case study: A negative routine rubella test was misinterpreted by the doctor as being positive, and the mother requested pregnancy termination. The error was corrected, but the mother insisted on termination of her pregnancy. She explained that once the possibility of an anomaly had been raised in her mind, albeit in error, she could not dispel the fear that her baby might be abnormal.

False positive screening or diagnostic tests may do considerable harm, both through inappropriate medical interventions, and through undermining the mother's confidence. Diagnostic tests should be offered only if we have good evidence that the benefits outweigh the harms.

Tests of the baby's growth and wellbeing range from simple measures such as symphysis–fundal height measurement and mothers' reports of the baby's movements, to ultrasound visualisation, analysis of heart rate

A Cochrane Pocketbook: Pregnancy and Childbirth   G.J. Hofmeyr et al.
Copyright © 2008, Z. Alfievic, C. A. Crowther, L. Duley, A. M. Gulmezoglu, G. ML. Gyte , E. D. Hodnett, G. J. Hofmeyr, J. P. Neilson

patterns, doppler studies of the baby's blood flow patterns, electrocardiographic studies and scalp blood sampling.

SYMPHYSIS–FUNDAL HEIGHT MEASUREMENT IN PREGNANCY: not enough data to provide reliable evidence. (Neilson JP) CD000944 (in RHL 11)

BACKGROUND: In many settings, symphysis–fundal height measurement has replaced clinical assessment of fetal size by abdominal palpation because the latter has been reported to perform poorly.

OBJECTIVES: To assess the effects of routine use of symphysis–fundal height measurements (tape measurement of the distance from the pubic symphysis to the uterine fundus) during antenatal care on pregnancy outcome.

METHODS: Standard PCG methods (see page xvii). Search date: August 2002.

MAIN RESULTS: One trial involving 1639 women was included. No obvious differences were detected in any of the outcomes measured.

AUTHOR'S CONCLUSIONS: There is not enough evidence to evaluate the use of symphysis–fundal height measurements during antenatal care.

☺ **ULTRASOUND FOR FETAL ASSESSMENT IN EARLY PREGNANCY:** reduced the rates of undiagnosed multiple pregnancy and labour inductions for post-dates pregnancy. (Neilson JP) CD000182 (in RHL 11)

BACKGROUND: Advantages of early pregnancy ultrasound screening are thought to be more accurate calculation of gestational age, earlier identification of multiple pregnancies, and diagnosis of non-viable pregnancies and certain fetal malformations.

OBJECTIVES: To assess the use of routine (screening) ultrasound compared with the selective use of ultrasound in early pregnancy (ie before 24 weeks).

METHODS: Standard PCG methods (see page xvii). Search date: June 2001.

MAIN RESULTS: Nine trials were included. The quality of the trials was generally good. Routine ultrasound examination was associated with earlier detection of multiple pregnancies (twins undiagnosed at 26 weeks, odds ratio 0.08, 95% confidence interval 0.04 to 0.16) and reduced rates of induction of labour for post-term pregnancy (odds ratio 0.61, 95% confidence interval 0.52 to 0.72). There were no differences detected for substantive clinical outcomes such as perinatal mortality (odds ratio 0.86, 95% confidence interval 0.67 to 1.12). Where detection of fetal abnormality was a specific aim of the examination, the number of terminations of pregnancy for fetal anomaly increased.

AUTHOR'S CONCLUSIONS: Routine ultrasound in early pregnancy appears to enable better gestational age assessment, earlier detection of multiple pregnancies and earlier detection of clinically unsuspected fetal malformation at a time when termination of pregnancy is possible. However, the benefits for other substantive outcomes are less clear.

4.2 Prenatal diagnosis

4.2.1 Procedures

AMNIOCENTESIS AND CHORIONIC VILLUS SAMPLING FOR PRENATAL DIAGNOSIS: the risk of pregnancy loss was least for second trimester amniocentesis, followed by transabdominal then transcervical chorion villus sampling, then early amniocentesis; second trimester amniocentesis had fewer failures than chorion villus sampling, but results are more delayed. (Alfirevic Z, Sundberg K, Brigham S) CD003252 (in RHL 11)

BACKGROUND: A major disadvantage of second trimester amniocentesis is that the result is usually available only after 18 weeks' gestation. Chorionic villus sampling (CVS) and early amniocentesis can be done between 9 and 14 weeks and offer an earlier alternative.

OBJECTIVES: To assess comparative safety and accuracy of second trimester amniocentesis, early amniocentesis, transcervical and transabdominal CVS.

METHODS: Standard PCG methods (see page xvii). Search date: March 2003.

MAIN RESULTS: A total of 14 randomised studies have been included. In a low risk population with a background pregnancy loss of around 2%, a second trimester amniocentesis will increase this risk by another 1%. This difference did not reach statistical significance, but the increase in spontaneous miscarriages following second trimester amniocentesis compared with controls (no amniocentesis) did (2.1% versus 1.3%; relative risk (RR) 1.02 to 2.52). Early amniocentesis is not a safe early alternative to second trimester amniocentesis because of increased pregnancy loss (7.6% versus 5.9%; RR 1.29, 95% CI 1.03 to 1.61) and higher incidence of talipes compared to CVS (1.8% versus 0.2%; RR 6.43, 95% CI 1.68 to 24.64).

Compared with second trimester amniocentesis, transcervical CVS carries a significantly higher risk of pregnancy loss (14.5% versus 11%; RR 1.40, 95% CI 1.09 to 1.81) and spontaneous miscarriage (12.9% versus 9.4%; RR 1.50, 95% CI 1.07 to 2.11). One study compared transabdominal CVS with second trimester amniocentesis and found no significant difference in the total pregnancy loss between the two procedures (6.3% versus 7%). Transcervical CVS is more technically demanding than transabdominal CVS with more failures to obtain sample and more multiple insertions.

AUTHORS' CONCLUSIONS: Second trimester amniocentesis is safer than transcervical CVS and early amniocentesis. If earlier diagnosis is required, transabdominal CVS is preferable to early amniocentesis or transcervical CVS. In circumstances where transabdominal CVS may be technically difficult the preferred options are transcervical CVS in the first trimester or second trimester amniocentesis.

INSTRUMENTSFORCHORIONICVILLUSSAMPLINGFORPRENATAL DIAGNOSIS: forceps were more efficient than cannulae for transcervical chorion villus sampling. (Alfirevic Z, von Dadelszen P) CD000114

BACKGROUND: Chorionic villus sampling (CVS) is the method of choice for obtaining fetal tissue for prenatal diagnosis before 15 weeks of pregnancy. CVS can be performed using either a transabdominal or transcervical approach. The type of instrument used could have a significant impact on the success rate of the procedure. An ability to manoeuvre the instrument within the uterine cavity without puncturing the gestational sac and to see the tip of the instrument on ultrasound scanning are particularly important.
OBJECTIVES: To assess the effects of instruments used to obtain chorionic tissue in early pregnancy by the transabdominal or transcervical route (chorionic villus sampling). The outcomes of interest were technical difficulties during the procedure, quality and quantity of obtained tissue, maternal adverse effects, pregnancy outcome and cost-effectiveness.
METHODS: Standard PCG methods (see page xvii). Search date: November 2002.

MAIN RESULTS: There were no trials comparing instruments for transabdominal CVS. Forceps and cannula were evaluated in five transcervical CVS trials involving 472 women. When a cannula was used, operators obtained an inadequate sample (less than five mg) more often (relative risk (RR) 4.21, 95% confidence interval (CI) 2.15 to 8.25). Compared with forceps, cannulae had to be re-inserted more often (RR 2.98, 95% CI 1.62 to 5.47). Also, inserting a cannula was more painful (RR 1.93, 95% CI 1.11 to 3.37). One study reported the cost of the procedures and found CVS with cannula to be more expensive (weighted mean difference $183.7, 95% confidence interval 152.62 to 214.78).

When different types of cannulae were compared, the Portex cannula was more likely to result in an inadequate sample and a difficult or painful procedure when compared with either the silver or aluminium cannula respectively.

AUTHORS' CONCLUSIONS: Although there is some evidence to support the use of small forceps for transcervical chorionic villus sampling, the evidence is not strong enough to support change in practice for clinicians who have become familiar with aspiration cannulae.

4.2.2 Genetic disorders

Advances in genetic diagnostic tests are progressively increasing the range of genetic disorders which can be diagnosed, raising complex ethical dilemmas.

PRE-CONCEPTION AND ANTENATAL SCREENING FOR THE FRAGILE SITE ON THE X-CHROMOSOME: no randomised trials to provide reliable evidence. (Kornman L, Chambers H, Nisbet D, Liebelt J) CD001806

BACKGROUND: Fragile X is the most common cause of mental retardation after Down syndrome. It is the commonest inherited cause of mental retardation, and results from a dynamic mutation in a gene on the long arm of the X chromosome. Various strategies are used for prenatal screening.

OBJECTIVES: To determine whether pre-conceptual or antenatal screening for fragile X carrier status in apparently low risk women confers any additional benefit over the existing practice of offering testing to women thought to be at increased risk.

METHODS: Standard PCG methods (see page xvii). Search date: November 2002.
MAIN RESULTS: No trials were included.

AUTHORS' CONCLUSIONS: No information is available from randomised trials to indicate whether routine pre-conceptual or antenatal screening for fragile X carrier status confers any benefit over testing women thought to be at increased risk.

4.2.3 Counselling

The technical and emotional complexities of inheritance make skilled counselling the cornerstone of genetic diagnostic programs.

Case report: A pregnant woman whose father had Huntington's chorea (a dominantly inherited, disabling degeneration of brain cells) wished to prevent the possibility of giving birth to an affected child without discovering whether she was destined to develop the condition. While it was technically possible to identify the relevant genetic sequence in her baby with certainty, it was necessary to instead do 'linkage' testing to determine whether her baby had inherited the relevant gene from his affected grandfather. This would give him the same 50% risk of being affected as his mother had. She thus accepted the risk of termination of a normal pregnancy rather than an accurate diagnosis which would have revealed whether she herself was affected.

There are no Cochrane reviews of this topic.

4.2.4 Fetal surgery

Operating on unborn babies has been limited to specialised centres, with generally disappointing results.

There are no Cochrane reviews of this topic

4.3 Impaired growth and wellbeing of the unborn baby

'...for we live, move, have a being, and are subject to the actions of the elements, and the malices of diseases, in the other World, the truest

Microcosm, the Womb of our mother.' Browne T. *Religio medici*. London: MacMillan, 1926: 63.

The care of pregnant women is unique with respect to the need to consider the interests of two individuals simultaneously. At times, the mother and baby have conflicting needs, and difficult decisions must be taken. To care for a mother with eclampsia at 24 weeks of pregnancy, the birth of her baby may be expedited before he or she is viable. To reduce the risk of harm to a baby thought to be compromised, the mother may be subjected to the risks of caesarean section.

To make the best decisions, particular attention must be paid to assessing the wellbeing of the baby as an individual. Because such assessments are indirect they are imprecise, and clinicians are faced with the dilemma of choosing between the risk of failing to intervene when a baby may be compromised, or intervening unnecessarily when tests of wellbeing are falsely positive.

4.3.1   Screening and diagnosis

> **FETAL MOVEMENT COUNTING FOR ASSESSMENT OF FETAL WELLBEING:** not enough data to provide reliable evidence. (Mangesi L, Hofmeyr GJ) CD004909

BACKGROUND: Fetal movement counting is a method by which a woman quantifies the movements she feels to assess the condition of the baby. The purpose is to try to reduce perinatal mortality by alerting caregivers when the baby might have become compromised. This method may be used routinely, or only in women who are considered at increased risk of complications in the baby. Some clinicians believe that fetal movement counting is a good method as it allows the clinician to make appropriate interventions in good time. On the other hand, fetal movement counting may cause anxiety to women.
OBJECTIVES: To assess outcomes of pregnancy where fetal movement counting was done routinely, selectively or was not done at all; and to compare different methods of fetal movement counting.
METHODS: Standard PCG methods (see page xvii). Search date: September 2006

MAIN RESULTS: Four studies, involving 71 370 women, were included in this review; 68 654 in one cluster-randomised trial. All four trials compared formal fetal movement counting. Two trials compared different types of counting with each other; one with no formal instruction, and one with hormonal analysis. Women in the formal fetal movement counting group had significantly fewer visits to the hospital antenatally than those women randomised to hormone analysis (relative risk (RR) 0.26, 95% confidence interval (CI) 0.20 to 0.35), whereas there were fewer Apgar scores less than seven in five minutes for women randomised to hormone analysis (RR 1.72, 95% CI 1.01 to 2.93).

There was a significantly higher compliance with the Cardiff 'count to ten' method than with the formal fetal movement counting method (RR 0.25, 95% CI 0.19 to 0.32).

All other outcomes reported were non-significant.

AUTHORS' CONCLUSIONS: This review does not provide enough evidence to influence practice. In particular, no trials compared fetal movement counting with no fetal movement counting. Robust research is needed in this area.

BIOCHEMICAL TESTS OF PLACENTAL FUNCTION FOR ASSESSMENT IN PREGNANCY: were not found to improve outcome. (Neilson JP) CD000108

BACKGROUND: Biochemical tests of placental or feto-placental function were widely used in the 1960s and 1970s in high-risk pregnancies to try to predict, and thus try to avoid, adverse fetal outcome.

OBJECTIVES: To assess the effects of performing biochemical tests of placental function in high-risk, low-risk, or unselected pregnancies.

METHODS: Standard PCG methods (see page xvii). Search date: February 2003.

MAIN RESULTS: A single eligible trial of poor quality was identified. It involved 622 women with high-risk pregnancies who had had plasma (o)estriol estimations. Women were allocated to have their (o)estriol results revealed or concealed on the basis of hospital record number (with attendant risk of selection bias). There were no obvious differences in perinatal mortality (relative risk (RR) 0.88, 95% confidence interval (CI) 0.36 to 2.13) or planned delivery (RR 0.97, 95% CI 0.81 to 1.15) between the two groups.

AUTHORS' CONCLUSIONS: The available trial data do not support the use of (o)estriol estimation in high-risk pregnancies. The single small trial available does not have the power to exclude a beneficial effect but this is probably of historical interest since biochemical testing has been superseded by biophysical testing in antepartum fetal assessment.

BIOPHYSICAL PROFILE FOR FETAL ASSESSMENT IN HIGH-RISK PREGNANCIES: not enough data to support its use. (Lalor JG, Fawole B, Alfirevic Z, Devane D) CD000038

BACKGROUND: A biophysical profile (BPP) includes ultrasound monitoring of fetal movements, fetal tone and fetal breathing, ultrasound assessment of liquor volume with or without assessment of the fetal heart rate. The BPP is performed in an effort to identify babies that may be at risk of poor pregnancy outcome, so that additional assessments of wellbeing may be performed, or labour may be induced or a caesarean section performed to expedite birth.

OBJECTIVES: To assess the effects of the BPP when compared with conventional monitoring (CTG only or MBPP) on pregnancy outcome in high-risk pregnancies.

METHODS: Standard PCG methods (see page xvii). Search date: October 2007.

MAIN RESULTS: We included five trials, involving 2974 women. Most trials were not of high quality. Although the overall incidence of adverse outcomes was low, available evidence from randomised controlled trials does not support the use of BPP as a test of fetal wellbeing in high-risk pregnancies. We found no significant differences between the groups in perinatal deaths (relative risk (RR) 1.33, 95% confidence interval (CI) 0.60 to 2.98) or in Apgar score less than seven at five minutes (RR 1.27, 95% CI 0.85 to 1.92).Combined data from the two high-quality trials suggest an increased risk of caesarean section in the BPP group (RR 1.60, 95% CI 1.05 to 2.44, n = 280, interaction test P = 0.03). However, the number of participating women was relatively small (n = 280). Therefore, additional evidence is required in order to be definitive regarding the efficacy of this test in high-risk pregnancies. Furthermore, the impact of the BPP on other interventions, length of hospitalisation, serious short-term and long-term neonatal morbidity and parental satisfaction, requires further evaluation.

AUTHORS' CONCLUSIONS: At present, there is insufficient evidence from randomised trials to support the use of BPP as a test of fetal wellbeing in high-risk pregnancies.

CARDIOTOCOGRAPHY FOR ANTEPARTUM FETAL ASSESSMENT: in intermediate or high risk women showed a reduction in utilisation of services; a trend to increased rather than decreased perinatal mortality; there were no recent trials. (Pattison N, McCowan L) CD001068

BACKGROUND: Cardiotocography is a form of fetal assessment which simultaneously records fetal heart rate, fetal movements and uterine contractions to investigate hypoxia.

OBJECTIVES: To assess the effects of antenatal cardiotocography on perinatal morbidity and mortality and maternal morbidity.

METHODS: Standard PCG methods (see page xvii). Search date: November 1998.

MAIN RESULTS: Four studies involving 1588 pregnancies were included. All trials were conducted on high or intermediate risk pregnancies. Antenatal cardiotocography appeared to have no significant effect on perinatal mortality or morbidity. There was a trend to an increase in perinatal deaths in the cardiotocography group (odds ratio 2.85, 95% confidence interval 0.99 to 7.12). There was no increase in the incidence of interventions such as elective caesarean section or induction of labour. The one trial which examined an effect on antenatal patient management showed a significant reduction in hospital admissions and a reduction in inpatient stay in the cardiotocography group.

AUTHORS' CONCLUSIONS: There is not enough evidence to evaluate the use of antenatal cardiotocography for fetal assessment. All of the trials included in this review date from the introduction of antenatal cardiotocography and may be difficult to relate to current practice.

☺ **FETAL VIBROACOUSTIC STIMULATION FOR FACILITATION OF TESTS OF FETAL WELL-BEING:** reduced the rate of non-reactive cardiotocograph tests. (Tan KH, Smyth R) CD002963

BACKGROUND: Acoustic stimulation of the fetus has been suggested to improve the efficiency of antepartum fetal heart rate testing.

OBJECTIVES: To assess the merits or adverse effects of the use of fetal vibroacoustic stimulation in conjunction with tests of fetal well-being.

METHODS: Standard PCG methods (see page xvii). Search date: July 2003.

MAIN RESULTS: A total of nine trials with a total of 4838 participants were included. Fetal vibroacoustic stimulation reduced the incidence of non-reactive antenatal cardiotocography test (seven trials; relative risk (RR) 0.62, 95% confidence interval (CI) random 0.52 to 0.74) and reduced the overall mean cardiotocography testing time (three trials; weighted mean difference (WMD) −9.94 minutes, 95% CI −9.37 minutes to −10.50 minutes). Vibroacoustic stimulation compared with mock stimulation evoked significantly more fetal movements when used in conjunction with fetal heart rate testing (one trial, RR 0.23, 95% CI 0.18 to 0.30).

AUTHORS' CONCLUSIONS: Vibroacoustic stimulation offers benefits by decreasing the incidence of non-reactive cardiotocography and reducing the testing time. Further randomised trials should be encouraged to determine not only the optimum intensity, frequency, duration and position of the vibroacoustic stimulation, but also to evaluate the efficacy, predictive reliability, safety and perinatal outcome of these stimuli with cardiotocography and other tests of fetal well-being.

⊗ **FETAL MANIPULATION FOR FACILITATING TESTS OF FETAL WELLBEING:** did not reduce the rate of non-reactive fetal heart rate tests. (Tan KH, Sabapathy A) CD003396

BACKGROUND: Manual fetal manipulation has been suggested to improve the efficiency of antepartum fetal heart rate testing.

OBJECTIVES: To assess the merits or adverse effects of the use of manual fetal manipulation in conjunction with tests of fetal wellbeing.

METHODS: Standard PCG methods (see page xvii). Search date: October 2007.

MAIN RESULTS: Only three trials with a total of 1100 women with 2130 episodes of participation were included. Manual fetal manipulation did not decrease the incidence of non-reactive antenatal cardiotocography test (odds ratio 1.28, 95% confidence interval 0.94 to 1.74).

AUTHORS' CONCLUSIONS: Manual fetal manipulation has not been shown to reduce the incidence of non-reactive cardiotocography. Trials of manual fetal manipulation should take into consideration that there have not been any benefits demonstrated as yet.

AMNIOTIC FLUID INDEX VERSUS SINGLE DEEPEST VERTICAL POCKET AS A SCREENING TEST FOR PREVENTING ADVERSE PREGNANCY OUTCOME: (Nabhan AF, Abdelmoula YA) Protocol [see page xviii] CD006593

ABRIDGED BACKGROUND: Amniotic fluid provides a supportive environment for fetal development. It is maintained in a dynamic equilibrium; its volume is the sum of fluid (from fetal urine and lung fluid) flowing into and out (to fetal swallowing and intramembranous absorption) of the amniotic space. Amniotic fluid volume (AFV) is an important parameter in the assessment of fetal wellbeing. Oligohydramnios, a decreased AFV, occurs as a result of fetal anomalies, intrauterine growth restriction, prolonged (post-term) pregnancies, and pre-eclampsia. Oligohydramnios is associated with increased fetal and neonatal morbidity and mortality. Therefore, the prenatal diagnosis of oligohydramnios is important in the management of pregnancy.

Ultrasonography is non-invasive and hence it is used widely for the follow up of pregnancy.. Several methods are used to assess amniotic fluid. The AFI and the single deepest pocket are the more commonly employed techniques for assessing adequacy of amniotic fluid. Many authorities practice planned delivery, either by induction of labor or caesarean delivery, following the diagnosis of a decreased AFV at term. However, there is no clear consensus on the best method to assess amniotic fluid.

OBJECTIVES: To compare the use of amniotic fluid index with the 2×1 cm single deepest vertical pocket as a screening tool for decreased amniotic fluid volume for the prevention of adverse pregnancy outcome.

⊗ **MATERNAL GLUCOSE ADMINISTRATION FOR FACILITATING TESTS OF FETAL WELLBEING:** did not reduce the rate of non-reactive fetal heart rate tests. (Tan KH, Sabapathy A) CD003397

BACKGROUND: Antenatal maternal glucose administration has been suggested to improve the efficiency of antepartum fetal heart rate testing.

OBJECTIVES: To assess the merits or adverse effects of antenatal maternal glucose administration in conjunction with tests of fetal wellbeing.
METHODS: Standard PCG methods (see page xvii). Search date: June 2006.
MAIN RESULTS: A total of two trials with a total of 708 participants were included. Antenatal maternal glucose administration did not decrease the incidence of non-reactive antenatal cardiotocography tests.

AUTHORS' CONCLUSIONS: Antenatal maternal glucose administration has not been shown to reduce non-reactive cardiotocography. More trials are needed to further substantiate this and to determine not only the optimum dose, but also to evaluate the efficacy, predictive reliability, safety and perinatal outcome of glucose administration in conjunction with cardiotocography and also other tests of fetal wellbeing.

> ☺ **DOPPLER ULTRASOUND FOR FETAL ASSESSMENT IN HIGH RISK PREGNANCIES:** reduced labour inductions and admission to hospital; there was a trend to reduced perinatal deaths. (Neilson JP, Alfirevic Z) CD000073

BACKGROUND: Abnormal waveforms from Doppler ultrasound may indicate poor fetal prognosis. It is also possible that Doppler ultrasound could encourage inappropriate early delivery.
OBJECTIVES: To assess the effects of Doppler ultrasound in high risk pregnancies on obstetric care and fetal outcomes.
METHODS: Standard PCG methods (see page xvii). Search date: June 2001.
MAIN RESULTS: 11 studies involving nearly 7000 women were included. The trials were generally of good quality. Compared to no Doppler ultrasound, Doppler ultrasound in high risk pregnancy (especially those complicated by hypertension or presumed impaired fetal growth) was associated with a trend to a reduction in perinatal deaths (odds ratio 0.71, 95% confidence interval 0.50 to 1.01). The use of Doppler ultrasound was also associated with fewer inductions of labour (odds ratio 0.83, 95% confidence interval 0.74 to 0.93) and fewer admissions to hospital (odds ratio 0.56, 95% 0.43 to 0.72), without reports of adverse effects. No difference was found for fetal distress in labour (odds ratio 0.81, 95% confidence interval 0.59 to 1.13) or caesarean delivery (odds ratio 0.94, 95% 0.82 to 1.06).

AUTHORS' CONCLUSIONS: The use of Doppler ultrasound in high risk pregnancies appears to improve a number of obstetric care outcomes and appears promising in helping to reducing perinatal deaths.

4.3.2 Conservative management of compromised babies

'For the [foetus], which has in it the intrinsic principle of life, is governed thereby, and constantly draws its proper nourishment, as if immovably rooted to the uterus, night and day.' Galen C. *Hygiene*. Springfield, Ilinois: Charles C Thomas, 1951: 29.

⊗ ABDOMINAL DECOMPRESSION IN NORMAL PREGNANCY: did not improve pregnancy outcomes. (Hofmeyr GJ, Kulier R) CD001062

BACKGROUND: Abdominal decompression was developed as a means of pain relief during labour. It has also been used for complications of pregnancy, and in healthy pregnant women in an attempt to improve fetal wellbeing and intellectual development.

OBJECTIVES: To assess the effects of prophylactic abdominal decompression on admission for pre-eclampsia, fetal growth, perinatal morbidity and mortality and childhood development.

METHODS: Standard PCG methods (see page xvii). Search date: October 2007.

MAIN RESULTS: Three studies were included. There was no difference between the abdominal decompression groups and the control groups for low birth weight (relative risk 0.69, 95% confidence interval 0.27 to 1.77) and perinatal mortality (relative risk 2.47, 95% confidence interval 0.77 to 7.92). There were no differences in admission for pre-eclampsia, Apgar score and childhood development.

AUTHORS' CONCLUSIONS: There is no evidence to support the use of abdominal decompression in normal pregnancies. Future research should be directed towards the use of abdominal decompression during labour, and during complicated pregnancies.

ABDOMINAL DECOMPRESSION FOR SUSPECTED FETAL COMPROMISE/PRE-ECLAMPSIA: showed benefits which need to be confirmed by methodologically more sound trials. (Hofmeyr GJ) CD000004

BACKGROUND: Abdominal decompression was developed as a means of pain relief during labour. It has also been used for complications of pregnancy, and in healthy pregnant women in an attempt to improve fetal wellbeing and intellectual development.

OBJECTIVES: To assess the effects of antenatal abdominal decompression for maternal hypertension or impaired fetal growth on perinatal outcome.

METHODS: Standard PCG methods (see page xvii). Search date: October 2004.

MAIN RESULTS: Three studies were included, all with the possibility of containing serious bias.

Therapeutic abdominal decompression was associated with the following reductions: persistent pre-eclampsia (relative risk 0.36, 95% confidence interval 0.18 to 0.72); fetal distress in labour (relative risk 0.37, 95% confidence interval 0.19 to 0.71); low birthweight (relative risk 0.50, 95% confidence interval 0.40 to 0.63); Apgar scores less than six at one minute (relative risk 0.26, 95% confidence interval 0.12 to 0.56); and perinatal mortality (relative risk 0.39, 95% confidence interval 0.22 to 0.71).

AUTHOR'S CONCLUSIONS: Due to the methodological limitations of the studies, the effects of therapeutic abdominal decompression are not clear. The apparent improvements in birthweight and perinatal mortality warrant further evaluation of abdominal decompression where there is impaired fetal growth and possibly for women with pre-eclampsia.

BED REST IN HOSPITAL FOR SUSPECTED IMPAIRED FETAL GROWTH: not enough data to provide reliable evidence. (Say L, Gülmezoglu AM, Hofmeyr GJ) CD000034

BACKGROUND: Bed rest in hospital or at home is widely advised for many complications of pregnancy. The increased clinical supervision needs to be balanced with the risk of thrombosis, the stress on the pregnant women, as well as the costs to families and health services.

OBJECTIVES: To assess the effects of bed rest in hospital for women with suspected impaired fetal growth.

METHODS: Standard PCG methods (see page xvii). Search date: October 2007.

MAIN RESULTS: One study involving 107 women was included. Allocation of treatment was by odd or even birth date. There were differences in baseline fetal weights and birthweights, but these were not statistically significant (mean estimated fetal weight deviation at enrolment was −21.7% for the bed rest group and −20.7% for the ambulatory group; mean birthweight was −19.7% for the bed rest group and −20.6% for the ambulatory group). No differences were detected between bed rest and ambulatory management for fetal growth parameters (relative risk 0.43, 95% confidence interval: 0.15 to 1.27) and neonatal outcomes.

AUTHORS' CONCLUSIONS: There is not enough evidence to evaluate the use of a bed rest in hospital policy for women with suspected impaired fetal growth.

BETAMIMETICS FOR SUSPECTED IMPAIRED FETAL GROWTH: not enough data to provide reliable evidence. (Say L, Gülmezoglu AM, Hofmeyr GJ) CD000036

BACKGROUND: Betamimetic drugs may promote fetal growth by increasing the availability of nutrients and by decreasing vascular resistance. They may also induce adverse effects via their effects on carbohydrate metabolism.

OBJECTIVES: To assess the effects of betamimetic therapy for suspected impaired fetal growth on fetal growth and perinatal outcome.

METHODS: Standard PCG methods (see page xvii). Search date: October 2007.

MAIN RESULTS: Two studies of 118 women were included. No statistically significant differences were found between the betamimetic groups and the control groups for low birthweight (relative risk 1.17, 95% confidence interval 0.75 to 1.83), other anthropometric measures or neonatal morbidity and mortality.

AUTHORS' CONCLUSIONS: Larger, well-designed studies are needed to evaluate the effects of betamimetics on fetal growth. Since there is potential for adverse effects due to the pharmacological characteristics of this group of drugs, data related to any potential harms should be collected in addition to beneficial effects.

CALCIUM CHANNEL BLOCKERS FOR POTENTIAL IMPAIRED
FETAL GROWTH: not enough data to provide reliable evidence.
(Say L, Gülmezoglu AM, Hofmeyr GJ) CD000049

BACKGROUND: Calcium channel blockers may increase the blood flow to the fetus or may improve fetal–placental cellular energy generation. This could enhance fetal growth.
OBJECTIVES: To assess the effects of calcium channel blockers on fetal growth and neonatal morbidity and mortality in pregnancies where impaired fetal growth is suspected.
METHODS: Standard PCG methods (see page xvii). Search date: November 2006.
MAIN RESULTS: One study of 100 women (all smokers) was included. Mean birthweight was significantly higher in women receiving flunarizine compared to the control group. No other significant differences were found.

AUTHORS' CONCLUSIONS: There is not enough evidence to evaluate the use of calcium channel blockers for impaired fetal growth. The apparent beneficial effect of calcium channel blockers on birthweight warrants further investigation.

HORMONES FOR SUSPECTED IMPAIRED FETAL GROWTH:
there were no randomised trials to provide reliable evidence.
(Say L, Gülmezoglu AM, Hofmeyr GJ) CD000109

BACKGROUND: It has been suggested that oestrogens may improve fetal growth due to an increase in nutritional supply to the fetus from greater uterine blood flow.
OBJECTIVES: To assess the effects of hormone administration for suspected impaired fetal growth and perinatal outcome.
METHODS: Standard PCG methods (see page xvii). Search date: November 2006.
MAIN RESULTS: No studies were included since none of the potentially relevant trials reported clinical outcomes.

AUTHORS' CONCLUSIONS: There is not enough evidence to evaluate the clinical use of hormone administration for suspected impaired fetal growth.

> **MATERNAL NUTRIENT SUPPLEMENTATION FOR SUSPECTED IMPAIRED FETAL GROWTH:** not enough data to provide reliable evidence. (Say L, Gülmezoglu AM, Hofmeyr GJ) CD000148

BACKGROUND: One way of attempting to improve fetal growth has been nutrient supplementation for the mother when fetal growth is impaired. Different nutrients such as carbohydrates and amino acids have been suggested as treatments for impaired fetal growth.

OBJECTIVES: To assess the effects of nutrient administration for suspected fetal growth impairment on fetal growth and perinatal outcome.

METHODS: Standard PCG methods (see page xvii). Search date: August 2004.

MAIN RESULTS: Three studies involving 121 women were included. The trials were small and/or had methodological limitations. Carnite was associated with shorter pregnancy duration after enrolment (weighted mean difference −2.12, 95% confidence interval −3.58 to 0.66 weeks). No other differences were found.

AUTHORS' CONCLUSIONS: There is not enough evidence to evaluate the use of nutrient therapy for suspected impaired fetal growth. The studies were too small to assess clinical outcomes adequately.

> **MATERNAL OXYGEN ADMINISTRATION FOR SUSPECTED IMPAIRED FETAL GROWTH:** reduced perinatal mortality but groups not well matched; confirmation from larger trials is needed. (Say L, Gülmezoglu AM, Hofmeyr GJ) CD000137

BACKGROUND: Fetal hypoxaemia is often a feature of fetal growth impairment. It has been suggested that perinatal outcome after suspected impaired fetal growth might be improved by giving mothers continuous oxygen until delivery.

OBJECTIVES: To assess the effects of maternal oxygen therapy in suspected impaired fetal growth on fetal growth and perinatal outcome.

METHODS: Standard PCG methods (see page xvii). Search date: November 2006.

MAIN RESULTS: Three studies involving 94 women were included. Oxygenation compared with no oxygenation was associated with a lower perinatal mortality rate (relative risk 0.50, 95% confidence interval 0.32 to 0.81). However, higher gestational age in the oxygenation groups may have accounted for the difference in mortality rates.

AUTHORS' CONCLUSIONS: There is not enough evidence to evaluate the benefits and risks of maternal oxygen therapy for suspected impaired fetal growth. Further trials of maternal hyperoxygenation seem warranted.

PLASMA VOLUME EXPANSION FOR SUSPECTED IMPAIRED FETAL GROWTH: there were no randomised trials to provide reliable evidence. (Say L, Gülmezoglu AM, Hofmeyr GJ) CD000167

BACKGROUND: Failure of the normal expansion of plasma volume in the mother is associated with impaired fetal growth and pre-eclampsia.
OBJECTIVES: To assess the effects of plasma volume expansion for suspected impaired fetal growth.
METHODS: Standard PCG methods (see page xvii). Search date: November 2006.
MAIN RESULTS: No studies were included.

AUTHORS' CONCLUSIONS: There is not enough evidence to evaluate the use of plasma volume expansion for suspected impaired fetal growth.

TRANSCUTANEOUS ELECTROSTIMULATION FOR SUSPECTED PLACENTAL INSUFFICIENCY (DIAGNOSED BY DOPPLER STUDIES): there were no randomised trials to provide reliable evidence (Say L, Gülmezoglu AM, Hofmeyr GJ) CD000079

BACKGROUND: Transcutaneous electrostimulation is thought to be able to improve blood flow and so it has been suggested that it may help to promote fetal growth.
OBJECTIVES: To assess the effects of transcutaneous electrostimulation in suspected placental insufficiency on the promotion of fetal growth.
METHODS: Standard PCG methods (see page xvii). Search date: November 2006.
MAIN RESULTS: No studies were included.

AUTHORS' CONCLUSIONS: There is not enough evidence to evaluate the use of transcutaneous electrostimulation in the management of women with suspected placental insufficiency.

MATERNAL HYDRATION FOR INCREASING AMNIOTIC FLUID VOLUME IN OLIGOHYDRAMNIOS AND NORMAL AMNIOTIC FLUID VOLUME: increased amniotic fluid volume; the clinical benefits have not been assessed. (Hofmeyr GJ, Gülmezoglu AM) CD000134

BACKGROUND: Oligohydramnios (reduced amniotic fluid) may be responsible for malpresentation problems, umbilical cord compression, concentration of meconium in the liquor and difficult or failed external cephalic version. Simple maternal hydration has been suggested as a way of increasing amniotic fluid volume in order to reduce some of these problems.

OBJECTIVES: To assess the effects of maternal hydration on amniotic fluid volume and measures of pregnancy outcome.

METHODS: Standard PCG methods (see page xvii). Search date: January 2004.

MAIN RESULTS: Two studies of 78 women were included. The women were asked to drink two litres of water before having a repeat ultrasound examination. Maternal hydration in women with and without oligohydramnios was associated with an increase in amniotic volume (weighted mean difference for women with oligohydramnios 2.01, 95% confidence interval 1.43 to 2.60; and weighted mean difference for women with normal amniotic fluid volume 4.5, 95% confidence interval 2.92 to 6.08). Intravenous hypotonic hydration in women with oligohydramnios was associated with an increase in amniotic fluid volume (weighted mean difference 2.3, 95% confidence interval 1.36 to 3.24). Isotonic intravenous hydration had no measurable effect. No clinically important outcomes were assessed in any of the trials.

AUTHORS' CONCLUSIONS: Simple maternal hydration appears to increase amniotic fluid volume and may be beneficial in the management of oligohydramnios and prevention of oligohydramnios during labour or prior to external cephalic version. Controlled trials are needed to assess the clinical benefits and possible risks of maternal hydration for specific clinical purposes.

4.4 Blood group incompatibilities – prevention and treatment

In 1939 Levine and Stetson found atypical agglutinins, active against the father's erythrocytes, in the serum of a woman who had given birth to an oedematous stillborn baby. There followed a series of discoveries which led to understanding, diagnosing, treating and preventing the condition. For women with access to health services, the risks of 'erythroblastosis fetalis' (breakdown of the baby's red blood cells) have virtually been eliminated by administering anti-D immunoglobulin to Rhesus (D) negative women after the birth of a rhesus positive baby.

For women who become immunised, amniocentesis, cordocentesis, ultrasound examination and Doppler studies are used to assess the wellbeing of the baby. Anaemic babies may be transfused before or after birth, and jaundice curbed by phototherapy or exchange transfusion.

> The removal of as much as possible of the baby's own blood should theoretically help diminish the damage resulting from the presence of this free and bound [maternal anti-Rh agglutinins] in the circulation and in the tissues. Such reasoning led to the trial of replacement transfusion... Diamond LK. Replacement transfusion as a treatment of erythroblastosis fetalis. *Pediatrics* 1948; 2: 520–4.

☺ **ANTI-D ADMINISTRATION AFTER CHILDBIRTH FOR PREVENTING RHESUS ALLOIMMUNISATION:** significantly reduced the incidence of (RhD) alloimmunisation six months after birth and in a subsequent pregnancy. (Crowther C, Middleton P) CD000021

BACKGROUND: The development of Rhesus immunisation and its prophylactic use since the 1970s has meant that severe Rhesus D (RhD) alloimmunisation is now rarely seen.
OBJECTIVES: To assess the effects of giving anti-D to Rhesus negative women, with no anti-D antibodies, who had given birth to a Rhesus positive infant.
METHODS: Standard PCG methods (see page xvii). Search date: June 2007. Initial analyses included all trials. Other analyses assessed the effect of trial quality, ABO compatibility and dose.

MAIN RESULTS: Six eligible trials compared postpartum anti-D prophylaxis with no treatment or placebo. The trials involved over 10 000 women, but trial quality varied. Anti-D lowered the incidence of RhD alloimmunisation six months after birth (relative risk (RR) 0.04, 95% confidence interval (CI) 0.02 to 0.06), and in a subsequent pregnancy (RR 0.12, 95% CI 0.07 to 0.23). These benefits were seen, regardless of the ABO status of the mother and baby, when anti-D was given within 72 hours of birth. Higher doses (up to 200 micrograms) were more effective than lower doses (up to 50 micrograms) in preventing RhD alloimmunisation in a subsequent pregnancy.

AUTHORS' CONCLUSIONS: Anti-D, given within 72 hours after childbirth, reduces the risk of RhD alloimmunisation in Rhesus negative women who have given birth to a Rhesus positive infant. However the evidence on the optimal dose is limited.

ANTI-D ADMINISTRATION IN PREGNANCY FOR PREVENTING RHESUS ALLOIMMUNISATION: may reduce rhesus immunisation; confirmation from more robust trials is needed. (Crowther CA, Middleton P) CD000020

BACKGROUND: During pregnancy, a Rhesus negative (Rh-negative) woman may develop antibodies when her fetus is Rhesus positive (Rh-positive). These may harm Rh-positive babies.

OBJECTIVES: To assess the effects of antenatal anti-D immunoglobulin on the incidence of Rhesus D alloimmunisation when given to Rh-negative women without anti-D antibodies.

METHODS: Standard PCG methods (see page xvii). Search date: June 2007.

MAIN RESULTS: Two average to poor-quality trials, involving over 4500 women, compared anti-D prophylaxis with no treatment. When women received anti-D at 28 and 34 weeks' gestation, relative risk (RR) of immunisation during pregnancy was 0.42 (95% confidence interval (CI) 0.15 to 1.17); after the birth of a Rh-positive infant the RR was 0.42 (95% CI 0.15 to 1.17); and within 12 months after birth of a Rh-positive infant the RR was 0.41 (95% CI 0.16 to 1.04). While none of these differences were statistically significant, the risk difference (RD) between anti-D and no treatment was significant (RD −0.01, 95% CI −0.01 to 0.00), suggesting reduced incidence of immunisation after anti-D prophylaxis.

In the higher dose trial (100 µg; 500 international units (IU) anti-D), there was a non-significant reduction in immunisation at two to 12 months following birth of a Rh-positive infant in women who had received anti-D (RR 0.14, 95% CI 0.02 to 1.15). However, women receiving anti-D were significantly less likely to register a positive Kleihauer test (which detects fetal cells in maternal blood) in pregnancy (RR 0.60, 95% CI 0.41 to 0.88) and at the birth of a Rh-positive infant (RR 0.60, 95% CI 0.46 to 0.79). No data were available for the risk of Rhesus D alloimmunisation in a subsequent pregnancy. No differences were seen for neonatal jaundice.

AUTHORS' CONCLUSIONS: The risk of Rhesus D alloimmunisation during or immediately after a first pregnancy is about 1%. Administration of 100 µg (500 IU) anti-D to women in their first pregnancy can reduce this risk to about 0.2% without, to date, any adverse effects. Although unlikely to confer benefit in the current pregnancy, fewer women may have Rhesus D antibodies in any subsequent pregnancy, but the effects of this needs to be tested in studies of robust design.

ANTENATAL INTERVENTIONS FOR FETOMATERNAL ALLOIMMUNE THROMBOCYTOPENIA: not enough data to provide reliable evidence. (Rayment R, Brunskill SJ, Stanworth S, Soothill PW, Roberts DJ, Murphy MF) CD004226

BACKGROUND: Fetomaternal alloimmune thrombocytopenia occurs when the mother produces antibodies against a platelet alloantigen that the fetus has inherited from the father. A consequence of this can be a reduced number of platelets (thrombocytopenia) in the fetus, which can result in bleeding whilst in the womb or shortly after birth. In severe cases this bleeding may lead to long-lasting disability or death. Antenatal management of fetomaternal alloimmune thrombocytopenia centres on preventing severe thrombocytopenia in the fetus. Available management options include administration of intravenous immunoglobulins or corticosteroids to the mother or intrauterine transfusion of antigen compatible platelets to the fetus. All options are costly and need to be assessed in terms of potential risk and benefit to both the mother and an individual fetus.

OBJECTIVES: To determine the optimal antenatal treatment of fetomaternal alloimmune thrombocytopenia to prevent fetal and neonatal haemorrhage and death.

METHODS: Standard PCG methods (see page xvii). Search date: February 2004.

MAIN RESULTS: One study met the inclusion criteria (54 pregnant women). This trial compared intravenous immunoglobulins plus corticosteroid (dexamethasone) with intravenous immunoglobulins alone.

No significant differences were reported between the treatment and control groups, in any outcome measured: mean platelet count at birth (weighted mean difference (WMD) 14.10 x 10^9/l, 95% confidence interval (CI) −30.26 to 58.46), mean gestational age at birth (WMD −0.50 weeks, 95% CI −2.69 to 1.69), mean rise in platelet count from first to second fetal blood screen (WMD −3.50 x 10^9/l, 95% CI −24.62 to 17.62) and mean rise in platelet count from birth to first fetal blood screen (WMD 24.40 x 10^9/l (95% CI −14.17 to 62.97)). This trial had adequate methodological quality; however the method used to calculate sample size was inappropriate: therefore the power calculation was not sufficient to determine any significance in differences between the treatment groups.

AUTHORS' CONCLUSIONS: There are insufficient data from randomised controlled trials to determine the optimal antenatal management of fetomaternal alloimmune thrombocytopenia. Future trials should consider the dose of intravenous immunoglobulins, the timing of initial treatment, monitoring of response to treatment by fetal blood sampling, laboratory measures to define pregnancies with a high risk of intercranial haemorrhage, management of non-responders and long-term follow up of children.

ANTENATAL PHENOBARBITAL FOR REDUCING NEONATAL JAUNDICE AFTER RED CELL ISOIMMUNIZSATION: not enough data to provide reliable evidence (Thomas JT, Muller P, Wilkinson C) CD005541

BACKGROUND: Neonates from isoimmunized pregnancies have increased morbidity from neonatal jaundice. The increased bilirubin from haemolysis often needs phototherapy, exchange transfusion or both after birth. Various trials in pregnant women who were not isoimmunized but had other risk factors for neonatal jaundice have shown a reduction in need for phototherapy and exchange transfusion by the use of antenatal phenobarbital. A recent retrospective case-controlled study showed reduction in the need for exchange transfusion for the neonates from isoimmunized pregnancies.

OBJECTIVES: To assess the effects of antenatal phenobarbital in red cell isoimmunized pregnancies in reducing the incidence of phototherapy and exchange transfusion for the neonate.

METHODS: Standard PCG methods (see page xvii). Search date: June 2006.

MAIN RESULTS: No trials met the inclusion criteria for this review.

AUTHORS' CONCLUSIONS: The use of antenatal phenobarbital to reduce neonatal jaundice in red cell isoimmunized pregnant women has not been evaluated in randomized controlled trials.

4.5   Death of the unborn baby

Death of an unborn baby may occur in the context of conditions which affect the placental blood flow or the baby, such as hypertensive disorders, intrauterine infection, placental abruption or diabetes, or be unexpected. Even extensive tests may fail to discover the cause of death. For the parents, an unexplained death may be more difficult to come to terms with, a situation analgous to an unexplained ('cot') death in childhood.

Options for care where the baby has died during pregnancy may include induction of labour or expectant management. Delaying delivery avoids the risks of labour induction, but may be emotionally unacceptable for the woman. Delay for more than four weeks carries a small risk of developing a coagulopathy.

There are no Cochrane reviews of this topic.

Chapter 5: Pregnancy Complications

5.1 Prelabour rupture of membranes

Charles Dickens's character David Copperfield was born with intact membranes. Being born with a 'caul' was considered a favourable omen.

More usually, the membranes rupture or are ruptured during labour. Rupture of the membranes (ROM) may occur before labour, when it is usually followed within hours by the spontaneous onset of labour. Failure of this to happen is called prelabour rupture of membranes, which may occur before (preterm) or at term. Vaginal speculum examination may be used to confirm the diagnosis.

Little attention has been paid to distinguishing between rupture of hindwaters as opposed to the forewaters, in terms of prognosis and management.

5.1.1 Preterm prelabour rupture of membranes

For preterm, prelabour rupture of membranes, with no evidence of infection, the option of expectant management arises.

The relationship between preterm labour, rupture of membranes and amnionitis (infection of the amniotic fluid) is complex. While established amnionitis is treated with antibiotics and expediting the birth of the baby, the place of routine antibiotic treatment for preterm and term prelabour ruptured membranes has been the subject of several trials.

> ☺ **ANTIBIOTICS FOR PRETERM RUPTURE OF MEMBRANES:** antibiotics (e.g. erythromycin) reduce the risks associated with preterm ROM; co-amoxyclav should be avoided. (Kenyon S, Boulvain M, Neilson J) CD001058 (in RHL 11)

A Cochrane Pocketbook: Pregnancy and Childbirth   G.J. Hofmeyr et al.
Copyright © 2008, Z. Alfiervic, C. A. Crowther, L. Duley, A. M. Gulmezoglu, G. ML. Gyte , E. D. Hodnett, G. J. Hofmeyr, J. P. Neilson

BACKGROUND: Premature birth carries substantial neonatal morbidity and mortality. One cause, associated with preterm rupture of membranes (and), is often subclinical infection. Maternal antibiotic therapy might lessen infectious morbidity and delay labour, but could suppress labour without treating underlying infection.

OBJECTIVES: To evaluate the immediate and long-term effects of administering antibiotics to women with prelabour rupture of membranes (PROM) before 37 weeks, on maternal infectious morbidity, fetal and neonatal morbidity and mortality, and longer-term childhood development.

METHODS: Standard PCG methods (see page xvii). Search date: August 2004.

In addition, trials, in which no placebo was used, were included for the outcome of perinatal death alone.

DATA COLLECTION AND ANALYSIS: We extracted data from each report without blinding of either the results or the treatments that women received. We sought unpublished data from a number of authors.

MAIN RESULTS: 22 trials involving over 6000 women and their babies were included.

The use of antibiotics following PROM is associated with a statistically significant reduction in chorioamnionitis (relative risk (RR) 0.57, 95% confidence interval (CI) 0.37 to 0.86). There was a reduction in the numbers of babies born within 48 hours (RR 0.71, 95% CI 0.58 to 0.87) and seven days of randomisation (RR 0.80, 95% CI 0.71 to 0.90). The following markers of neonatal morbidity were reduced: neonatal infection (RR 0.68, 95% CI 0.53 to 0.87), use of surfactant (RR 0.83, 95% CI 0.72 to 0.96), oxygen therapy (RR 0.88, 95% CI 0.81 to 0.96) and abnormal cerebral ultrasound scan prior to discharge from hospital (RR 0.82, 95% CI 0.68 to 0.98). Co-amoxiclav was associated with an increased risk of neonatal necrotising enterocolitis (RR 4.60, 95% CI 1.98 to 10.72).

AUTHORS' CONCLUSIONS: Antibiotic administration following PROM is associated with a delay in delivery and a reduction in major markers of neonatal morbidity. This data support the routine use of antibiotics in PROM.

The choice as to which antibiotic would be preferred is less clear as, by necessity, fewer data are available. Co-amoxiclav should be avoided in women at risk of preterm delivery because of the increased risk of neonatal necrotising enterocolitis. From the available evidence, erythromycin would seem a better choice.

> **AMNIOINFUSION FOR PRETERM RUPTURE OF MEMBRANES:** not enough data to provide reliable evidence. (Hofmeyr GJ) CD000942

BACKGROUND: Preterm rupture of membranes places a fetus at risk of cord compression and amnionitis. Amnioinfusion aims to prevent or relieve umbilical cord compression by infusing a solution into the uterine cavity.

OBJECTIVES: To assess the effects of amnioinfusion for preterm rupture of membranes on maternal and perinatal outcomes.

METHODS: Standard PCG methods (see page xvii). Search date: May 2001.

MAIN RESULTS: One trial of 66 women was included. It had some methodological flaws. No significant differences between amnioinfusion and no amnioinfusion were detected for caesarean section (relative risk 0.32, 95% confidence interval 0.07 to 1.40), low Apgar scores (relative risk 0.28, 95% confidence interval 0.03 to 2.33) or neonatal death (relative risk 0.55, 95% confidence interval 0.05 to 5.77). In the amnioinfusion group, the number of severe fetal heart rate decelerations per hour during the first stage of labour were reduced (weighted mean difference −1.20, 95% confidence interval −1.83 to −0.57). These outcomes are consistent with those found in the Cochrane review on amnioinfusion for cord compression.

AUTHOR'S CONCLUSIONS: There is not enough evidence concerning the use of amnioinfusion for preterm rupture of membranes.

5.1.2 Term prelabour rupture of membranes

> **ANTIBIOTICS FOR PRELABOUR RUPTURE OF MEMBRANES AT OR NEAR TERM:** not enough data to provide reliable evidence. (Flenady V, King J) CD001807 (in RHL 11)

BACKGROUND: Prelabour rupture of the membranes at or near term (term PROM) increases the risk of infection for the woman and her baby. The routine use of antibiotics for women at the time of term PROM may reduce this risk. However, due to increasing problems with bacterial resistance and the risk of maternal anaphylaxis with antibiotic use, it is important to assess the evidence addressing risks and benefits in order to ensure judicious use of antibiotics. This review was undertaken to assess the balance of risks and benefits to the mother and infant of antibiotic prophylaxis for prelabour rupture of the membranes at or near term.

OBJECTIVES: To assess the effects of antibiotics, administered prophylactically to women with prelabour rupture of the membranes at 36 weeks or beyond, on maternal, fetal and neonatal outcomes.

METHODS: Standard PCG methods (see page xvii). Search date: September 2005.

MAIN RESULTS: The results of two trials, involving a total of 838 women, are included in this review. The use of antibiotics resulted in a statistically significant reduction in maternal infectious morbidity (chorioamnionitis or endometritis): RR 0.43 (95% CI 0.23, 0.82), RD −4% (95% CI −7%, −1%), NNT 25 (95% CI 14 −100). No statistically significant differences were shown for outcomes of neonatal morbidity.

AUTHORS' CONCLUSIONS: No clear practice recommendations can be drawn from the results of this review on this clinically important question, related to a paucity of reliable data. Further well designed randomised controlled trials are needed to assess the effects of routine use of maternal antibiotics for women with prelabour rupture of the membranes at or near term.

5.2   Preterm birth

Preterm birth is a major cause of parental death and disability. Rates of preterm birth have been remarkably unresponsive to improvements in medical care over the last 50 years, including the widespread use of betastimulant tocolytics since the 1970s. The survival of babies born early has improved dramatically with access to intensive neonatal care. Preterm birth is defined as birth before 37 weeks' gestation. The earlier in gestation the birth occurs, the greater the mortality and morbidity risks.

Spontaneous preterm birth may follow one of two clinical patterns. Unexpected rupture of the membranes followed by a relatively painless birth suggests incompetence of the cervix. Birth following early 'normal' labour may be due to various complications such as clinical or subclinical infection of the amniotic fluid, membranes and placenta or placental abruption (antepartum bleeding may or may not be a feature), or may be unexplained. Elective preterm birth follows a planned decision to end the pregnancy due to illness of the mother or baby such as pre-eclampsia, intrauterine growth restriction or antepartum haemorrhage.

5.2.1 Prediction/prevention of preterm birth

Strategies which aim to reduce the risk of spontaneous preterm birth include bedrest, cervical cerclage (either following the diagnosis of cervical incompetence in a previous pregnancy, or through routine cervical surveillance clinically or with ultrasound), psychosocial interventions, routine or selective treatment with antibiotics, use of progesterone or treatments to suppress uterine contractions either prophylactically, selectively or in established preterm labour.

SPECIALISED ANTENATAL CLINICS FOR WOMEN WITH A PREGNANCY AT HIGH RISK OF PRETERM BIRTH (EXCLUDING MULTIPLE PREGNANCY) TO IMPROVE MATERNAL AND INFANT OUTCOMES:
(Whitworth M, Quenby S) Protocol [see page xviii] CD006760

ABRIDGED BACKGROUND: Despite research over the past few decades, no decrease in the incidence of preterm birth has occurred, although there have been improved survival and outcomes for premature infants.

Amongst the risk factors for preterm birth, previous preterm delivery is a strong predictor and the earlier the birth the more likely it is to be repeated at the same gestation. Other risk factors include cervical weakness, cervical trauma and stress. Specialised clinics for women with a history of spontaneous preterm delivery have been advocated, with non-randomised cohort data suggesting improved perinatal outcomes with the provision of intensive antenatal education, continuity of carer and individualised care. The package of care offered in such clinics may include promising prophylactic interventions for labour prevention including progesterone, clindamycin or cervical cerclage. However, stress has been associated with enhanced risk of preterm delivery and there is evidence that whilst some pregnant women welcome referral to a specialist clinic during pregnancy, others experience it as unsettling.

OBJECTIVES: To assess, using the best available evidence, the value of specialised antenatal clinics for women with a pregnancy at high risk of preterm delivery when compared with 'standard' antenatal clinics.

BED REST IN SINGLETON PREGNANCIES FOR PREVENTING PRETERM BIRTH: not enough data to provide reliable evidence. (Sosa C, Althabe F, Belizán J, Bergel E) CD003581 (in RHL 11)

BACKGROUND: Bed rest in hospital or at home is widely recommended for the prevention of preterm birth. This advice is based on the observation that hard work and hard physical activity during pregnancy could be associated with preterm birth and with the idea that bed rest could reduce uterine activity. However, bed rest may have some adverse effects on other outcomes.

OBJECTIVES: To evaluate the effect of prescription of bed rest in hospital or at home for preventing preterm birth in pregnant women at high risk of preterm birth.

METHODS: Standard PCG methods (see page xvii). Search date: July 2003.

MAIN RESULTS: One study met the inclusion criteria (1266 women). This trial has uncertain methodological quality due to lack of reporting. 432 women were prescribed bed rest at home and a total of 834 women received a placebo (412) or no intervention (422). Preterm birth before 37 weeks was similar in both groups (7.9% in the intervention group versus 8.5% in the control group), and the relative risk was 0.92 with a 95% confidence interval from 0.62 to 1.37. No other results were available.

AUTHORS' CONCLUSIONS: There is no evidence, either supporting or refuting the use of bed rest at home or in hospital, to prevent preterm birth. Although bed rest in hospital or at home is widely used as the first step of treatment, there is no evidence that this practice could be beneficial. Due to the potential adverse effects that bed rest could have on women and their families, and the increased costs for the healthcare system, clinicians should not routinely advise women to rest in bed to prevent preterm birth. Potential benefits and harms should be discussed with women facing an increased risk of preterm birth. Appropriate research is mandatory. Future trials should evaluate

the effectiveness of bed rest, and the effectiveness of the prescription of bed rest, to prevent preterm birth.

> **CERVICAL STITCH (CERCLAGE) FOR PREVENTING PREGNANCY LOSS IN WOMEN:** was not effective in women at low or moderate risk, or with short cervices as measured with ultrasound. (Drakeley AJ, Roberts D, Alfirevic Z) CD003253 (in RHL 11)

BACKGROUND: A cervical stitch has been used to prevent preterm deliveries in women with previous second trimester pregnancy losses, or other risk factors such as short cervix on digital or ultrasound examination.

OBJECTIVES: To assess the effectiveness and safety of prophylactic cerclage (before the cervix has dilated) and emergency cerclage (where cervices have started to shorten and dilate and then labour is halted) and to determine whether a particular technique of stitch insertion is better than others.

METHODS: Standard PCG methods (see page xvii). Search date July 2002.

MAIN RESULTS: Six trials with a total of 2175 women were analysed. Prophylactic cerclage was compared with no cerclage in four trials. There was no overall reduction in pregnancy loss and preterm delivery rates, although a small reduction in births under 33 weeks' gestation was seen in the largest trial (relative risks 0.75, 95% confidence interval 0.58 to 0.98). Cervical cerclage was associated with mild pyrexia, increased use of tocolytic therapy and hospital admissions but no serious morbidity. Two trials examined the role of therapeutic cerclage when ultrasound examination revealed a short cervix. Pooled results failed to show a reduction in total pregnancy loss, early pregnancy loss or preterm delivery before 28 and 34 weeks in women assigned to cervical cerclage.

AUTHORS' CONCLUSIONS: The use of a cervical stitch should not be offered to women at low or medium risk of mid trimester loss, regardless of cervical length by ultrasound. The role of cervical cerclage for women who have a short cervix on ultrasound remains uncertain as the numbers of randomised women are too few to draw firm conclusions. There is no information available as to the effect of cervical cerclage or its alternatives on the family unit and long term outcome.

ANTIBIOTICS FOR TREATING BACTERIAL VAGINOSIS IN PREGNANCY: given before 20 weeks may reduce the risk of preterm birth. (McDonald HM, Brocklehurst P, Gordon A) CD000262 (in RHL 11)

BACKGROUND: Bacterial vaginosis is an imbalance of the normal vaginal flora with an overgrowth of anaerobic bacteria and a lack of the normal lactobacillary flora. Bacterial vaginosis during pregnancy has been associated with poor perinatal outcome and, in particular, preterm birth (PTB). Identification and treatment may reduce the risk of PTB and its consequences.

OBJECTIVES: To assess the effects of antibiotic treatment of bacterial vaginosis in pregnancy.

METHODS: Standard PCG methods (see page xvii). Search date: May 2006.

MAIN RESULTS: We included 15 trials of good quality, involving 5888 women. Antibiotic therapy was effective at eradicating bacterial vaginosis during pregnancy (Peto odds ratio (OR) 0.17, 95% confidence interval (CI) 0.15 to 0.20; 10 trials, 4357 women). Treatment did not reduce the risk of PTB before 37 weeks (Peto OR 0.91, 95% CI 0.78 to 1.06; 15 trials, 5888 women), or the risk of preterm prelabour rupture of membranes (PPROM) (Peto OR 0.88, 95% CI 0.61 to 1.28; four trials, 2579 women).

However, treatment before 20 weeks' gestation may reduce the risk of preterm birth less than 37 weeks (Peto OR 0.63, 95% CI 0.48 to 0.84; five trials, 2387 women).

In women with a previous PTB, treatment did not affect the risk of subsequent PTB (Peto OR 0.83, 95% CI 0.59 to 1.17, five trials of 622); however, treatment may decrease the risk of PPROM (Peto OR 0.14, 95% CI 0.05 to 0.38) and low birthweight (Peto OR 0.31, 95% CI 0.13 to 0.75)(two trials, 114 women). In women with abnormal vaginal flora (intermediate flora or bacterial vaginosis) treatment may reduce the risk of PTB before 37 weeks (Peto OR 0.51, 95% CI 0.32 to 0.81; two trials, 894 women). Clindamycin did not reduce the risk of PTB before 37 weeks (Peto OR 0.80, 95% CI 0.60 to 1.05; six trials, 2406 women).

AUTHORS' CONCLUSIONS: Antibiotic treatment can eradicate bacterial vaginosis in pregnancy. This review provides little evidence that screening and treating all pregnant women with asymptomatic bacterial vaginosis will prevent PTB and its consequences. However, there is

some suggestion that treatment before 20 weeks' gestation may reduce the risk of PTB. This needs to be further verified by future trials.

RISK SCORING SYSTEMS FOR PREDICTING PRETERM BIRTH WITH THE AIM OF REDUCING ASSOCIATED ADVERSE OUTCOMES: (Darcy M-A, Watson LF, Rayner J, Rowlands S) Protocol [see page xviii] CD004902

ABRIDGED BACKGROUND: Identification of pregnancies that are at greater than average risk of adverse outcome is a fundamental concept in antenatal care, and has been implicit in obstetric teaching for many years. A number of investigators have been interested in whether some sort of systematic, objective measure of the level of risk would enable correct classification of the pregnancy more often than subjective clinical impression. Preterm birth is a major public health problem worldwide. The main purpose of screening for an increased risk of preterm birth is to enable high level antenatal care, aimed at prevention or delay of preterm birth in those identified as being at increased risk, or transfer in utero to a hospital with neonatal intensive care available.

OBJECTIVES: To determine whether the use of a risk-screening tool designed to predict preterm birth (in combination with appropriate consequent interventions) reduces the incidence of preterm birth and very preterm birth, and associated adverse outcomes.

FETAL FIBRONECTIN TESTING FOR REDUCING THE RISK OF PRETERM BIRTH: (Berghella V, Hayes E, Visintine J, Baxter J) Protocol [see page xviii] CD006843

ABRIDGED BACKGROUND: Despite extensive research efforts, the incidence of preterm birth is increasing in many countries. The interventions that have been shown to effectively reduce the risk of preterm birth or improve outcomes for babies born preterm in asymptomatic women have been: smoking cessation counseling for smokers; antibiotics for asymptomatic bacteriuria; intramuscular progesterone for women with prior preterm birth now carrying a singleton gestation; ultrasound-indicated cerclage in women with both a prior preterm birth and shortening of cervical length less than 25 mm before 24 weeks in the current singleton pregnancy; and history-indicated cerclage in women with three or more prior preterm births or second trimester losses. In symptomatic women, corticosteroids given to mother prior to preterm birth are effective in preventing neonatal mortality. The fetal fibronectin test assesses risk of preterm labour and preterm birth by measuring the amount of fetal fibronectin in cervicovaginal secretions. **OBJECTIVES:** To assess the effectiveness of management based on fetal fibronectin testing for preventing preterm birth.

MAGNESIUM SUPPLEMENTATION IN PREGNANCY: not enough data to provide reliable evidence. (Makrides M, Crowther CA) CD000937

BACKGROUND: Many women, especially those from disadvantaged backgrounds, have intakes of magnesium below recommended levels. Magnesium supplementation during pregnancy may be able to reduce fetal growth retardation and pre-eclampsia, and increase birth weight.

OBJECTIVES: The objective of this review was to assess the effects of magnesium supplementation during pregnancy on maternal, neonatal and paediatric outcomes.

METHODS: Standard PCG methods (see page xvii). Search date: June 2001.

MAIN RESULTS: Seven trials involving 2689 women were included. Six of these trials randomly allocated women to either an oral magnesium supplement or a control group, whist the largest trial with 985 women had a cluster design where randomisation was according to study centre. The analysis was conducted with and without the cluster trial.

In the analysis of all trials, oral magnesium treatment from before the 25th week of gestation was associated with a lower frequency of preterm birth (relative risk (RR) 0.73, 95% confidence interval (CI) 0.57 to 0.94), a lower frequency of low birth weight (RR 0.67, 95% CI 0.46 to 0.96) and fewer small for gestational age infants (RR 0.70, 95% CI 0.53 to 0.93) compared with placebo. In addition, magnesium treated women had less hospitalisations during pregnancy (RR 0.66, 95% CI 0.49 to 0.89) and fewer cases of antepartum haemorrhage (RR 0.38, 95% CI 0.16 to 0.90) than placebo treated women.

In the analysis excluding the cluster randomised trial, the effects of magnesium treatment on the frequencies of preterm birth, low birth weight and small for gestational age were not different from placebo.

Of the seven trials included in the review, only one was judged to be of high quality. Poor quality trials are likely to have resulted in a bias favouring magnesium supplementation.

AUTHORS' CONCLUSIONS: There is not enough high quality evidence to show that dietary magnesium supplementation during pregnancy is beneficial.

> **PRENATAL ADMINISTRATION OF PROGESTERONE FOR PRE-VENTING PRETERM BIRTH:** reduced births less than 37 weeks, but unclear if this translates into improved health outcomes and only limited information regarding the potential harms. (Dodd JM, Flenady V, Cincotta R, Crowther CA) CD004947 (in RHL 11)

BACKGROUND: Preterm birth is the major complication of pregnancy associated with perinatal mortality and morbidity and occurs in up to 6% to 10% of all births. Administration of progesterone for the prevention of preterm labour has been advocated.

OBJECTIVES: To assess the benefits and harms of progesterone administration during pregnancy in the prevention of preterm birth.

METHODS: Standard PCG methods (see page xvii). Search date: March 2005.

MAIN RESULTS: For all women administered progesterone, there was a reduction in the risk of preterm birth less than 37 weeks (six studies, 988 participants, relative risk (RR) 0.65, 95% confidence interval (CI) 0.54 to 0.79) and preterm birth less than 34 weeks (one study, 142 participants, RR 0.15, 95% CI 0.04 to 0.64). Infants born to mothers administered progesterone were less likely to have birthweight less than 2500 grams (four studies, 763 infants, RR 0.63, 95% CI 0.49 to 0.81) or intraventricular haemorrhage (one study, 458 infants, RR 0.25, 95% CI 0.08 to 0.82). There was no difference in perinatal death between women administered progesterone and those administered placebo (five studies, 921 participants, RR 0.66, 95% CI 0.37 to 1.19). There were no other differences reported for maternal or neonatal outcomes.

AUTHORS' CONCLUSIONS: Intramuscular progesterone is associated with a reduction in the risk of preterm birth less than 37 weeks' gestation, and infant birthweight less than 2500 grams. However, other important maternal and infant outcomes have been poorly reported to date, with most outcomes reported from a single trial only (Meis, 2003). It is unclear if the prolongation of gestation translates into improved maternal and longer-term infant health outcomes. Similarly,

information regarding the potential harms of progesterone therapy to prevent preterm birth is limited. Further information is required about the use of vaginal progesterone in the prevention of preterm birth.

HOME UTERINE MONITORING FOR DETECTING PRETERM LABOUR: (Urquhart C, Currell R, Callow E, Harlow F) Protocol [see page xviii] CD006172

ABRIDGED BACKGROUND: Preterm birth is a major cause of perinatal mortality and morbidity. Home uterine activity monitoring is one of the methods that has been used to try to predict preterm birth in the belief that early detection of increased contraction frequency would allow early intervention with tocolytic drugs to inhibit labour and prolong pregnancy. Monitoring at home could allow mothers to avoid prolonged or additional hospital admissions, and to be cared for at home. On the other hand, some mothers might become more anxious during the monitoring, particularly if they were remote from hospital, and greater awareness might in itself lead to more frequent presentation at hospital.

OBJECTIVES: The objective of the review is to determine whether home uterine activity monitoring is effective in improving the outcomes for women and their infants considered to be at high risk of preterm birth when compared with conventional or other care packages which do not include home uterine monitoring.

PROPHYLACTIC ORAL BETAMIMETICS FOR PREVENTING PRETERM LABOUR IN SINGLETON PREGNANCIES: not enough data to provide reliable evidence. (Whitworth M, Quenby S) CD006395

BACKGROUND: Preterm birth occurs in up to 6% to 10% of all births and is the major complication of pregnancy associated with perinatal mortality and morbidity. Previous preterm delivery is a strong predictor for preterm labour, and the earlier the birth, the more likely it is to be repeated at the same gestation. In the acute setting, betamimetics can decrease contraction frequency or delay preterm birth by 24 to 48 hours.

OBJECTIVES: To assess the effectiveness of prophylactic oral betamimetics for the prevention of preterm labour and birth for women with singleton pregnancies at high risk of preterm delivery.

METHODS: Standard PCG methods (see page xvii). Search date: October 2007.

MAIN RESULTS: One trial (64 singleton pregnancies) was included. The trial compared the oral betamimetic agent isoxuprine with placebo. No difference was seen for perinatal mortality rate (relative risk (RR) 4.74, 95% confidence interval (CI) 0.50 to 45.00). There was no evidence of an effect of oral betamimetic agents in reduction of spontaneous onset of preterm labour (RR 1.07, 95% CI 0.14 to 8.09) or preterm birth less than 37 weeks' gestation. There was no significant association between the use of oral betamimetics and side effects sufficient to stop therapy (RR 2.51, 95% CI 0.59 to 10.76). No differences were found for infant outcomes; birthweight less than 2500 grams (RR 1.74, 95% CI 0.44 to 6.87) or neonatal death (RR 4.74, 95% CI 0.50 to 45.00). This trial had adequate methodological quality; however the sample size was inappropriate to determine any significance in neonatal outcome differences between the treatment groups.

AUTHORS' CONCLUSIONS: There is insufficient evidence to support or refute the use of prophylactic oral betamimetics for preventing preterm birth in women at high risk of preterm labour with a singleton pregnancy.

ANTENATAL LOWER GENITAL TRACT INFECTION SCREENING AND TREATMENT PROGRAMMES FOR PREVENTING PRETERM DELIVERY: (Swadpanich U, Lumbiganon P, Prasertcharoensook W, Laopaiboon M) Protocol [see page xviii] CD006178

ABRIDGED BACKGROUND: A wide spectrum of causes and demographic factors have been implicated in the birth of preterm infants. Many micro-organisms cause both symptomatic and asymptomatic infection and may result in preterm prelabour rupture of membranes, preterm labour, or both. For example, Gardnerella vaginalis, Bacteroides species, Mobiluncus species, Ureaplasma urealyticum, Mycoplasma hominis, Chlamydia trachomatis, Trichomonas vaginalis, Neisseria gonorrhoeae, Group B streptococci, Staphylococcus aureus, syphilis, HIV, enteropharyngeal bacteria and Peptostreptococcus species have been associated with an increased risk of preterm birth.

OBJECTIVES: To assess the effectiveness and complications of antenatal lower genital tract infection screening and treatment programmes in reducing preterm birth and subsequent morbidity.

TREATING PERIODONTAL DISEASE FOR PREVENTING PRE-TERM BIRTH IN PREGNANT WOMEN: (Crowther CA, Thomas N, Middleton P, Chua M, Esposito M) Protocol [see page xviii] CD005297 (Oral Health Group)

ABRIDGED BACKGROUND: Between 30 and 50% of preterm births are thought to be caused by maternal infections. Maternal oral infection with specific organisms associated with periodontitis may be linked to preterm labour.

OBJECTIVES: To assess the effects of treating periodontal disease in pregnant women in order to prevent preterm birth, with the primary aim of reducing fetal, infant, childhood and maternal morbidity and mortality. Any reduction in preterm births should result in reduced fetal, infant, childhood and maternal morbidity and mortality. The primary hypothesis of the review is that treatment during pregnancy for periodontal disease (performed by a dentist, dental hygienist or therapist) will reduce the incidence of preterm birth.

PROBIOTICS FOR PREVENTING PRETERM LABOUR: reduce genital infections, but no evidence regarding preterm birth. (Othman M, Neilson JP, Alfirevic ZA) CD005941

BACKGROUND: Preterm birth causes 60% to 80% of neonatal deaths. Survivors can experience life-long complications. The risk of preterm labour in the presence of maternal infection is thought to be 30% to 50%. Probiotics are defined as live micro-organisms which, when administered in an adequate amount, confer a health benefit on the host. They have been shown to displace and kill pathogens and modulate the immune response by interfering with the inflammatory cascade that leads to preterm labour and delivery. During pregnancy, local treatment restoring normal vaginal flora and acidity without systemic effects could be preferable to other treatment in preventing preterm labour.

OBJECTIVES: To evaluate the effectiveness and the safety of probiotics for preventing preterm labour and birth.

METHODS: Standard PCG methods (see page xvii). Search date: June 2006.

MAIN RESULTS: We assessed four trials for inclusion in the review. One trial started in February 2005 and is still ongoing. We excluded one trial because there were no data to be extracted from the article. Of the two trials included in the review, one enrolled women after 34 weeks of pregnancy using oral fermented milk as probiotic, while the other study utilised commercially available yogurt to be used vaginally by women diagnosed with bacterial vaginosis in early pregnancy. Reduction in genital infection was the only prespecified clinical outcome for which the data were available; pooled results showed an 81% reduction in the risk of genital infection with the use of probiotics (risk ratio 0.19; 95% confidence interval 0.08 to 0.48).

AUTHORS' CONCLUSIONS: Although the use of probiotics appears to treat vaginal infections in pregnancy, there are currently insufficient data from trials to assess impact on preterm birth and its complications.

5.2.2   Prenatal treatment for babies born preterm

Prenatal strategies which aim to benefit the infant at risk of preterm birth include antenatal corticosteroids, thyrotrophin releasing hormone, phenobarbital, vitamin K and magnesium sulphate and delayed cord clamping.

In 1972 Liggins and Howie first reported the effectiveness of prenatal steroid treatment for reducing the morbidity and mortality associated with human preterm birth. Recently, attention has been focussed on fine-tuning antenatal corticosteroid treatment to maximise benefits and minimise harms. Several other treatments to improve the outcomes for babies born early have been disappointing.

> ☺ **ANTENATAL CORTICOSTEROIDS FOR ACCELERATING FETAL LUNG MATURATION FOR WOMEN AT RISK OF PRETERM BIRTH:** reduced neonatal death and morbidity. (Roberts D, Dalziel S) CD004454 (in RHL 11)

BACKGROUND: Respiratory distress syndrome (RDS) is a serious complication of preterm birth and the primary cause of early neonatal mortality and disability.

OBJECTIVES: To assess the effects on fetal and neonatal morbidity and mortality, on maternal mortality and morbidity and on the child in later life of administering corticosteroids to the mother before anticipated preterm birth.

METHODS: Standard PCG methods (see page xvii). Search date: October 2005.

MAIN RESULTS: 21 studies (3885 women and 4269 infants) are included. Treatment with antenatal corticosteroids does not increase risk to the mother of death, chorioamnionitis or puerperal sepsis. Treatment with antenatal corticosteroids is associated with an overall reduction in neonatal death (relative risk (RR) 0.69, 95% confidence interval (CI) 0.58 to 0.81, 18 studies, 3956 infants), RDS (RR 0.66, 95% CI 0.59 to 0.73, 21 studies, 4038 infants), cerebroventricular haemorrhage (RR 0.54, 95% CI 0.43 to 0.69, 13 studies, 2872 infants), necrotising enterocolitis (RR 0.46, 95% CI 0.29 to 0.74, eight studies, 1675 infants), respiratory support, intensive care admissions (RR 0.80, 95% CI 0.65 to 0.99, two studies, 277 infants) and systemic infections in the first 48 hours of life (RR 0.56, 95% CI 0.38 to 0.85, five studies, 1319 infants). Antenatal corticosteroid use is effective in women with premature rupture of membranes and pregnancy related hypertension syndromes.

AUTHORS' CONCLUSIONS: The evidence from this new review supports the continued use of a single course of antenatal corticosteroids to accelerate fetal lung maturation in women at risk of preterm birth. A single course of antenatal corticosteroids should be considered routine for preterm delivery with few exceptions. Further information is required concerning optimal dose to delivery interval, optimal corticosteroid to use, effects in multiple pregnancies and to confirm the long-term effects into adulthood.

☺ **REPEAT DOSES OF PRENATAL CORTICOSTEROIDS FOR WOMEN AT RISK OF PRETERM BIRTH FOR PREVENTING NEONATAL RESPIRATORY DISEASE:** reduced neonatal morbidity, but not enough data on long-term outcomes. (Crowther CA, Harding JE) CD003935 (in RHL 11)

BACKGROUND: It is not clear whether there is benefit in repeating the dose of prenatal corticosteroids for women who remain at risk of preterm birth after an initial course.

OBJECTIVES: To assess the effectiveness and safety of a repeat dose(s) of prenatal corticosteroids.

METHODS: Standard PCG methods (see page xvii). Search date: February 2007.

MAIN RESULTS: Five trials, involving over 2000 women between 23 and 33 weeks' gestation, are included. Treatment with repeat dose(s) of corticosteroid was associated with a reduction in occurrence (relative risk (RR) 0.82, 95% confidence interval (CI) 0.72 to 0.93, four trials, 2155 infants) and severity of any neonatal lung disease (RR 0.60, 95% CI 0.48 to 0.75, three trials, 2139 infants) and serious infant morbidity (RR 0.79, 95% CI 0.67 to 0.93, four trials, 2157 infants). Mean birthweight was not significantly different between treatment groups (weighted mean difference (WMD) −62.07 g, 95% CI −129.10 to 4.96, four trials, 2273 infants), although in one trial, treatment with repeat dose(s) of corticosteroid was associated with a reduction in birthweight Z score (WMD −0.13, 95% CI −26 to 0.00, one trial, 1144 infants), and in two trials, with an increased risk of being small for gestational age at birth (RR 1.63, 95% CI 1.12 to 2.37, two trials, 602 infants). No statistically significant differences were seen for any of the other primary outcomes that included other measures of respiratory morbidity, fetal and neonatal mortality, periventricular haemorrhage, periventricular leukomalacia and maternal infectious morbidity. Treatment with repeat dose(s) of corticosteroid was associated with a significantly increased risk of caesarean section (RR 1.11, 95% CI 1.01 to 1.22, four trials, 1523 women).

AUTHORS' CONCLUSIONS: Repeat dose(s) of prenatal corticosteroids reduce the occurrence and severity of neonatal lung disease and the risk of serious health problems in the first few weeks of life. These short-term benefits for babies support the use of repeat dose(s) of prenatal corticosteroids for women at risk of preterm birth. However, these benefits are associated with a reduction in some measures of weight, and head circumference at birth, and there is still insufficient evidence on the longer-term benefits and risks.

DIFFERENT CORTICOSTERIODS AND REGIMENS FOR ACCELERATING FETAL LUNG MATURATION FOR WOMEN AT RISK OF PRETERM BIRTH: (Brownfoot F, Crowther CA, Middleton P). Protocol [see page xviii] CD006764

ABRIDGED BACKGROUND: Preterm infants (less than 37 weeks' gestation), especially those born before 32 weeks' gestation, are at high risk of respiratory distress syndrome (RDS). RDS develops as a consequence of surfactant deficiency and immature lung development. In the fetal lung, the action of corticosteroids leads to an increase in protein production, biosynthesis of phospholipids and the appearance of surfactant. Despite their widespread use, there is currently variation in clinical practice as to the type of corticosteroid used, the dose given, the route of administration and the frequency of administration of corticosteroid doses.

OBJECTIVES: To assess the effects on fetal and neonatal morbidity and mortality, on maternal morbidity and mortality and on the child in later life of administering different types of corticosteroids (betamethasone or dexamethasone), different corticosteroid dose regimens and mode of administration.

⊗ **THYROTROPIN-RELEASING HORMONE ADDED TO CORTI-COSTEROIDS FOR WOMEN AT RISK OF PRETERM BIRTH FOR PREVENTING NEONATAL RESPIRATORY DISEASE:** increased adverse outcomes. (Crowther CA, Alfirevic Z, Haslam RR) CD000019

BACKGROUND: Thyrotropin-releasing hormone (TRH) added to prenatal corticosteroids has been suggested as a way to further reduce breathing problems and neonatal lung disease in infants born preterm.

OBJECTIVES: To assess the effect of giving prenatal TRH in addition to corticosteroids to women at risk of very preterm birth for the prevention of neonatal respiratory disease.

METHODS: Standard PCG methods (see page xvii). Search date: July 2003.

MAIN RESULTS: Over 4600 women were recruited into the 13 included trials. Five trials were rated of high quality. Overall, prenatal TRH, in addition to corticosteroids, did not reduce the risk of neonatal respiratory disease or chronic oxygen dependence, and did not improve any of the fetal, neonatal or childhood outcomes assessed by intention to treat analyses.

Indeed, the data showed prenatal TRH to have adverse effects for women and their infants. All side-effects monitored were more likely to occur in women receiving TRH. In the infants, prenatal TRH increased the risk of needing ventilation (relative risk (RR) 1.16, 95% confidence interval (CI) 1.03 to 1.29, three trials, 1969 infants), having a low Apgar score at five minutes (RR 1.48, 95% CI 1.14 to 1.92, three trials, 1969 infants) and, for the two trials providing data, was associated with poorer outcomes at childhood follow up.

Sensitivity analyses by trial quality, or subgroups with differing times from entry to birth, or different dose regimens of TRH, did not change these findings.

AUTHORS' CONCLUSIONS: Prenatal thyrotropin-releasing hormones, in addition to corticosteroids, given to women at risk of very preterm birth do not improve infant outcomes and can cause maternal side-effects.

PHENOBARBITAL PRIOR TO PRETERM BIRTH FOR PREVENTING NEONATAL PERIVENTRICULAR HAEMORRHAGE: not enough high quality data to provide reliable evidence. (Crowther CA, Henderson-Smart DJ) CD000164

BACKGROUND: Preterm infants are at risk of periventricular haemorrhage. Phenobarbital might prevent ischaemic injury or reduce fluctuations in blood pressure and blood flow in the brain.

OBJECTIVES: To assess the benefits and harms of giving phenobarbital to women at risk of imminent very preterm birth with the primary aim of preventing periventricular haemorrhage in the infant.

METHODS: Standard PCG methods (see page xvii). Search date: October 2002.

MAIN RESULTS: Over 1750 women were entered into the nine trials included. Analyses of all included trials showed a significant reduction in the rates of all grades of periventricular haemorrhage (PVH) (RR 0.65, 95% CI 0.50 to 0.83, nine trials, 1591 women) and severe grades of PVH (three and four) (RR 0.41, 95% CI 0.20 to 0.85, eight trials, 1527 women) in infants whose mothers had been given prenatal phenobarbital. These results were influenced by trials of poor quality which contributed excessive weight in the analysis due to their higher rates of severe PVH. When only the two higher quality trials were included, these beneficial effects disappeared for all grades of PVH (RR 0.90, 95% CI 0.75 to 1.08, two trials, 945 women), and severe grades of PVH (RR 1.05, 95% CI 0.60 to 1.83, two trials, 945 women).

No difference was found in the incidence of neurodevelopmental abnormalities at paediatric follow up assessed between 18 to 36 months of age.

Maternal sedation was more likely in women receiving phenobarbital (RR 2.06, 95% CI 1.79 to 2.37, one trial, 576 women).

AUTHORS' CONCLUSIONS: The evidence in this review does not support the use of prophylactic maternal phenobarbital administration to prevent periventricular haemorrhage or to protect from neurological disability in preterm infants. Phenobarbital administration leads to maternal sedation. If any future trials are carried out, they should measure neurodevelopmental status at follow up.

> **VITAMIN K PRIOR TO PRETERM BIRTH FOR PREVENTING NEO-NATAL PERIVENTRICULAR HAEMORRHAGE:** was not shown to be effective. (Crowther CA, Henderson-Smart DJ) CD000229

BACKGROUND: Preterm infants are at risk of periventricular haemorrhage. This can be a sign of brain damage that might lead to neurodevelopmental abnormalities, including cerebral palsy. It has been suggested that vitamin K might improve coagulation in preterm infants.

OBJECTIVES: To assess the effects of vitamin K administered to women at risk of imminent very preterm birth to prevent periventricular haemorrhage and associated neurological injury in the infant.

METHODS: Standard PCG methods (see page xvii). Search date: September 2000.

The primary outcomes were neonatal mortality, neonatal neurological morbidity, as measured by the presence of periventricular haemorrhage (PVH) on ultrasound during the first week of life, and long term neurodevelopment. Secondary outcomes included other neonatal morbidity and any maternal side effects.

MAIN RESULTS: Five trials were included, involving more than 420 women. The trials were of variable quality. Antenatal vitamin K was associated with a non-significant trend to a reduction in all grades of periventricular haemorrhage (relative risk (RR) 0.82, 95% confidence interval (CI) 0.67–1.00) and in severe PVH (grades three and four) (RR 0.75, 95% CI 0.45–1.25) for babies receiving prenatal vitamin K compared with control babies. This trend disappeared when poorer quality trials were excluded. Information on neurodevelopment was only given for a small sample of children in one trial with discrepancy in results given in the two reports.

AUTHORS' CONCLUSIONS: Vitamin K administered to women prior to very preterm birth has not been shown to significantly prevent periventricular haemorrhages in preterm infants.

MAGNESIUM SULPHATE FOR WOMEN AT RISK OF PRETERM BIRTH FOR NEUROPROTECTION OF THE FETUS: reduced gross motor dysfunction in early childhood; more research is needed. (Doyle LW, Crowther CA, Middleton P, Marret S) CD004661

BACKGROUND: Epidemiological and basic science evidence suggests that magnesium sulphate before birth may be neuroprotective for the fetus.

OBJECTIVES: To assess the effectiveness and safety of magnesium sulphate as a neuroprotective agent when given to women considered at risk of preterm birth.

METHODS: Standard PCG methods (see page xvii). Search date: October 2006.

MAIN RESULTS: Four trials (3701 babies) were eligible for this review. No statistically significant effect of antenatal magnesium sulphate therapy was detected on any major paediatric outcome, including mortality (e.g. paediatric mortality relative risk (RR) 0.97; 95% confidence interval (CI) 0.74 to 1.28; four trials; 3701 infants), and neurological outcomes in the first few years of life, including cerebral palsy (RR 0.77; 95% CI 0.56 to 1.06; four trials; 3701 infants), neurological impairments or disabilities. There were also no significant effects of antenatal magnesium therapy on combined rates of mortality with neurological outcomes. There was a significant reduction in the rate of substantial gross motor dysfunction (RR 0.56; 95% CI 0.33 to 0.97; two trials; 2848 infants). There were higher rates of minor maternal side-effects in the magnesium groups, but no significant effects on major maternal complications.

AUTHORS' CONCLUSIONS: The role for antenatal magnesium sulphate therapy as a neuroprotective agent for the preterm fetus is not yet established. Given the possible beneficial effects of magnesium

sulphate on gross motor function in early childhood, outcomes later in childhood should be evaluated to determine the presence or absence of later potentially important neurological effects, particularly on motor or cognitive function. Further information will be available from one of the studies where outcomes are being evaluated again at eight to nine years of age, and from another trial currently in progress.

SEE ALSO: EARLY VERSUS DELAYED UMBILICAL CORD CLAMPING IN PRETERM INFANTS (PAGE 278).

5.2.3   Treatment of preterm labour

Treatment to suppress preterm labour may postpone birth for long enough to allow meaningful growth and maturation of the baby, or at least to allow steroid treatment to take effect (24 to 48 hours). A range of pharmaceutical and non-pharmaceutical treatment strategies have been used.

BETAMIMETICS FOR INHIBITING PRETERM LABOUR: reduced births within 48 hours; considerable side-effects. (Anotayanonth S, Subhedar NV, Neilson JP, Harigopal S) CD004352

BACKGROUND: Preterm birth is a major contributor to perinatal mortality and morbidity worldwide. Tocolytic agents are drugs used to inhibit uterine contractions. The most widely used tocolytic agents are betamimetics, especially in resource-poor countries.

OBJECTIVES: To assess the effects of betamimetics given to women with preterm labour.

METHODS: Standard PCG methods (see page xvii). Search date: May 2006.

MAIN RESULTS: Seventeen randomized controlled trials are included. Eleven trials, involving 1320 women, compared betamimetics with placebo. Betamimetics decreased the number of women in preterm labour giving birth within 48 hours (relative risk (RR) 0.63; 95% confidence interval (CI) 0.53 to 0.75) but there was no decrease in the number of births within seven days after carrying out a sensitivity analysis of studies with adequate allocation of concealment. No benefit was demonstrated for betamimetics on perinatal death (RR 0.84; 95% CI 0.46 to 1.55, seven trials, n = 1332) or neonatal death (RR 1.00; 95% CI 0.48 to 2.09, five trials, n = 1174). No significant effect was demonstrated for respiratory distress syndrome (RR 0.87; 95% CI 0.71 to 1.08, eight trials, n = 1239). A few trials reported the following outcomes, with no difference detected: cerebral palsy, infant death and necrotizing enterocolitis. Betamimetics were significantly associated with the following: withdrawal from treatment due to adverse effects; chest pain; dyspnea; tachycardia; palpitation; tremor; headaches; hypokalemia; hyperglycemia; nausea or vomiting; and nasal stuffiness; and fetal tachycardia. Other betamimetics were compared with ritodrine in five trials (n = 948) and hexoprenaline compared with salbutamol in one trial (n = 140). Trials were small, varied and of insufficient quality to delineate any consistent patterns of effect.

AUTHORS' CONCLUSIONS: Betamimetics help to delay delivery for women transferred to tertiary care or completed a course of antenatal corticosteroids. However, multiple adverse effects must be considered. The data are too few to support the use of any particular betamimetics.

☺ **CALCIUM CHANNEL BLOCKERS FOR INHIBITING PRETERM LABOUR:** improved several substantive perinatal outcomes; were more effective than other tocolytics. (King JF, Flenady VJ, Papatsonis DNM, Dekker GA, Carbonne B) CD002255 (in RHL 11)

BACKGROUND: Preterm birth is a major contributor to perinatal mortality and morbidity and affects approximately six to seven per cent of births in developed countries. Tocolytics are drugs used to suppress uterine contractions. The most widely tested tocolytics are betamimetics. Although they have been shown to delay delivery, betamimetics have not been shown to improve perinatal outcome, and they have a high frequency of unpleasant and even fatal maternal side effects. There is growing interest in calcium channel blockers as a potentially effective and well tolerated form of tocolysis.

OBJECTIVES: To assess the effects on maternal, fetal and neonatal outcomes of calcium channel blockers, administered as a tocolytic agent, to women in preterm labour.

METHODS: Standard PCG methods (see page xvii). Search date: June 2002.

MAIN RESULTS: 12 randomised controlled trials involving 1029 women were included. When compared with any other tocolytic agent (mainly betamimetics), calcium channel blockers reduced the number of women giving birth within seven days of receiving treatment (relative risk (RR) 0.76; 95% confidence interval (CI) 0.60 to 0.97) and prior to 34 weeks' gestation (RR 0.83; 95% CI 0.69 to 0.99). Calcium channel blockers also reduced the requirement for women to have treatment ceased for adverse drug reaction (RR 0.14; 95% CI 0.05 to 0.36), the frequency of neonatal respiratory distress syndrome (RR 0.63; 95% CI 0.46 to 0.88), necrotising enterocolitis (RR 0.21; 95% CI 0.05 to 0.96), intraventricular haemorrhage (RR 0.59 95% CI 0.36 to 0.98) and neonatal jaundice (RR 0.73; 95% CI 0.57 to 0.93).

AUTHORS' CONCLUSIONS: When tocolysis is indicated for women in preterm labour, calcium channel blockers are preferable to other tocolytic agents, mainly betamimetics. Further research should address the effects of different dosage regimens and formulations of calcium channel blockers on maternal and neonatal outcomes.

CYCLO-OXYGENASE (COX) INHIBITORS FOR TREATING PRE-TERM LABOUR: not enough data to provide reliable evidence. (King J, Flenady V, Cole S, Thornton S) CD001992

BACKGROUND: Preterm birth is a major cause of perinatal mortality and morbidity. Cyclo-oxygenase (COX) inhibitors inhibit uterine contractions, are easily administered and have fewer maternal side-effects compared to conventional tocolytics. However, adverse effects have been reported on the fetus and newborn as a result of exposure to COX inhibitors.

OBJECTIVES: To assess the effects on maternal, fetal and neonatal outcomes of COX inhibitors administered as a tocolytic agent to women in preterm labour when compared with (i) placebo or no intervention and (ii) other tocolytics. In addition, to compare the effects of non-selective COX inhibitors with COX-2 selective inhibitors.

METHODS: Standard PCG methods (see page xvii). Search date: August 2004.

MAIN RESULTS: This review includes outcome data from 13 trials with a total of 713 women. The non-selective COX inhibitor indomethacin was used in 10 trials. When compared with placebo, COX inhibition (indomethacin only) resulted in a reduction in birth before 37 weeks' gestation (relative risk (RR) 0.21; one trial, 36 women), an increase in gestational age (weighted mean difference (WMD) 3.53 weeks) and birthweight (WMD 716.34 g; two trials, 67 women). Compared to any other tocolytic, COX inhibition resulted in a reduction in birth before 37 weeks' gestation (RR 0.53; three trials, 168 women) and a reduction in maternal drug reaction requiring cessation of treatment (RR 0.07; five trials and 355 women). A comparison of non-selective COX inhibitors versus any COX-2 inhibitor (two trials, 54 women) did not demonstrate any differences in maternal or neonatal outcomes.

Due to small numbers, all estimates of effect are imprecise and need to be interpreted with caution. Potential adverse effects of COX inhibition on the fetus, newborn or mother could not be adequately assessed due to insufficient data.

AUTHORS' CONCLUSIONS: There is insufficient information on which to base decisions about the role of COX inhibition for women in preterm labour. Further well designed trials are needed.

HYDRATION FOR TREATMENT OF PRETERM LABOUR: not enough data to provide reliable evidence. (Stan C, Boulvain M, Hirsbrunner-Amagbaly P, Pfister R) CD003096

BACKGROUND: Hydration has been proposed as a treatment for women with preterm labour. Theoretically, hydration may reduce uterine contractility by increasing uterine blood flow and by decreasing pituitary secretion of antidiuretic hormone and oxytocin.

OBJECTIVES: To evaluate the effectiveness of intravenous or oral hydration to avoid preterm birth and its consequences in women with preterm labour.

METHODS: Standard PCG methods (see page xvii). Search date: June 2007.

MAIN RESULTS: Two studies, including a total of 228 women with preterm labour and intact membranes, compared intravenous hydration with bed rest alone. Risk of preterm delivery, before 37 weeks (relative risk (RR): 1.09; 95% confidence interval (CI): 0.71–1.68), before 34 weeks (RR: 0.72; 95% CI: 0.20–2.56) or before 32 weeks (RR: 0.76; 95% CI: 0.29–1.97), was similar between groups. Admission to neonatal intensive care unit occurred with similar frequency in both groups

(RR: 0.99; 95% CI: 0.46–2.16). Cost of treatment was slightly higher (US$39) in the hydration group. This difference was not statistically significant and only includes hospital costs during a visit of less than 24 hours. No studies evaluated oral hydration.

AUTHORS' CONCLUSIONS: The data are too few to support the use of hydration as a specific treatment for women presenting with preterm labour. The two small studies available do not show any advantage of hydration compared to bed rest alone. Intravenous hydration does not seem to be beneficial, even during the period of evaluation soon after admission, in women with preterm labour. Women with evidence of dehydration may, however, benefit from the intervention.

⊗ **MAGNESIUM SULPHATE FOR PREVENTING PRETERM BIRTH IN THREATENED PRETERM LABOUR:** was ineffective at delaying birth or preventing preterm birth; increased adverse outcomes for the baby. (Crowther CA, Hiller JE, Doyle LW) CD001060

BACKGROUND: Magnesium sulphate is used to inhibit uterine activity in women in preterm labour to prevent preterm birth.

OBJECTIVES: To assess the effectiveness and safety of magnesium sulphate therapy given to women in threatened preterm labour with the aim of preventing preterm birth and its sequelae.

METHODS: Standard PCG methods (see page xvii). Search date: May 2002. Types of outcome measures: measures of effectiveness, complications, women's satisfaction with their care and health service use.

MAIN RESULTS: Over 2000 women were recruited into the 23 included trials. Only nine trials were rated of high quality for the concealment of allocation. In the magnesium sulphate versus control (all studies) no difference was seen for the risk of birth within 48 hours of treatment for women given magnesium sulphate compared with controls when using a random effects model (relative risk (RR) 0.85, 95% confidence interval (CI) 0.58–1.25, 11 trials, 881 women). No benefit was seen for magnesium sulphate on the risk of giving birth preterm (<37 weeks) or very preterm (<34 weeks). The risk of death (fetal and paediatric) was higher for infants exposed to magnesium sulphate (RR 2.82, 95% CI 1.20–6.62, seven trials, 727 infants). There were only two fetal deaths, both in the magnesium sulphate group in one study. The six other trials reported there were no fetal deaths. No differences for total paediatric mortality were shown in the six trials with data.

No beneficial effect was seen from using magnesium sulphate on the risk of other neonatal morbidity. A non-significant reduction in the risk of cerebral palsy was reported at follow up at 18 months corrected age (RR 0.14, 95% CI 0.01–2.60, one trial, 99 children).

AUTHORS' CONCLUSIONS: Magnesium sulphate is ineffective at delaying birth or preventing preterm birth, and its use is associated with an increased mortality for the infant. Any further trials should be of high quality, large enough to assess serious morbidity and mortality, compare different dose regimens and provide neurodevelopmental status of the child.

NITRIC OXIDE DONORS FOR THE TREATMENT OF PRETERM LABOUR: not enough data to provide reliable evidence. (Duckitt K, Thornton S) CD002860

BACKGROUND: A number of tocolytics have been advocated for the treatment of threatened preterm labour in order to delay delivery. The rationale is that a delay in delivery may be associated with improved neonatal morbidity or mortality. Nitric oxide donors, such as nitroglycerine, have been used to relax the uterus. This review addresses their efficacy, side effects and influence on neonatal outcome.

OBJECTIVES: To determine whether nitric oxide donors administered in threatened preterm labour are associated with a delay in delivery, adverse side effects or improved neonatal outcome.

METHODS: Standard PCG methods (see page xvii). Search date: March 2002.

MAIN RESULTS: Five randomised controlled trials (466 women) were included. Nitroglycerine was the NO donor used in all these trials. Nitric oxide donors did not delay delivery or improve neonatal outcome when compared with placebo, no treatment or alternative tocolytics such as ritodrine, albuterol and magnesium sulphate. There was, however, a reduction in number of deliveries less than 37 weeks when compared with alternative tocolytics but the numbers of deliveries before 32 and 34 weeks were not influenced. Side effects (other than headache) were reduced in women who received nitric oxide donors rather than other tocolytics. However, women were significantly more likely to experience headache when NO donors had been used.

AUTHORS' CONCLUSIONS: There is currently insufficient evidence to support the routine administration of nitric oxide donors in the treatment of threatened preterm labour.

OXYTOCIN RECEPTOR ANTAGONISTS FOR INHIBITING PRETERM LABOUR: may increase adverse outcomes for the baby. (Papatsonis D, Flenady V, Cole S, Liley H) CD004452 (in RHL 11)

BACKGROUND: Preterm birth, defined as birth before 37 completed weeks, is the single most important cause of perinatal mortality and morbidity in high-income countries. Oxytocin receptor antagonists have been proposed as effective tocolytic agents for women in preterm labour to postpone the birth, with fewer side-effects than other tocolytic agents.

OBJECTIVES: To assess the effects on maternal, fetal and neonatal outcomes of tocolysis with oxytocin receptor antagonists for women with preterm labour compared with placebo or no intervention and compared with any other tocolytic agent.

METHODS: Standard PCG methods (see page xvii). Search date: September 2004.

MAIN RESULTS: Six trials (1695 women) were included. Compared with placebo, atosiban did not reduce the incidence of preterm birth or improve neonatal outcome. In one trial (583 infants), atosiban was associated with an increase in infant deaths at 12 months of age compared with placebo (relative risk (RR) 6.15; 95% confidence intervals (CI) 1.39 to 27.22). However, this trial randomised significantly more women to atosiban before 26 weeks' gestation. Use of atosiban resulted in lower infant birthweight (weighted mean difference −138.31 gm; 95% CI −248.76 to −27.86) and more maternal adverse drug reactions (RR 4.02; 95% CI 2.05 to 7.85, two trials, 613 women).

Compared with betamimetics, atosiban increased the numbers of infants born under 1500 g (RR 1.96; 95% CI 1.15 to 3.35, two trials, 575 infants). Atosiban was associated with fewer maternal drug reactions requiring treatment cessation (RR 0.04; 95% CI 0.02 to 0.11, number needed to treat 6; 95% CI 5 to 7, four trials, 1035 women).

AUTHORS' CONCLUSIONS: This review failed to demonstrate the superiority of atosiban over betamimetics or placebo in terms of tocolytic efficacy or infant outcomes. The finding of an increase in infant deaths in one placebo controlled trial warrants caution. A recent Cochrane review suggests that calcium channel blockers (mainly nifedipine) are associated with better neonatal outcome and fewer maternal side-effects than betamimetics. However, a randomised comparison of nifedipine with placebo is not available. Further well-designed randomised controlled trials of tocolytic therapy are needed. Such trials should incorporate a placebo arm.

PROPHYLACTIC ANTIBIOTICS FOR INHIBITING PRETERM LABOUR WITH INTACT MEMBRANES: may increase adverse outcomes for the baby. (King J, Flenady V) CD000246 (in RHL 11)

BACKGROUND: The contribution of subclinical genital tract infection to the aetiology of preterm birth is gaining increasing recognition, but the role of prophylactic antibiotic treatment in the management of preterm labour is uncertain. Since rupture of the membranes is an important factor in the progression of preterm labour, it is important to see if the routine administration of antibiotics confers any benefit, prior to membrane rupture.

OBJECTIVES: To assess the effects of prophylactic antibiotics, administered to women in preterm labour with intact membranes, on maternal and neonatal outcomes.

METHODS: Standard PCG methods (see page xvii). Search date: May 2002.

MAIN RESULTS: This review has been updated (2002) to include data from the 'ORACLE II 2001' trial (six times larger than the previous 10 trials combined), which now dominates the results of this review. Meta-analysis of the 11 included trials (7428 women enrolled) shows a reduction in maternal infection with the use of prophylactic antibiotics (relative risk 0.74, 95% confidence interval 0.64 to 0.87) but fails to demonstrate a benefit or harm for any of the prespecified neonatal outcomes.

AUTHORS' CONCLUSIONS: This review fails to demonstrate a clear overall benefit from prophylactic antibiotic treatment for preterm labour with intact membranes on neonatal outcomes and raises concerns about increased neonatal mortality for those who received antibiotics. This treatment cannot therefore be currently recommended

for routine practice. Further research may be justified (when sensitive markers for subclinical infection become available) in order to determine if there is a subgroup of women who could experience benefit from antibiotic treatment for preterm labour prior to membrane rupture, and to identify which antibiotic or combination of antibiotics is most effective.

PROGESTATIONAL AGENTS FOR TREATING THREATENED OR ESTABLISHED PRETERM LABOUR: (Su LL, Samuel M, Chong YS) Protocol [see page xviii] CD006770

ABRIDGED BACKGROUND: Progesterone is known to have an inhibitory effect on uterine contractility and is thought to play a key role in the maintenance of pregnancy until term. The use of progestational agents for the treatment of threatened or established preterm labour has not been extensively studied.

OBJECTIVES: The principal objective of this review is to determine if the use of progestational agents is effective as a form of treatment or co-treatment for women with threatened or established preterm labour with intact membranes.

COMBINATION OF TOCOLYTIC AGENTS FOR INHIBITING PRETERM LABOUR: (JM Nardin, G Carroli, Z Alfirevic) Protocol CD006169

ABRIDGED BACKGROUND: A variety of tocolytic treatments have been used to inhibit uterine activity in women in preterm labour. In vitro studies have demonstrated that simultaneous blockage of different pathways could result in an additive or even synergistic effect capable of potentiating the uterine relaxation induced by each single drug and, most importantly, allow a reduction ofpe therapeutic concentration needed for each single drug.

OBJECTIVES: To assess the effects on maternal, fetal and neonatal outcomes of any combination of tocolytic drugs for the treatment of preterm labour when compared to any other treatment, no treatment or placebo.

5.2.4 Maintenance tocolytic therapy after an episode of preterm labour

Several pharmacological and non-pharmacological treatments have been tried for the prevention of recurrent preterm labour.

> **MAGNESIUM MAINTENANCE THERAPY FOR PREVENTING PRE-TERM BIRTH AFTER THREATENED PRETERM LABOUR:** not enough data to provide reliable evidence. (Crowther CA, Moore V) CD000940

BACKGROUND: Magnesium maintenance therapy is one of the types of tocolytic therapy used after an episode of threatened preterm labour (and usually an initial dose of tocolytic therapy) in an attempt to prevent the onset of further preterm contractions.

OBJECTIVES: To assess the effects of magnesium maintenance therapy on preventing preterm birth after threatened preterm labour.

METHODS: Standard PCG methods (see page xvii). Search date: August 2002.

MAIN RESULTS: Three trials, which recruited 303 women, were included. Two trials were of poor quality and none included any long-term follow up of infants. No differences in the incidence of preterm birth or peri-natal mortality were seen when magnesium maintenance therapy was compared with placebo or no treatment; or alternative therapies (rito-drine or terbutaline). The relative risk (RR) for preterm birth (less than 37 weeks) for magnesium compared with placebo or no treatment was 0.85, 95% confidence interval (CI) 0.47 to 1.51; and 0.98, 95% CI 0.56 to 1.72 for magnesium compared with alternative therapies. The RR for perinatal mortality for magnesium compared with placebo or no treat-ment, and also compared with alternative treatments, was 5.00, 95% CI 0.25 to 99.16. Women taking magnesium preparations were less likely to report palpitations or tachycardia than women receiving alternative therapies (RR 0.22, 95% CI 0.11 to 0.44) but were much more likely to experience diarrhoea (RR 10.67, 95% CI 3.35 to 33.99).

AUTHORS' CONCLUSIONS: There is not enough evidence to show any difference between magnesium maintenance therapy and either pla-cebo or no treatment, or alternative therapies (ritodrine or terbu-taline), in preventing preterm birth after an episode of threatened preterm labour.

> **MAINTENANCE THERAPY WITH CALCIUM CHANNEL BLOCK-ERS FOR PREVENTING PRETERM BIRTH AFTER THREATENED PRETERM LABOUR:** not enough data to provide reliable evidence. (Gaunekar NN, Crowther CA) CD004071

BACKGROUND: Calcium channel blocker maintenance therapy is one of the types of tocolytic therapy used after an episode of threatened preterm labour (and usually an initial dose of tocolytic therapy) in an attempt to prevent the onset of further preterm contractions.

OBJECTIVES: To assess the effects of calcium channel blockers as maintenance therapy on preventing preterm birth after threatened preterm labour.

METHODS: Standard PCG methods (see page xvii). Search date: March 2004.

MAIN RESULTS: One trial of 74 women was included. No difference in the incidence of preterm birth was found when calcium channel blocker (nifedipine) maintenance therapy was compared with no treatment. Twenty-five women out of 37 in each group gave birth before 37 weeks (relative risk 1.00, 95% confidence interval 0.73 to 1.37). The trial did not report stillbirths and neonatal deaths prior to discharge. Neurological follow up of the infants was not addressed.

AUTHORS' CONCLUSIONS: The role of maintenance therapy with calcium channel blockers for preventing preterm birth is not clear. Well designed randomised trials of sufficient size with relevant outcomes are required.

⊗ **ORAL BETAMIMETICS FOR MAINTENANCE THERAPY AFTER THREATENED PRETERM LABOUR:** have not shown benefit. (Dodd JM, Crowther CA, Dare MR, Middleton P) CD003927

BACKGROUND: Some women, who have threatened to give birth prematurely, subsequently settle. They may then take oral tocolytic maintenance therapy to prevent preterm birth and to prolong gestation.

OBJECTIVES: To assess the effects of oral betamimetic maintenance therapy after threatened preterm labour for preventing preterm birth.

METHODS: Standard PCG methods (see page xvii). Search date: June 2005.

MAIN RESULTS: 11 randomised controlled trials (RCTs) were included. No differences were seen for admission to the neonatal intensive care unit when betamimetics were compared with placebo (relative risk (RR) 1.29, 95% confidence interval (CI) 0.64 to 2.60; one RCT of terbutaline with 140 women) or with magnesium (RR 0.80, 95% CI 0.43 to 1.46; one RCT of 137 women). The rate of preterm birth (less than 37 weeks) showed no significant difference in four RCTs, two comparing ritodrine with placebo/no treatment and two comparing terbutaline with placebo/no treatment (RR 1.08, 95% CI 0.88 to 1.32, 384 women). No differences between betamimetics and placebo, no treatment or other tocolytics were seen for perinatal mortality and morbidity outcomes. Some adverse effects such as tachycardia were more frequent in the betamimetics groups than the groups allocated to placebo, no treatment or another type of tocolytic.

AUTHORS' CONCLUSIONS: Available evidence does not support the use of oral betamimetics for maintenance therapy after threatened preterm labour.

MAINTENANCE THERAPY WITH OXYTOCIN ANTAGONISTS FOR INHIBITING PRETERM BIRTH AFTER THREATENED PRETERM LABOUR: (Papatsonis D, Flenady V) Protocol [see page xviii] CD005938

ABRIDGED BACKGROUND: For those women with preterm labour who are treated with tocolytic agents and remain undelivered after 48 hours' maintenance, treatment with a tocolytic agent is sometimes used to further delay delivery and to prolong pregnancy. Oxytocin antagonists (commonly atosiban) are used as a tocolytic agent in several countries and have been registered in Europe as a tocolytic agent.

OBJECTIVES: To assess the efficacy and safety of maintenance treatment with oxytocin antagonists, after a period of threatened preterm labour, in preventing preterm birth and other adverse outcomes.

⊗ TERBUTALINE PUMP MAINTENANCE THERAPY AFTER THREATENED PRETERM LABOR FOR PREVENTING PRETERM BIRTH: did not have measurable benefits. (Nanda K, Cook LA, Gallo MF, Grimes DA) CD003933

BACKGROUND: Women with preterm labor that is arrested with tocolytic therapy are at increased risk of recurrent preterm labor. Terbutaline pump maintenance therapy has been given to such women to decrease the risk of recurrent preterm labor, preterm birth, and its consequences.

OBJECTIVES: To determine the effectiveness and safety of terbutaline pump maintenance therapy after threatened preterm labor in preventing preterm birth and its complications.

METHODS: Standard PCG methods (see page xvii). Search date: April 2007.

MAIN RESULT: We included two studies. Terbutaline pump maintenance therapy did not appear to offer any advantages over the saline placebo pump or oral terbutaline maintenance therapy in preventing preterm births by prolonging pregnancy or its complications among women with arrested preterm labor. The weighted mean difference (WMD) for gestational age at birth was -0.14 weeks (95% confidence interval (CI) -1.66 to 1.38) for terbutaline pump therapy compared with saline placebo pump for both trials combined and 1.40 weeks (95% CI -1.13 to 3.93) for terbutaline pump versus oral terbutaline therapy for the first trial. The second trial reported a relative risk (RR) of 1.17 (95% CI 0.79 to 1.73) of preterm birth (less than 37 completed weeks) and a RR of 0.97 (95% CI 0.51 to 1.84) of very preterm birth (less than 34 completed weeks) for terbutaline pump compared with saline placebo pump. Terbutaline pump therapy also did not result in a higher rate of therapy continuation or a lower rate of infant complications. No data were reported on long-term infant outcomes, costs, or maternal assessment of therapy.

AUTHORS' CONCLUSIONS: Terbutaline pump maintenance therapy has not been shown to decrease the risk of preterm birth by prolonging pregnancy. Furthermore, the lack of information on the safety of the therapy, as well as its substantial expense, argues against its role in the management of arrested preterm labor. Future use should only be in the context of well-conducted, adequately powered randomized controlled trials.

5.2.5 Mode of birth for infants born preterm

Intuition suggests that preterm babies may be born more safely by caesarean section. On the other hand, it is possible that labour and vaginal birth may enhance the baby's adaptation to extrauterine life. Vaginal birth is in general safest for the mother.

> **ELECTIVE CAESAREAN SECTION VERSUS EXPECTANT MANAGE-MENT FOR DELIVERY OF THE SMALL BABY:** not enough data to provide reliable evidence. (Grant A, Glazener CMA) CD000078

BACKGROUND: Elective caesarean delivery for women in labour with a small or immature baby might reduce the chances of fetal or neonatal death, but it might also increase the risk of maternal morbidity.

OBJECTIVES: To assess the effects of a policy of elective caesarean delivery versus expectant management for small babies.

METHODS: Standard PCG methods (see page xvii). Search date: June 2006.

MAIN RESULTS: Six studies involving 122 women were included. All trials reported recruiting difficulties. Babies in the elective group were less likely to have respiratory distress syndrome (odds ratio (OR) 0.43, 95% confidence interval (CI) 0.18 to 1.06) although they were more likely to have a low cord pH immediately after delivery (OR 10.82, 95% CI 1.60 to 73.24). They were less likely to have neonatal seizures (0/39 versus 2/42) and there were fewer deaths (2/62 versus 6/60) but these differences did not reach statistical significance. However, their mothers were more likely to have serious morbidity (OR 6.44, 95% CI 1.48 to 27.89).

AUTHORS' CONCLUSIONS: There is not enough evidence to evaluate the use of a policy for elective caesarean delivery for small babies. Randomised trials in this area are likely to continue to experience recruitment problems. However, it still may be possible to investigate elective caesarean delivery in small babies with cephalic presentations.

5.3   Prolonged pregnancy

Pregnancy beyond 41 or 42 weeks' gestation may be associated with placental insufficiency, reduced amniotic fluid volume, meconium staining of the amniotic fluid, macrosomia (a large baby) and increasing perinatal mortality. For these reasons, strategies have developed to prevent women's pregnancies progressing beyond 41 or 42 weeks.

INDUCTION OF LABOUR FOR IMPROVING BIRTH OUTCOMES FOR WOMEN AT OR BEYOND TERM: labour induction at 41 or more weeks reduced perinatal deaths slightly. (Gülmezoglu AM, Crowther CA, Middleton P) CD004945 (in RHL 11)

BACKGROUND: As a pregnancy continues beyond term the risks of babies dying inside the womb or in the immediate newborn period increase. Whether a policy of labour induction at a predetermined gestational age can reduce this increased risk is the subject of this review.

OBJECTIVES: To evaluate the benefits and harms of a policy of labour induction at term or post-term compared to awaiting spontaneous labour or later induction of labour.

METHODS: Standard PCG methods (see page xvii). Search date: June 2006.

Trials comparing cervical ripening methods, membrane stripping/sweeping or nipple stimulation without any commitment to delivery within a certain time were excluded. Outcomes are analysed in two main categories: gestational age and cervix status.

MAIN RESULTS: We included 19 trials reporting on 7984 women. A policy of labour induction at 41 completed weeks or beyond was associated with fewer (all-cause) perinatal deaths (1/2986 versus 9/2953; relative risk (RR) 0.30; 95% confidence interval (CI) 0.09 to 0.99). The risk difference is 0.00 (95% CI 0.01 to 0.00). If deaths due to congenital abnormality are excluded, no deaths remain in the labour induction group and seven deaths remain in the no-induction group. There was no evidence of a statistically significant difference in the risk of caesarean section (RR 0.92; 95% CI 0.76 to 1.12; RR 0.97; 95% CI 0.72 to 1.31) for women induced at 41 and 42 completed weeks respectively. Women induced at 37 to 40 completed weeks were more likely to have a caesarean section with expectant management than those in the labour induction group (RR 0.58; 95% CI 0.34 to 0.99). There were fewer babies with meconium aspiration syndrome (41+: RR 0.29; 95% CI 0.12 to 0.68, four trials, 1325 women; 42+: RR 0.66; 95% CI 0.24 to 1.81, two trials, 388 women).

AUTHORS' CONCLUSIONS: A policy of labour induction after 41 completed weeks or later compared to awaiting spontaneous labour either indefinitely or at least one week is associated with fewer perinatal deaths. However, the absolute risk is extremely small. Women should be appropriately counselled on both the relative and absolute risks.

5.4 Multiple pregnancy

Multiple pregnancies which result from multiple ovulation are considerably more common in certain families and ethnic groups, older women and following assisted reproduction. They are dichorionic, with separate placental circulations. Monozygotic twins (resulting from one fertilised egg splitting) are less common, and have more complications, particularly preterm birth. The rate of complications increases with earlier splitting of the zygote from developmentally separate placentae (dichorionic) to single placenta (monochorionic, often with shared placental circulations), to single amniotic sac (monoamniotic) to conjoined twins.

Women with a multiple pregnancy are more likely to experience pre-eclampsia, preterm labour and have an operative birth than women with a singleton. For their infants there are increased risks of preterm birth, poor intrauterine growth, perinatal mortality and cerebral palsy. Care for women with a multiple pregnancy has included strategies to decrease the problems these women and their infants face. Parents of twins may benefit from extra support, such as that provided by multiple pregnancy peer support groups.

Clinical signs suggesting multiple pregnancy include a fundal height greater than expected by dates, a globular uterus with multiple small parts palpable, and an abdominal girth exceeding 100cm. Without routine ultrasound examination, in at least one in five women the multiple pregnancy will not be identified before the first birth.

During birth of the first twin, the head of the second twin may be manually guided towards the pelvis. Tocolytics may be needed to facilitate correction of the lie of the second twin or to suppress contractions if the second twin is undeliverable vaginally and a caesarean section is needed. Once the second twin is in a suitable position for vaginal birth, oxytocin infusion may be used to shorten the delay between births.

Hazards of labour include inadvertent administration of a third stage uterotonic drug before birth of all the babies, and postpartum haemorrhage.

SPECIALISED ANTENATAL CLINICS FOR WOMEN WITH A MULTIPLE PREGNANCY TO IMPROVE MATERNAL AND INFANT OUTCOMES: no randomised trials to provide reliable evidence. (Dodd JM, Crowther CA) CD005300

BACKGROUND: Regular antenatal care for women with a multiple pregnancy is accepted practice, and while most women have an increase in the number of antenatal visits, there is no consensus as to what constitutes optimal care. 'Specialised' antenatal clinics have been advocated as a way of improving outcomes for women and their infants.

OBJECTIVES: To assess, using the best available evidence, the benefits and harms of 'specialised' antenatal clinics compared with 'standard' antenatal care for women with a multiple pregnancy.

METHODS: Standard PCG methods (see page xvii). Search date: October 2006.

MAIN RESULTS: There are no included studies.

AUTHORS' CONCLUSIONS: There is no information available from randomised controlled trials to support the role of 'specialised' antenatal clinics for women with a multiple pregnancy compared with 'standard' antenatal care in improving maternal and infant health outcomes. The value of 'specialised' multiple pregnancy clinics in improving health outcomes for women and their infants requires evaluation in appropriately powered and designed randomised controlled trials.

HOSPITALISATION AND BED REST FOR MULTIPLE PREGNANCY: increased the rate of very preterm births; may reduce the rate of low birth weight infants. (Crowther CA) CD000110

BACKGROUND: Bed rest used to be widely advised for women with a multiple pregnancy.

OBJECTIVES: The objective was to assess the effect of bed rest in hospital for women with a multiple pregnancy for prevention of preterm birth and other fetal, neonatal and maternal outcomes.

METHODS: Standard PCG methods (see page xvii). Search date: August 2000.

Prespecified sensitivity analyses have been carried out to evaluate the effect of trial quality, the effects of hospitalisation for bed rest in women with an uncomplicated twin pregnancy, in women with a triplet pregnancy and in women with a twin pregnancy complicated by cervical effacement and dilatation prior to labour.

MAIN RESULTS: Six trials were included which involved over 600 women and 1400 babies.

(1) Analyses of all trials.

Routine bed rest in hospital for multiple pregnancy did not reduce the risk of preterm birth, or perinatal mortality. There was a trend to a decreased number of low birth weight infants born to women in the routinely hospitalised group, which became significant when the trial using alternate allocation was excluded (odds ratio (OR) 0.79; 95% confidence interval (CI) 0.63–0.99). No differences were seen in the number of very low birth weight infants. No support for the policy was found in other neonatal outcomes. No information is available on developmental outcomes for infants in any of the trials. Women's views about the care they received were reported rarely.

(2) Analyses of hospitalisation for bed rest in women with an uncomplicated twin pregnancy.

The risk of preterm birth was not reduced. Indeed significantly more women gave birth very preterm (< 34 weeks, gestation) (OR 1.84; 95% CI 1.01–3.34). No differences were seen in perinatal mortality, or in other neonatal outcomes.

Women receiving hospitalisation for bed rest had a decreased risk of developing hypertension (OR 0.55; 95% CI 0.32–0.97), although this effect was no longer apparent when the trial using alternate allocation was excluded.

(3) Analyses of hospitalisation for bed rest in women with a triplet pregnancy.

Most of the comparisons made between the hospitalised and control groups suggest beneficial treatment effects from routine hospitalisation for bed rest. However all the differences observed between the experimental and control groups were compatible with chance variation.

(4) Analyses of hospitalisation for bed rest in women with a twin pregnancy complicated by cervical effacement and dilatation prior to labour.

No differences were seen in the risk of preterm birth, perinatal mortality, fetal growth or in other neonatal outcomes.

AUTHOR'S CONCLUSIONS: There is currently not enough evidence to support a policy of routine hospitalisation for bed rest in multiple pregnancy. No reduction in the risk of preterm birth or perinatal death is evident, although there is a suggestion that fetal growth is improved.

For women with an uncomplicated twin pregnancy the results of this review suggest that it may be harmful in that the risk of very preterm birth is increased. Until further evidence is available to the contrary, the policy cannot be recommended for routine clinical practice.

REDUCTION OF THE NUMBER OF FETUSES FOR WOMEN WITH TRIPLET AND HIGHER ORDER MULTIPLE PREGNANCIES: no randomised trials to provide reliable evidence. (Dodd JM, Crowther CA) CD003932

BACKGROUND: When couples are faced with the dilemma of a higher order multiple pregnancy there are three options. Termination of the entire pregnancy has generally not been acceptable to women, especially for those with a past history of infertility. Attempting to continue with all the fetuses is associated with inherent problems of preterm birth, survival and long term morbidity. The other alternative relates to reduction in the number of fetuses by selective termination. The acceptability of these options for the couple will depend on their social background and underlying beliefs. This review focused on reduction in the number of fetuses.

OBJECTIVES: To assess a policy of multifetal reduction with a policy of expectant management of women with a triplet or higher order multiple pregnancy.

METHODS: Standard PCG methods (see page xvii). Search date: October 2004.

MAIN RESULTS: There were no randomised controlled trials identified.

AUTHORS' CONCLUSIONS: There are insufficient data available to support a policy of pregnancy reduction procedures for women with a triplet or higher order multiple pregnancy. While randomised controlled trials will provide the most reliable evidence about the risks and benefits of fetal reduction procedures, reduction in the number of fetuses by selective termination may not be acceptable to women, especially for those with a past history of infertility. The acceptability of this option, and willingness to undergo randomisation, will depend on the couple's social background and beliefs, and consequently recruitment to such a trial may prove exceptionally difficult.

☺ **INTERVENTIONS FOR THE TREATMENT OF TWIN–TWIN TRANSFUSION SYNDROME:** endoscopic laser coagulation of anastomotic vessels improves perinatal outcome. (Roberts D, Neilson JP, Kilby M, Gates S) CD002073

BACKGROUND: Twin–twin transfusion syndrome, a condition affecting monochorionic twin pregnancies, is associated with a high risk of perinatal mortality and morbidity. A number of treatments have been introduced to treat the condition but it is unclear which intervention improves maternal and fetal outcome.

OBJECTIVES: The objective of this review was to evaluate the impact of treatment modalities in twin–twin transfusion syndrome.

METHODS: Standard PCG methods (see page xvii). Search date: October 2007.

MAIN RESULTS: Two studies (213 women) were included. This review shows that laser coagulation of anastomotic vessels results in less death of both infants per pregnancy (relative risk (RR) 0.33; 95% confidence interval (CI) 0.16 to 0.67, one trial), less perinatal death (RR 0.59; 95% CI 0.0.40 to 0.87 adjusted for cluster, one trial) and less neonatal death (RR 0.29; 95% CI 0.14 to 0.61 adjusted for cluster, one trial) than in pregnancies treated with amnioreduction. There is no difference in perinatal outcome between amnioreduction and septostomy. A third study is awaiting assessment. More babies were alive without neurological abnormality at the age of six months in the laser group than the amnioreduction groups (RR 1.66; 95% CI 1.17 to 2.35 adjusted for clustering, one trial). This difference did not persist beyond six months of age. There was no significant difference in the babies alive at six months with neurological abnormality treated by laser coagulation or amnioreduction (RR 0.58; 95% CI 0.18 to 1.86 adjusted for clustering, one trial).

AUTHORS' CONCLUSIONS: Endoscopic laser coagulation of anastomotic vessels should be considered in the treatment of all stages of twin–twin transfusion syndrome to improve perinatal outcome. Further research on the effect of treatment on milder forms of twin–twin transfusion syndrome (Quintero stage 1 and 2) are required. The long-term outcomes of survivors from the studies included in this review are required.

PROPHYLACTIC ORAL BETAMIMETICS FOR REDUCING PRE-TERM BIRTH IN WOMEN WITH A TWIN PREGNANCY: increased the mean birthweights, but there was not enough data to provide reliable evidence. (Yamasmit W, Chaithongwongwatthana S, Tolosa JE, Limpongsanurak S, Pereira L, Lumbiganon P) CD004733

BACKGROUND: Twin pregnancies are associated with a high risk of neonatal mortality and morbidity due to an increased rate of preterm birth. Betamimetics can decrease contraction frequency or delay preterm birth in singleton pregnancies by 24 to 48 hours. The efficacy of oral betamimetics in women with a twin pregnancy is unproven.

OBJECTIVES: To assess the effects of prophylactic oral betamimetics administered to women with twin pregnancies.

METHODS: Standard PCG methods (see page xvii). Search date: May 2004.

MAIN RESULTS: Five trials (344 twin pregnancies) were included. All trials compared oral betamimetics to placebo. Betamimetics reduced the incidence of preterm labour (one trial, 50 twin pregnancies, relative risk (RR) 0.40; 95% confidence interval (CI) 0.19 to 0.86). However, betamimetics did not reduce preterm birth less than 37 weeks' gestation (four trials, 276 twin pregnancies, RR 0.85; 95% CI 0.65 to 1.10) or less than 34 weeks' gestation (one trial, 144 twin pregnancies, RR 0.47; 95% CI 0.15 to 1.50). Mean neonatal birthweight in the betamimetic group was significantly higher than in the placebo group (three trials, 478 neonates, weighted mean difference 111.2 grams; 95% CI 22.2 to 200.2). Nevertheless, there was no evidence of an effect of betamimetics in reduction of low birthweight (two trials, 366 neonates, RR 1.19; 95% CI 0.77 to 1.85) or small-for-gestational age neonates (two trials, 178 neonates, RR 0.92; 95% CI 0.52 to 1.65). Two trials (388 neonates) showed that betamimetics significantly reduced the incidence of respiratory distress syndrome but the difference was not significant when the analysis was adjusted for correlation of babies from twins. Three trials (452 neonates) showed no evidence of an effect of betamimetics in reducing neonatal mortality (RR 0.80; 95% CI 0.35 to 1.82).

AUTHORS' CONCLUSIONS: There is insufficient evidence to support or refute the use of prophylactic oral betamimetics for preventing preterm birth in women with a twin pregnancy.

ELECTIVE DELIVERY OF WOMEN WITH A TWIN PREGNANCY
FROM 37 WEEKS' GESTATION: not enough data to provide reliable
evidence. (Dodd JM, Crowther CA) CD003582

BACKGROUND: The optimal timing of birth for women with an otherwise uncomplicated twin pregnancy at term is uncertain, with clinical support for both elective delivery at 37 weeks, as well as expectant management (awaiting the spontaneous onset of labour).

OBJECTIVES: To assess a policy of elective delivery from 37 weeks' gestation compared with an expectant approach for women with an otherwise uncomplicated twin pregnancy.

METHODS: Standard PCG methods (see page xvii). Search date: October 2004.

MAIN RESULTS: A single randomised controlled trial comparing elective induction of labour at 37 weeks for women with a twin pregnancy with expectant management was identified. A total of 36 women were recruited to the trial, with 17 women allocated to the induction of labour group and 19 women to the expectant management group. For primary outcomes, there were no statistically significant differences between elective induction of labour and expectant management with regard to all caesarean births (relative risk (RR) 0.56, 95% confidence interval (CI) 0.16 to 1.90), caesarean birth for fetal distress (RR 0.37, 95% CI 0.02 to 8.53), or perinatal death (RR not estimable). For secondary outcomes, there were no statistically significant differences between the two interventions with regard to haemorrhage requiring blood transfusion (RR 0.37, 95% CI 0.02 to 8.53), meconium stained liquor (RR 0.10, 95% CI 0.01 to 1.77), Apgar score of less than seven at five minutes (RR not estimable) and infant birth weight less than 2500 g (RR 0.95, 95% CI 0.49 to 1.82).

AUTHORS' CONCLUSIONS: The small trial identified was underpowered to detect the outcome measures of interest. Consequently, there are insufficient data available to support a practice of elective delivery from 37 weeks' gestation for women with an otherwise uncomplicated twin pregnancy at term.

PLANNED CAESAREAN SECTION FOR WOMEN WITH A TWIN
PREGNANCY: (Hofmeyr GJ, Barrett JF, Crowther CA) Protocol [see
page xviii] CD006553

ABRIDGED BACKGROUND: Infants from a twin pregnancy are at a higher risk of perinatal/neonatal mortality than infants from a singleton pregnancy. Some of this is due to a higher risk of preterm birth. However, even among twin babies that are greater than 2500 g at birth, there is a higher risk of death than among singletons of the same birthweight. Some of the higher risk of adverse perinatal outcome in twins compared with singletons may be due to restricted fetal growth which, in turn, may result in a higher risk of adverse events occurring during pregnancy, during labour or during birth. It is possible that some of these adverse outcomes may be avoided by an appropriately timed delivery by caesarean section (CS).

OBJECTIVES: To assess, from the best available evidence, the effects on mortality and morbidity for mother and baby of a policy of planned caesarean section versus planned vaginal birth for twin pregnancy.

CAESAREAN DELIVERY FOR THE SECOND TWIN: was not shown to be of benefit. (Crowther CA) CD000047

BACKGROUND: The optimal mode of birth for a second twin in breech position is controversial, with support for both caesarean and vaginal birth.

OBJECTIVES: To assess the effects of caesarean birth compared with vaginal birth of a second twin not presenting cephalically.

METHODS: Standard PCG methods (see page xvii). Search date: January 2007.

MAIN RESULTS: One trial involving 60 pairs of twins was included. Maternal febrile morbidity were increased in women allocated to the caesarean group (relative risk (RR) 3.67, 95% confidence interval (CI) 1.15–11.69), and there was a trend to an increased need for use of general anaesthesia (RR 2.40, 95% CI 0.98–5.88). No differences were detected in neonatal outcome.

AUTHOR'S CONCLUSIONS: Caesarean section for the birth of a second twin not presenting cephalically is associated with increased maternal febrile morbidity with, as yet, no identified improvement in neonatal outcome. This policy should not be adopted except within the context of further controlled trials.

5.5   Antepartum haemorrhage

Vaginal bleeding in the second half of pregnancy or during labour is called antepartum haemorrhage and can be life threatening for the woman and her baby. Pregnant women are advised to report any vaginal bleeding without delay. It is important to distinguish, usually by careful vaginal speculum examination, between bleeding from a local cause and that from inside the uterus.

Uterine bleeding may be due to attachment of the placenta to the lower segment of the uterus (placenta praevia), separation of a normally situated placenta (placental abruption), rupture of the uterus, or may be 'unexplained'.

Placental abruption or 'accidental' haemorrhage is particularly dangerous because much or all of the bleeding may be concealed in the uterus, stimulating hypertonic contractions lethal to the baby, generating a coagulopathy and leading to underestimation of the blood loss from the mother's circulation. Cardiotocography may exhibit a characteristic uterine contraction pattern with no relaxation phase between contractions, as well as giving an indication of the baby's condition.

The main risk of placenta praevia is rapid maternal blood loss, which may be provoked by digital vaginal examination.

> **INTERVENTIONS FOR SUSPECTED PLACENTA PRAEVIA:** not enough data to provide reliable evidence, particularly on home versus hospital care, and cervical cerclage. (Neilson JP) CD001998 (in RHL 11)

BACKGROUND: Because placenta praevia is implanted unusually low in the uterus, it may cause major, and/or repeated, antepartum haemorrhage. The traditional policy of care of women with symptomatic placenta praevia includes prolonged stay in hospital and delivery by caesarean section.
OBJECTIVES: To assess the impact of any clinical intervention applied specifically because of a perceived likelihood that a pregnant woman might have placenta praevia.
METHODS: Standard PCG methods (see page xvii). Search date: August 2002.

MAIN RESULTS: Three trials were included, involving a total of 114 women. Both tested interventions (home versus hospitalisation and cervical cerclage versus no cerclage) were associated with reduced lengths of stay in hospital antenatally: weighted mean difference (WMD) respectively −18.50 days (95% confidence interval (CI) −26.83 to −10.17), −4.80 days (95% CI −6.37 to −3.23). Otherwise, there was little evidence of any clear advantage or disadvantage to a policy of home versus hospital care. The one woman who had a haemorrhage severe enough to require immediate transfusion and delivery was in the home care group. Cervical cerclage may reduce the risk of delivery before 34 weeks (relative risk (RR) 0.45, 95% CI 0.23 to 0.87), or the birth of a baby weighing less than two kilograms (RR 0.34 95% CI 0.14 to 0.83) or having a low five minute Apgar score (RR 0.19 95% CI 0.04 to 1.00). In general, these possible benefits were more evident in the trial of lower methodological quality.

AUTHOR'S CONCLUSIONS: There are insufficient data from trials to recommend any change in clinical practice. Available data should, however, encourage further work to address the safety of more conservative policies of hospitalisation for women with suspected placenta praevia, and the possible value of insertion of a cervical suture.

INTERVENTIONS FOR TREATING PLACENTAL ABRUPTION: no randomised trials to provide reliable evidence. (Neilson JP) CD003247

BACKGROUND: Placental abruption is an important cause of maternal and fetal mortality and morbidity.

OBJECTIVES: To assess the effectiveness and safety of any intervention for the care of women and/or their babies following a diagnosis of placental abruption.

METHODS: Standard PCG methods (see page xvii). Search date: October 2002.

MAIN RESULTS: No studies that met the inclusion criteria were identified.

AUTHOR'S CONCLUSIONS: The clinical management of placental abruption has to rely on knowledge other than that obtained through randomised clinical trials.

5.6 Infection during pregnancy

Many infections have the propensity for harm to both the mother and the baby. Strategies used range from specific treatment of identified infections, to routine treatment of all pregnant women with antimicrobials.

PROPHYLACTIC ANTIBIOTIC ADMINISTRATION IN PREGNANCY TO PREVENT INFECTIOUS MORBIDITY AND MORTALITY: improved several perinatal outcomes; vaginal antibiotics appeared to increase neonatal sepsis. (Thinkhamrop J, Hofmeyr GJ, Adetoro O, Lumbiganon P) CD002250 (in RHL 11)

BACKGROUND: Some previous studies have suggested that prophylactic antibiotics given during pregnancy improved maternal and perinatal outcomes, some have shown no benefit and some have reported adverse effects.

OBJECTIVES: To determine the effect of prophylactic antibiotics during second and third trimester of pregnancy on maternal and perinatal outcomes.

METHODS: Standard PCG methods (see page xvii). Search date: January 2004.

MAIN RESULTS: The review included six randomized controlled trials which recruited 2184 women to detect the effect of prophylactic antibiotic administration on pregnancy outcomes in the second or third trimester. Antibiotic prophylaxis in unselected pregnant women reduced the risk of prelabour rupture of membranes (Peto odds ratio (OR) 0.32, 95% confidence interval (CI) 0.14 to 0.73). In women with a previous preterm birth there was a risk reduction in low birth weight (OR 0.48, 95% CI 0.27 to 0.84) and postpartum endometritis (OR 0.46, 95% CI 0.24 to 0.89). There was a risk reduction in preterm delivery (OR 0.48, 95% CI 0.28 to 0.81) in pregnant women with a previous preterm birth associated with bacterial vaginosis (BV) during the current pregnancy but there was no risk reduction in pregnant women with previous preterm birth without BV during pregnancy (OR 1.06, 95% CI 0.68 to 1.64). However, vaginal antibiotic prophylaxis during pregnancy did not prevent infectious pregnancy outcomes and there is a possibility of adverse effects such as neonatal sepsis (OR 8.07, 95% CI 1.36 to 47.77).

AUTHORS' CONCLUSIONS: Antibiotic prophylaxis given during the second or third trimester of pregnancy reduces the risk of prelabour rupture of membranes when given routinely to pregnant women. Beneficial effects on birth weight and the risk of postpartum endometritis were seen for high-risk women.

5.6.1   Genital tract infections

> **ANTIBIOTICS FOR GONORRHOEA IN PREGNANCY:** various antibiotics had similar effectiveness; not enough data to provide reliable evidence. (Brocklehurst P) CD000098 (in RHL 11)

BACKGROUND: Neisseria gonorrhoeae can be transmitted from the mother's genital tract to the newborn during birth and can cause gonococcal ophthalmia neonatorum as well as systemic neonatal infection. It can also cause endometritis and pelvic sepsis in the mother.

OBJECTIVES: To assess the effects of antibiotic regimens in the treatment of genital infection with gonorrhoea during pregnancy with respect to neonatal and maternal morbidity.

METHODS: Standard PCG methods (see page xvii). Search date: January 2007.

MAIN RESULTS: Two trials involving 346 women were included. The only outcome included in these trials was the incidence of 'cure' assessed by bacterial culture. Failure to achieve 'microbiological cure' was similar for each antibiotic regimen: amoxicillin plus probenecid compared with spectinomycin (Peto odds ratio (Peto OR) 2.29, 95% confidence interval (CI) 0.74 to 7.08), amoxicillin plus probenecid compared with ceftriaxone (Peto OR 2.29, 95% CI 0.74 to 7.08) and ceftriaxone compared with cefixime (Peto OR 1.22, 95% CI 0.16 to 9.01). Side-effects were uncommon for all the tested regimens.

AUTHOR'S CONCLUSIONS: The number of women included in each of the comparisons is small and therefore, although no differences were detected between the different antibiotic regimens, the trials were limited in their ability to detect important but modest differences. For women who are allergic to penicillin, this review provides some reassurance that treatment with ceftriaxone or spectinomycin appears to have similar effectiveness in producing microbiological cure.

ANTIBIOTICS FOR UREAPLASMA IN THE VAGINA IN PREGNANCY: not enough data to provide reliable evidence. (Raynes-Greenow CH, Roberts CL, Bell JC, Peat B, Gilbert GL) CD003767

BACKGROUND: Preterm birth is a significant obstetric problem in high-income countries. Genital infections including ureaplasmas are suspected of playing a role in preterm birth and preterm rupture of the membranes. Antibiotics are used to treat women with preterm prelabour rupture of the membranes, and results in prolongation of pregnancy and lowers the risks of maternal and neonatal infection. However, antibiotics may be beneficial earlier in pregnancy to eradicate potentially causative agents.

OBJECTIVES: To assess whether antibiotic treatment of pregnant women with ureaplasma in the vagina reduces the incidence of preterm birth and other adverse pregnancy outcomes.

METHODS: Standard PCG methods (see page xvii). Search date: April 2003.

MAIN RESULTS: One trial involving 1071 women was included. Of these, 644 randomly received antibiotic treatment (174 erythromycin estolate, 224 erythromycin sterate, and 246 clindamycin hydrochloride) and 427 received placebo. This trial did not report data on preterm birth. Incidence of low birthweight less than 2500 g was only evaluated for erythromycin (combined) (n = 398) compared to placebo (n = 427) and there was no statistically significant difference between those treated and those not treated (relative risk (RR) 0.70, 95% confidence interval (CI) 0.46 to 1.07). In regard to side-effects sufficient to stop treatment, data were available for all women, and there were no statistically significant differences between any antibiotic (combined) and the placebo group (RR 1.25, 95% CI 0.85 to 1.85).

AUTHORS' CONCLUSIONS: There is insufficient evidence to show whether giving antibiotics to women with ureaplasma in the vagina will prevent preterm birth.

INTERVENTIONS FOR TREATING GENITAL CHLAMYDIA TRACHOMATIS INFECTION IN PREGNANCY: amoxicillin, clindamycin and azithramycin were found to be acceptable alternatives to erythromycin. (Brocklehurst P, Rooney G) CD000054 (in RHL 11)

BACKGROUND: Chlamydia trachomatis is a sexually transmitted infection. Mother-to-child transmission can occur at the time of birth and may result in ophthalmia neonatorum or pneumonitis in the newborn.

OBJECTIVES: To assess the effects of antibiotics in the treatment of genital infection with Chlamydia trachomatis during pregnancy with respect to neonatal and maternal morbidity.

METHODS: Standard PCG methods (see page xvii). Search date: September 2006.

MAIN RESULTS: Eleven trials were included. Trial quality was generally good. Amoxicillin appeared to be as effective as erythromycin in achieving microbiological cure (odds ratio 0.54, 95% confidence interval 0.28 to 1.02). Amoxicillin was better tolerated than erythromycin (odds ratio 0.16, 95% confidence interval 0.09 to 0.30). Clindamycin and azithromycin also appear to be effective, although the numbers of women included in trials are small.

AUTHORS' CONCLUSIONS: Amoxicillin appears to be an acceptable alternative therapy for the treatment of genital chlamydial infections in pregnancy when compared with erythromycin. Clindamycin and azithromycin may be considered if erythromycin and amoxicillin are contra-indicated or not tolerated.

INTERVENTIONS FOR TRICHOMONIASIS IN PREGNANCY: metronidazole was effective in clearing trichomonas; in one trial, preterm birth was increased. (Gülmezoglu AM) CD000220 (in RHL 11)

BACKGROUND: Vaginitis due to Trichomonas vaginalis is one of the most common of sexually transmitted diseases. Trichomoniasis affects women during pregnancy as well but it is not clearly established whether it causes preterm birth and other pregnancy complications.

OBJECTIVES: To assess the effects of various treatments for trichomoniasis during pregnancy.

METHODS: Standard PCG methods (see page xvii). Search date: January 2004.

MAIN RESULTS: Two trials with 842 pregnant women were included. In both trials around 90% of women were cleared of trichomonas in the vagina after treatment. In the US trial women with asymptomatic trichomoniasis between 16 to 23 weeks were treated with metronidazole on two occasions at least two weeks apart. The trial was stopped before reaching its target recruitment because metronidazole was not effective in reducing preterm birth and there was a likelihood of harm (relative risk: 1.8; 95% confidence interval: 1.2 to 2.7). The South African trial recruited women later in pregnancy and did not have the design and power to address adverse clinical outcomes.

AUTHORS' CONCLUSIONS: Metronidazole, given as a single dose, is likely to provide parasitological cure for trichomoniasis, but it is not known whether this treatment will have any effect on pregnancy outcomes. The cure rate could probably be higher if more partners used the treatment.

THIRD TRIMESTER ANTIVIRAL PROPHYLAXIS FOR PREVENTING MATERNAL GENITAL HERPES SIMPLEX VIRUS (HSV) RECURRENCES AND NEONATAL INFECTION: reduced maternal infections, but no data on neonatal infections. (Hollier L, Wendel GD) CD00494

BACKGROUND: Genital herpes simplex virus (HSV) infection is one of the most common viral sexually transmitted infections. The majority of women with genital herpes will have a recurrence during pregnancy. Transmission of the virus from mother to fetus typically occurs by direct contact with virus in the genital tract during birth.

OBJECTIVES: To assess the effectiveness of antenatal antiviral prophylaxis for recurrent genital herpes on neonatal herpes and maternal recurrences at delivery.

METHODS: Standard PCG methods (see page xvii). Search date: January 2007.

MAIN RESULTS: Seven randomized controlled trials (1249 participants) which met our inclusion criteria compared acyclovir to placebo or no treatment (five trials) and valacyclovir to placebo (two trials). The effect of antepartum antiviral prophylaxis on neonatal herpes could not be estimated. There were no cases of symptomatic neonatal herpes in the included studies in either the treatment or placebo groups. Women who received antiviral prophylaxis were significantly less likely to have a recurrence of genital herpes at delivery (relative risk (RR) 0.28, 95% confidence interval (CI) 0.18 to 0.43, $I^2 = 0$%). Women who received antiviral prophylaxis were also significantly less likely to have a cesarean delivery for genital herpes (RR 0.30, 95% CI 0.20 to 0.45, $I^2 = 27.3$%). Women who received antiviral prophylaxis were significantly less likely to have HSV detected at delivery (RR 0.14, 95% CI 0.05 to 0.39, $I^2 = 0\%$).

AUTHORS' CONCLUSIONS: Women with recurrent genital herpes simplex virus should be informed that the risk of neonatal herpes is low. There is insufficient evidence to determine if antiviral prophylaxis reduces the incidence of neonatal herpes. Antenatal antiviral prophylaxis reduces viral shedding and recurrences at delivery and reduces the need for cesarean delivery for genital herpes. Limited information exists regarding the neonatal safety of prophylaxis. The risks, benefits, and alternatives to antenatal prophylaxis should be discussed with women who have a history and prophylaxis initiated for women who desire intervention.

☺ **INTRAPARTUM ANTIBIOTICS FOR GROUP B STREPTOCOCCAL COLONIZATION:** reduced neonatal infections. (Smaill F) CD000115

BACKGROUND: Group B streptococcal infection is common in pregnant women without causing harm. However it is also a significant cause of neonatal morbidity and mortality.

OBJECTIVES: To assess the effects of intrapartum administration of antibiotics to women on infant colonization with group B streptococcus, early onset neonatal group B streptococcus sepsis and neonatal death from infection.

METHODS: Standard PCG methods (see page xvii). Search date: 1999

MAIN RESULTS: Five trials were included. Overall quality was poor, with potential selection bias in all the identified studies. Intrapartum antibiotic treatment reduced the rate of infant colonization (odds ratio 0.10, 95% confidence interval 0.07 to 0.14) and early onset neonatal infection with group B streptococcus (odds ratio 0.17, 95% confidence interval 0.07 to 0.39). A difference in neonatal mortality was not seen (odds ratio 0.12, 95% confidence interval 0.01 to 2.00).

AUTHOR'S CONCLUSIONS: Intrapartum antibiotic treatment of women colonized with group B streptococcus appears to reduce neonatal infection. Effective strategies to detect maternal colonization with group B streptococcus and better data on maternal risk factors for neonatal group B streptococcus infection in different populations are required.

> **TOPICAL TREATMENT FOR VAGINAL CANDIDIASIS (THRUSH) IN PREGNANCY:** a seven-day course of topical imidazole appeared most beneficial. (Young GL, Jewell D) CD000225

BACKGROUND: Vaginal candidiasis (moniliasis or thrush) is a common and frequently distressing infection for many women. It is even more common in pregnancy. There is no evidence that thrush in pregnancy is harmful to the baby.

OBJECTIVES: To assess the effects of different methods of treating vaginal candidiasis in pregnancy.

METHODS: Standard PCG methods (see page xvii). Search date: March 2001.

MAIN RESULTS: 10 trials were included. Based on five trials, imidazole drugs were more effective than nystatin when treating vaginal candidiasis in pregnancy (odds ratio 0.21, 95% confidence interval 0.16 to 0.29). In turn, nystatin was as effective as hydrargaphen in one trial (odds ratio 0.29, 95% confidence interval 0.05–1.84). A trial of clotrimazole was more effective than placebo (odds ratio 0.14, 95% confidence interval 0.06 to 0.31). Single dose treatment was no more or less effective than three or four days treatment. However, two trials involving 81 women showed that treatment lasting for four days was less effective than treatment for seven days' (odds ratio 11.7, 95% confidence interval 4.21 to 29.15). Based on two trials, treatment for seven days was no more or less effective than treatment for 14 days (odds ratio 0.41, 95% confidence interval 0.16 to 1.05). Terconazole was as effective as clotrimazole (odds ratio 1.41, 95% confidence interval 0.28–7.10).

AUTHORS' CONCLUSIONS: Topical imidazole appears to be more effective than nystatin for treating symptomatic vaginal candidiasis in pregnancy. Treatments for seven days may be necessary in pregnancy rather than the shorter courses more commonly used in non-pregnant women.

> **VAGINAL CHLORHEXIDINE DURING LABOUR TO PREVENT EARLY-ONSET NEONATAL GROUP B STREPTOCOCCAL INFECTION:** reduced colonization but not disease; trial quality was poor. (Stade B, Shah V, Ohlsson A) CD003520 (in RHL 11)

BACKGROUND: Early-onset group B β -haemolytic streptococcus (GBS) infection accounts for approximately 30% of neonatal infections, has a high mortality rate and is acquired through vertical transmission from colonized mothers. Several trials have demonstrated the efficacy of intrapartum chemoprophylaxis (IPC) for preventing early-onset disease (EOD). Vaginal disinfection with chlorhexidine during labour has been proposed as another strategy for preventing GBS EOD in the preterm and term neonate. Chlorhexidine has been found to have no impact on antibiotic resistance, is inexpensive and is applicable to poorly equipped delivery sites.

OBJECTIVES: To determine the effectiveness of vaginal disinfection with chlorhexidine during labour for preventing early-onset GBS infection in preterm and term neonates.

METHODS: Standard PCG methods (see page xvii). Search date: September 2007

MAIN RESULTS: We identified no new trials eligible for inclusion in our update of this review. Five studies, including approximately 2190 term and preterm infants, met the inclusion criteria and reported on at least one of the outcomes of interest for this systematic review. When all studies were combined, there was a statistically significant (P = 0.005) reduction in colonization (typical RR 0.72; 95% CI 0.56 to 0.91; typical RD −0.16; 95% CI −0.26 to −0.05; NNT 6; 95% CI 4 to 20). There was no statistically significant between-study heterogeneity both for RR (chi² = 3.21 (P = 0.2), I² = 37.8%) and for RD (chi² = 1.66 (P = 0.44), I² = 0%). There was no statistically significant reduction in EOD including GBS sepsis, GBS pneumonia, GBS meningitis or mortality.

AUTHOR'S CONCLUSIONS: Vaginal chlorhexidine resulted in a statistically significant reduction in GBS colonization of neonates, but was not associated with reductions in other outcomes. The review currently does not support the use of vaginal disinfection with chlorhexidine in labour for preventing EOD. Results should be interpreted with caution as the methodological quality of the studies was poor.

VAGINAL CHLORHEXIDINE DURING LABOUR FOR PREVENTING MATERNAL AND NEONATAL INFECTIONS (EXCLUDING GROUP B STREPTOCOCCAL AND HIV): did not reduce perinatal infections.
(Lumbiganon P, Thinkhamrop J, Thinkhamrop B, Tolosa JE) CD004070

BACKGROUND: The incidence of chlorioamnionitis occurs in between eight and 12 women for every 1000 live births and 96% of the cases of chlorioamnionitis are due to ascending infection. Following spontaneous vaginal delivery, 1% to 4% of women develop postpartum endometritis. The incidence of neonatal sepsis is 0.5% to 1% of all infants born. Maternal vaginal bacteria are the main agents for these infections. It is reasonable to speculate that prevention of maternal and neonatal infections might be possible by washing the vagina and cervix with an antibacterial agent for all women during labour. Chlorhexidine belongs to the class of compounds known as the bis-biguanides. Chlorhexidine has antibacterial action against a wide range of aerobic and anaerobic bacteria, including those implicated in peripartal infections.

OBJECTIVES: To evaluate the effectiveness and side-effects of chlorhexidine vaginal douching during labour in reducing maternal and neonatal infections (excluding Group B Streptococcal and HIV).

METHODS: Standard PCG methods (see page xvii). Search date: April 2006.

MAIN RESULTS: Three studies (3012 participants) were included. There was no evidence of an effect of vaginal chlorhexidine during labour in preventing maternal and neonatal infections. Although the data suggest a trend in reducing postpartum endometritis, the difference was not statistically significant (relative risk 0.83; 95% confidence interval 0.61 to 1.13).

AUTHORS' CONCLUSIONS: There is no evidence to support the use of vaginal chlorhexidine during labour in preventing maternal and neonatal infections. There is a need for a well-designed randomized controlled trial using appropriate concentration and volume of vaginal chlorhexidine irrigation solution and with adequate sample size.

5.6.2 Urinary tract infection

Cystitis and acute pyelonephritis have characteristic symptoms. Empirical treatment is often started while awaiting the results of urine culture and sensitivity testing.

Routine screening for and treatment of asymptomatic bacteriuria has been recommended because of an association of the condition with preterm birth.

ANTIBIOTICS FOR ASYMPTOMATIC BACTERIURIA IN PREGNANCY:
cleared bacteria; reduced pyelonephritis; reduced low birthweight; but poor quality trials. (Smaill F, Vazquez JC) CD000490 (in RHL 11)

BACKGROUND: Asymptomatic bacteriuria occurs in 2% to 10% of pregnancies and, if not treated, up to 30% of mothers will develop acute pyelonephritis. Asymptomatic bacteriuria has been associated with low birthweight and preterm delivery.

OBJECTIVES: To assess the effect of antibiotic treatment for asymptomatic bacteriuria on persistent bacteriuria during pregnancy, the development of pyelonephritis and the risk of low birthweight and preterm delivery.

METHODS: Standard PCG methods (see page xvii). Search date: January 2007).

MAIN RESULTS: Fourteen studies were included. Overall the study quality was poor. Antibiotic treatment compared to placebo or no treatment was effective in clearing asymptomatic bacteriuria (risk ratio (RR) 0.25, 95% confidence interval (CI) 0.14 to 0.48). The incidence of pyelonephritis was reduced (RR 0.23, 95% CI 0.13 to 0.41). Antibiotic treatment was also associated with a reduction in the incidence of low birthweight babies (RR 0.66, 95% CI 0.49 to 0.89) but a difference in preterm delivery was not seen.

AUTHORS' CONCLUSIONS: Antibiotic treatment is effective in reducing the risk of pyelonephritis in pregnancy. A reduction in low birthweight is consistent with current theories about the role of infection in adverse pregnancy outcomes, but this association should be interpreted with caution given the poor quality of the included studies.

DURATION OF TREATMENT FOR ASYMPTOMATIC BACTERIURIA DURING PREGNANCY: not enough data to provide reliable evidence. (Villar J, Widmer M, Lydon-Rochelle MT, Gülmezoglu AM, Roganti A) CD000491

BACKGROUND: A Cochrane systematic review has shown that drug treatment of asymptomatic bacteriuria in pregnant women substantially decreases the risk of pyelonephritis and reduces the risk of preterm delivery. However, it is not clear whether single dose therapy is as effective as longer conventional antibiotic treatment.

OBJECTIVES: To assess the effects of different durations of treatment for asymptomatic bacteriuria in pregnancy.

METHODS: Standard PCG methods (see page xvii). Search date: July 2006.

MAIN RESULTS: 10 studies involving over 568 women were included. All were comparisons of single dose treatment with four to seven day treatments. The trials were generally of limited quality. The 'no cure rate' for asymptomatic bacteriuria in pregnant women was higher for one-day treatment than for seven-day treatment (relative risk (RR) 1.25, 95% confidence interval (CI) 0.93 to 1.67) although this difference was non-statistically significant. These results showed significant heterogeneity (P = 0.006). There was almost no difference in the recurrence of asymptomatic bacteriuria rate between both treatments (RR 1.14, 95% CI 0.77 to 1.67). No differences were detected for preterm births and pyelonephritis although sample size of trials was not appropriate. Single dose treatment was associated with a decrease in reports of 'any side-effects' (nausea, vomiting, diarrhoea) (RR 0.52, 95% CI 0.32 to 0.85).

AUTHORS' CONCLUSIONS: There is not enough evidence to evaluate whether single dose or longer duration doses are equivalent in treating asymptomatic bacteriuria in pregnant women. Because single dose treatment has lower cost and increased compliance, this comparison should be explored in a properly sized randomized controlled trial. WHO is currently conducting such a trial and the results will be available at the end of 2005.

TREATMENTS FOR SYMPTOMATIC URINARY TRACT INFECTIONS DURING PREGNANCY: antibiotics were all effective; not enough data to provide reliable evidence regarding relative effectiveness. (Vazquez JC, Villar J) CD002256

BACKGROUND: Urinary tract infections, including pyelonephritis, are serious complications that may lead to significant maternal and neonatal morbidity and mortality. There are a large number of drugs, and combinations of them, available to treat urinary tract infections, most of them tested in non-pregnant women. Attempting to define the optimal antibiotic regimen for pregnancy has, therefore, been problematic.

OBJECTIVES: To try to determine, from the best available evidence from randomized control trials, which agent is the most effective for the treatment of symptomatic urinary tract infections during pregnancy in terms of cure rates, recurrent infection, incidence of preterm delivery and premature rupture of membranes, admission to neonatal intensive care unit, need for change of antibiotic and incidence of prolonged pyrexia.

METHODS: Standard PCG methods (see page xvii). Search date: January 2006.

MAIN RESULTS: Nine studies were included, recruiting a total of 997 pregnant women. In most of the comparisons there were no significant differences between the treatments under study with regard to cure rates, recurrent infection, incidence of preterm delivery, admission to neonatal intensive care unit, need for change of antibiotic and incidence of prolonged pyrexia. Only when cefuroxime and cephradine were compared were there better cure rates (29/49 versus 41/52) and fewer recurrences (20/49 versus 11/52) in the cefuroxime group, but the sample size is insufficient to ensure that differences found in the effect of the drugs were real.

AUTHORS' CONCLUSIONS: Although antibiotic treatment is effective for the cure of urinary tract infections, there are insufficient data to recommend any specific treatment regimen for symptomatic urinary tract infections during pregnancy. All the antibiotics studied were shown to be very effective in decreasing the incidence of the different outcomes. Complications were very rare. All included trials had very small sample sizes to reliably detect important differences between treatments. Future studies should evaluate the most promising antibiotics, in terms of class, timing, dose, acceptability, maternal and neonatal outcomes and costs.

5.6.3   Other infections

ANTIBIOTIC REGIMENS FOR MANAGEMENT OF INTRAAMNI-OTIC INFECTION: not enough data to provide reliable evidence. (Hopkins L, Smaill F) CD003254 (in RHL 11)

BACKGROUND: Intraamniotic infection is associated with maternal morbidity and neonatal sepsis, pneumonia and death. Although antibiotic treatment is accepted as the standard of care, few studies have been conducted to examine the effectiveness of different antibiotic regimens for this infection and whether to administer antibiotics intrapartum or postpartum.

OBJECTIVES: To study the effects of different maternal antibiotic regimens for intraamniotic infection on maternal and perinatal morbidity and mortality.

METHODS: Standard PCG methods (see page xvii). Search date: May 2002.

The primary outcome was perinatal morbidity.

MAIN RESULTS: Two eligible trials (181 women) were included in this review. No trials were identified that compared antibiotic treatment with no treatment. Intrapartum treatment with antibiotics for intraamniotic infection was associated with a reduction in neonatal sepsis (relative risk (RR) 0.08; 95% confidence interval (CI) 0.00, 1.44) and pneumonia (RR 0.15; CI 0.01, 2.92) compared with treatment given immediately postpartum, but these results did not reach statistical significance (number of women studied = 45). There was no difference in the incidence of maternal bacteraemia (RR 2.19; CI 0.25, 19.48). There was no difference in the outcomes of neonatal sepsis (RR 2.16; CI 0.20, 23.21) or neonatal death (RR 0.72; CI 0.12, 4.16) between a regimen with and without anaerobic activity (number of women studied = 133). There was a trend towards a decrease in the incidence of postpartum endometritis in women who received treatment with ampicillin, gentamicin and clindamycin compared with ampicillin and gentamicin alone, but this did not reach statistical significance (RR 0.54; CI 0.19–1.49).

AUTHORS' CONCLUSIONS: The conclusions that can be drawn from this meta-analysis are limited due to the small number of studies. For none of the outcomes was a statistically significant difference seen between the different interventions. Current consensus is for the intrapartum administration of antibiotics when the diagnosis of intraamniotic infection is made; however, the results of this review neither support nor refute this although there was a trend towards improved neonatal outcomes when antibiotics were administered intrapartum. No recommendations can be made on the most appropriate antimicrobial regimen to choose to treat intraamniotic infection.

ANTIBIOTICS FOR SYPHILIS DIAGNOSED DURING PREGNANCY: not enough data to provide reliable evidence on optimal treatment regimens. (Walker GJA) CD001143 (in RHL 11)

BACKGROUND: Congenital syphilis is an increasing problem in many developing countries and in the transitional economies of Eastern Europe and the former Soviet Union. In several countries this increase has been aggravated by HIV/AIDS. While the effectiveness of penicillin in the treatment of syphilis in pregnant women and the prevention of congenital syphilis was established shortly after the introduction of penicillin in the 1940s, there is uncertainty about the optimal treatment regimens.

OBJECTIVES: To identify the most effective antibiotic treatment regimen (in terms of dose, length of course and mode of administration) of syphilis with and without concomitant infection with HIV for pregnant women infected with syphilis.

METHODS: Standard PCG methods (see page xvii). Search date: March 2006.

MAIN RESULTS: 29 studies met the criteria for detailed scrutiny. However, none of these met the pre-determined criteria for comparative groups and none included comparisons between randomly allocated groups of pregnant women.

AUTHOR'S CONCLUSIONS: While there is no doubt that penicillin is effective in the treatment of syphilis in pregnancy and the prevention of congenital syphilis, uncertainty remains about what are the optimal treatment regimens.

Further studies are needed to evaluate treatment failure cases with currently recommended regimens and this should include an assessment of the role of HIV infection in cases of prenatal syphilis treatment failure. The effectiveness of various antibiotic regimens for the treatment of primary and secondary syphilis in pregnant women needs to be assessed using randomised controlled trials which compare them with existing recommendations. This should include treatment with oral antibiotics which could be particularly relevant in resource-poor countries where the availability of safe needles and syringes cannot be guaranteed.

BACKGROUND: Observational studies have generally not provided evidence that delivery by caesarean section reduces perinatal hepatitis C virus (HCV) transmission. However, these studies have methodological weaknesses with potential for bias and their findings should be interpreted with caution.

OBJECTIVES: To assess the evidence from randomised controlled trials that a policy of delivery by planned caesarean section versus vaginal delivery reduces mother to infant HCV transmission.

METHODS: Standard PCG methods (see page xvii). Search date: October 2007.

MAIN RESULTS: We did not identify any randomised controlled trials.

AUTHORS' CONCLUSIONS: Currently, there is no evidence from randomised controlled trials upon which to base any practice recommendations regarding planned caesarean section versus vaginal delivery for preventing mother to infant hepatitis C virus transmission. In the absence of trial data, evidence to inform women and carers is only available from observational studies that are subject to biases. Systematic review of these studies is needed. There is a need to determine whether women and healthcare providers would support a large pragmatic randomised controlled trial to provide evidence regarding the benefits and harms of planned elective caesarean section versus planned vaginal birth for women with HCV infection.

BACKGROUND: Each year at least one million children worldwide die of pneumococcal infections. The development of bacterial resistance to antimicrobials adds to the difficulty of treatment of diseases and emphasizes the need for a preventive approach. Newborn vaccination schedules could substantially reduce the impact of pneumococcal disease in immunized children, but does not have an effect on the morbidity and mortality of infants less than three months of age. Pneumococcal vaccination during pregnancy may be a way of preventing pneumococcal disease during the first months of life before the pneumococcal vaccine administered to the infant starts to produce protection.

OBJECTIVES: To assess the effect of pneumococcal vaccination during pregnancy for preventing infant infection.

METHODS: Standard PCG methods (see page xvii). Search date: June 2004.

MAIN RESULTS: Three trials (280 participants) were included. There was no evidence that pneumococcal vaccination during pregnancy reduces the risk of neonatal infection (one trial, 149 pregnancies, relative risk (RR) 0.51; 95% confidence interval (CI) 0.18 to 1.41). Although the data suggest an effect in reducing pneumococcal colonization in infants by 16 months of age (one trial, 56 pregnancies, RR 0.33; 95% CI 0.11 to 0.98), there was no evidence of this effect in infants at two months of age (RR 0.28; 95% CI 0.02 to 5.11) or by seven months of age (RR 0.32; 95% CI 0.08 to 1.29).

AUTHORS' CONCLUSIONS: There is insufficient evidence to support whether pneumococcal vaccination during pregnancy could reduce infant infections.

PRENATAL EDUCATION FOR CONGENITAL TOXOPLASMOSIS: (Di Mario S, Basevi V, Gagliotti C, Spettoli D, Gori G, D'Amico R, Magrini N) Protocol [see page xviii] CD006171

ABRIDGED BACKGROUND: Congenital toxoplasmosis is a rare but potentially severe parasitic infection that can lead to intrauterine death or stillbirth, malformation, mental retardation, deafness and blindness of the infected infant. It is caused by Toxoplasma gondii (T. gondii). The susceptibility of pregnant women (that is the rate of seronegative pregnant women) to toxoplasmosis varies between countries. When infection does occur during pregnancy, T. gondii can be transmitted from the mother to the fetus (vertical transmission) and can lead to congenital toxoplasmosis. Primary prevention can involve the whole population, by educating the general public and filtering water, and veterinary public health intervention. Another possibility is primary prevention based on prenatal education of pregnant women or women of reproductive age to avoid toxoplasmosis in pregnancy.

OBJECTIVES: The primary objectives of this review are to assess the efficacy of prenatal education to reduce the rate of:

(1) new cases of congenital toxoplasmosis;
(2) toxoplasmosis seroconversion during pregnancy.

Secondary objectives are to assess the efficacy of prenatal education to increase the rate of:

(1) pregnant women's knowledge on risk factors for acquiring toxoplasmosis infection;
(2) pregnant women's awareness of the importance to avoid toxoplasmosis infection during pregnancy;
(3) pregnant women's behavior with respect to avoidance of risk factors for toxoplasmosis infection during pregnancy.

TREATMENTS FOR TOXOPLASMOSIS IN PREGNANCY: not enough data to provide reliable evidence. (Peyron F, Wallon M, Liou C, Garner P) CD001684

BACKGROUND: Toxoplasmosis is a widespread parasitic disease and usually causes no symptoms. However, infection of pregnant women may cause congenital infection, resulting potentially in mental retardation and blindness in the infant.

OBJECTIVES: The objective of this review was to assess whether or not treating toxoplasmosis in pregnancy reduces the risk of congenital toxoplasma infection.

METHODS: Standard PCG methods (see page xvii). Search date: February 2006.

We also inspected relevant reports of less robust experimental studies in which there were (non-randomly allocated) control groups, although it was not planned to include such data in the primary analysis.

MAIN RESULTS: Out of the 3332 papers identified, none met the inclusion criteria.

AUTHORS' CONCLUSIONS: Despite the large number of studies performed over the last three decades we still do not know whether

antenatal treatment in women with presumed toxoplasmosis reduces the congenital transmission of Toxoplasma gondii. Screening is expensive, so we need to evaluate the effects of treatment, and the impact of screening programmes. In countries where screening or treatment is not routine, these technologies should not be introduced outside the context of a carefully controlled trial.

☺ **VACCINES FOR WOMEN TO PREVENT NEONATAL TETANUS:** reduced neonatal deaths. (Demicheli V, Barale A, Rivetti A) CD002959

BACKGROUND: Tetanus is an acute, often fatal, disease caused by an exotoxin produced by Clostridium tetani. It occurs in newborn infants born to mothers who do not have sufficient circulating antibodies to protect the infant passively, by transplacental transfer. Prevention may be possible by the vaccination of pregnant or non-pregnant women, or both, with tetanus toxoid, and the provision of clean delivery services. Tetanus toxoid consists of a formaldehyde-treated toxin which stimulates the production of antitoxin.

OBJECTIVES: To assess the effectiveness of tetanus toxoid, administered to women of childbearing age or pregnant women, to prevent cases of, and deaths from, neonatal tetanus.

METHODS: Standard PCG methods (see page xvii). Search date: July 2007.

MAIN RESULTS: Two trials (10 560 infants) were included. One study (1919 infants) assessed the effectiveness of tetanus toxoid in preventing neonatal tetanus deaths. After a single dose, the relative risk (RR) was 0.57 (95% confidence interval (CI) 0.26 to 1.24), and the vaccine effectiveness was 43%. With a two or three dose course, the RR was 0.02 (95% CI 0.00 to 0.30); vaccine effectiveness was 98%. No effect was detected on causes of death other than tetanus. The RR of cases of neonatal tetanus after at least one dose of tetanus toxoid was 0.20 (95% CI 0.10 to 0.40); vaccine effectiveness was 80%. Another study, involving 8641 children, assessed the effectiveness of tetanus–diptheria toxoid in preventing neonatal mortality after one or two doses. The RR was 0.68 (95% CI 0.56 to 0.82); vaccine effectiveness was 32%. In preventing deaths at 4 to 14 days, the RR was 0.38 (95% CI 0.27 to 0.55), and vaccine effectiveness was 62% (95% CI 45% to 73%).

AUTHORS' CONCLUSIONS: Available evidence supports the implementation of immunisation practices on women of childbearing age or pregnant women in communities with similar, or higher, levels of risk of neonatal tetanus to the two study sites. More information is needed on possible interference of vaccination by malaria chemoprophylaxis on the roles of malnutrition and vitamin A deficiency, and on the quality of tetanus toxoid production and storage.

EFFECTS OF INTERVENTIONS FOR HELMINTHIC INFECTIONS IN PREGNANCY: (Haider BA, Bhutta ZA) Protocol [see page xviii] CD005547

ABRIDGED BACKGROUND: Helminthiasis is infestation of the human body with parasitic worms.

Intestinal helminths contribute to anaemia as they feed on blood and cause further haemorrhage by releasing anticoagulant compounds, thereby leading to iron deficiency anaemia. Globally, an estimated 44 million pregnancies are complicated by maternal hookworm infection alone, posing a serious threat to the health of mothers and fetuses. *Trichuris trichura* also causes intestinal blood loss, although much less so than hookworms on a per-worm basis. *Ascaris lumbricoides* interferes with the utilization of vitamin A, which is required for haematopoiesis.

Antihelminthic treatment is regarded as the most effective means of controlling mortality and morbidity due to intestinal helminth infections.

OBJECTIVES: To determine the effects of prophylactic administration of antihelminthics during the second or third trimester of pregnancy on maternal anaemia and pregnancy outcomes.

CHAPTER 6: INDUCTION OF LABOUR

Spontaneous labour, though sometimes inconvenient, has many advantages. Labour induction is considered when the benefits of earlier birth outweigh the risks of labour induction, taking into account the condition ('inducibility') of the mother's uterine cervix. One of the most common reasons for labour induction is prolonged pregnancy (see page 144).

6.1 Specific indications for labour induction

> ☺ **PLANNED EARLY BIRTH VERSUS EXPECTANT MANAGEMENT (WAITING) FOR PRELABOUR RUPTURE OF MEMBRANES AT TERM (37 WEEKS OR MORE):** reduced maternal infections and neonatal ICU admissions. (Dare MR, Middleton P, Crowther CA, Flenady VJ, Varatharaju B) CD005302 (in RHL 11)

BACKGROUND: Prelabour rupture of membranes at term is managed expectantly or by elective birth, but it is not clear if waiting for birth to occur spontaneously is better than intervening.

OBJECTIVES: To assess the effects of planned early birth versus expectant management for women with term prelabour rupture of membranes on fetal, infant and maternal wellbeing.

METHODS: Standard PCG methods (see page xvii). Search date: November 2004.

MAIN RESULTS: 12 trials (total of 6814 women) were included. Planned management was generally induction with oxytocin or prostaglandin, with one trial using homoeopathic caulophyllum. Overall, no differences were detected for mode of birth between planned and expectant groups: relative risk (RR) of caesarean section 0.94, 95% confidence interval (CI) 0.82 to 1.08 (12 trials, 6814 women); RR of operative vaginal birth 0.98, 95% 0.84 to 1.16 (seven trials, 5511 women). Significantly fewer women in the

A Cochrane Pocketbook: Pregnancy and Childbirth   G.J. Hofmeyr et al.
Copyright © 2008, Z. Alfiervic, C. A. Crowther, L. Duley, A. M. Gulmezoglu, G. ML. Gyte , E. D. Hodnett, G. J. Hofmeyr, J. P. Neilson

planned compared with expectant management groups had chorioamnionitis (RR 0.74, 95% CI 0.56 to 0.97; nine trials, 6611 women) or endometritis (RR 0.30, 95% CI 0.12 to 0.74; four trials, 445 women). No difference was seen for neonatal infection (RR 0.83, 95% CI 0.61 to 1.12; nine trials, 6406 infants). However, fewer infants under planned management went to neonatal intensive or special care compared with expectant management (RR 0.72, 95% CI 0.57 to 0.92, number needed to treat 20; five trials, 5679 infants). In a single trial, significantly more women with planned management viewed their care more positively than those expectantly managed (RR of 'nothing liked' 0.45, 95% CI 0.37 to 0.54; 5031 women).

AUTHORS' CONCLUSIONS: Planned management (with methods such as oxytocin or prostaglandin) reduces the risk of some maternal infectious morbidity without increasing caesarean sections and operative vaginal births. Fewer infants went to neonatal intensive care under planned management although no differences were seen in neonatal infection rates. Since planned and expectant management may not be very different, women need to have appropriate information to make informed choices.

PLANNED EARLY BIRTH VERSUS EXPECTANT MANAGEMENT FOR WOMEN WITH PRETERM PRELABOUR RUPTURE OF MEMBRANES AT 34 TO 37 WEEKS' GESTATION FOR IMPROVING PREGNANCY OUTCOME: (Buchanan SL, Crowther CA, Morris J) Protocol [see page xviii] CD004735

ABRIDGED BACKGROUND: Preterm prelabour rupture of the membranes (PPROM) occurs when there is rupture of the membranes prior to term and prior to the onset of labour. The clinician has to consider the potential risks and benefits of induction of labour against expectant management until term or complications arise which necessitate delivery.

OBJECTIVES: To assess the effect of planned early birth versus expectant management for women with preterm prelabour rupture of the membranes between 34 and 37 weeks' gestation for fetal, infant and maternal wellbeing.

MISOPROSTOL FOR INDUCTION OF LABOUR TO TERMINATE PREGNANCY IN THE SECOND OR THIRD TRIMESTER FOR WOMEN WITH A FETAL ANOMALY OR AFTER INTRAUTERINE FETAL DEATH: (Dodd JM, Crowther CA) Protocol [see page xviii] CD004901

ABRIDGED BACKGROUND: A woman may need to give birth prior to the spontaneous onset of labour in situations where the fetus has died in-utero (also called a stillbirth), or for the termination of pregnancy where the fetus, if born alive, would not survive or would have permanent handicap. When a baby dies before birth, the options for care are either to wait for labour to start spontaneously or to induce labour. Inducing labour may involve the use of the hormone oxytocin which causes the uterus to contract. Prostaglandins have been used as an alternative to oxytocin and are particularly useful where a woman's cervix is unfavourable or not ready to commence labour.

Misoprostol is a synthetic prostaglandin that is structurally related to prostaglandin E1 (PGE1).

OBJECTIVES: To compare, using the best available evidence, the benefits and harms of misoprostol to induce labour to terminate pregnancy in the second and third trimester for women with a fetal anomaly or after intrauterine fetal death when compared with other methods of induction of labour.

> ☺ **ELECTIVE DELIVERY IN DIABETIC PREGNANT WOMEN:** reduced macrosomia (large babies). (Boulvain M, Stan C, Irion O) CD001997

BACKGROUND: In pregnancies complicated by diabetes the major concerns during the third trimester are fetal distress and the potential for birth trauma associated with fetal macrosomia.

OBJECTIVES: To assess the effect of a policy of elective delivery, as compared to expectant management, in term diabetic pregnant women on maternal and perinatal mortality and morbidity.

METHODS: Standard PCG methods (see page xvii). Search date: July 2004.

MAIN RESULTS: The participants in the one trial included in this review were 200 insulin-requiring diabetic women. Most had gestational diabetes, except 13 women with type 2 pre-existing diabetes (class B). The trial compared a policy of active induction of labour at 38 completed weeks of pregnancy to expectant management until 42 weeks. The risk of caesarean section was not statistically different between groups (relative risk (RR) 0.81, 95% confidence interval (CI) 0.52–1.26). The risk of macrosomia was reduced in the active induction group (RR 0.56, 95% CI 0.32–0.98) and three cases of mild shoulder dystocia were reported in the expectant management group. No other perinatal morbidity was reported.

AUTHORS' CONCLUSIONS: The results of the single randomized controlled trial comparing elective delivery with expectant management at term in pregnant women with insulin-requiring diabetes show that induction of labour reduces the risk of macrosomia. The risk of maternal or neonatal morbidity was not different between groups, but, given the rarity of maternal and neonatal morbidity, the number of women included does not permit firm conclusions to be drawn. Women's views on elective delivery and on prolonged surveillance and treatment with insulin should be assessed in future trials.

See also: Elective delivery of women with a twin pregnancy from 37 weeks' gestation (page 195)

INDUCTION OF LABOUR FOR SUSPECTED FETAL MACROSOMIA: not enough data to provide reliable evidence. (Irion O, Boulvain M) CD000938

BACKGROUND: Women with a suspected macrosomic fetus are at risk of difficult operative delivery or caesarean section. Neonatal trauma may complicate the delivery. Induction of labour may reduce these risks by limiting the fetal growth and, therefore, decrease the birthweight. However, this intervention per se may be associated with an increased risk of caesarean section.

OBJECTIVES: To assess the effects of a policy of labour induction for suspected fetal macrosomia on method of delivery and maternal or perinatal morbidity.

METHODS: Standard PCG methods (see page xvii). Search date: September 2007.

MAIN RESULTS: We included three trials, involving 372 women. Compared to expectant management, induction of labour for suspected macrosomia has not been shown to reduce the risk of caesarean section (relative risk (RR) 0.96, 95% confidence interval (CI) 0.67 to 1.38) or instrumental delivery (RR 1.02, 95% CI 0.60 to 1.74). Perinatal morbidity was not statistically different between groups (shoulder dystocia: RR 1.06, 95% CI 0.44 to 2.56); one trial reported, however, two cases of brachial plexus injury and four cases of fracture in the expectant management group.

AUTHORS' CONCLUSIONS: Induction of labour for suspected fetal macrosomia in non-diabetic women has not been shown to alter the risk of maternal or neonatal morbidity, but the power of the included studies to show a difference in rare events is limited. Larger trials are needed to address this question.

> **ELECTIVE REPEAT CAESAREAN SECTION VERSUS INDUCTION OF LABOUR FOR WOMEN WITH A PREVIOUS CAESAREAN BIRTH:** no randomised trials to provide reliable evidence. (Dodd JM, Crowther CA) CD004906

BACKGROUND: When a woman has had a previous caesarean birth and requires induction of labour in a subsequent pregnancy, there are two options for her care: elective repeat caesarean or planned induction of labour. While there are risks and benefits for both elective repeat caesarean birth and planned induction of labour, current sources of information are limited to non-randomised cohort studies. Studies designed in this way have significant potential for bias and consequently conclusions based on these results are limited in their reliability and should be interpreted with caution.

OBJECTIVES: To assess, using the best available evidence, the benefits and harms of elective repeat caesarean section and planned induction of labour for women with a previous caesarean birth.

METHODS: Standard PCG methods (see page xvii). Search date: January 2006.

MAIN RESULTS: There were no randomised controlled trials identified.

AUTHORS' CONCLUSIONS: Planned elective repeat caesarean section and planned induction of labour for women with a prior caesarean birth are both associated with benefits and harms. Evidence for these care practices is drawn from non-randomised studies, associated with potential bias. Any results and conclusions must therefore be interpreted with caution. Randomised controlled trials are required to provide the most reliable evidence regarding the benefits and harms of both planned elective repeat caesarean section and planned induction of labour for women with a previous caesarean birth.

6.2   Techniques of labour induction – primary reviews

Once the decision has been taken to induce labour, the most appropriate method is required. The method chosen may be influenced by the clinical situation. For example, for an uncomplicated pregnancy with unfavourable cervix, a prostaglandin may be chosen. However, if there is concern about the baby's wellbeing, such as growth impairment, or there has been a previous caesarean section, a mechanical method which minimises the risk of uterine hyperstimulation may be chosen.

This series of reviews of methods of cervical ripening and labour induction used standardised methodology following a generic protocol. A strategy was developed to deal with the large volume and complexity of trial data relating to labour induction. This involved a two-stage method of data extraction. The initial data extraction was done centrally, and incorporated into the series of primary reviews arranged by methods of induction of labour. The data from the primary reviews will be incorporated into a series of secondary reviews, arranged by category of woman to reflect clinical scenarios. To avoid duplication of data in the primary reviews, the labour induction methods have been listed in a specific order, from one to 27. Each primary review includes comparisons between one of the methods (from two to 27) with only those methods above it on the list.

METHODS FOR CERVICAL RIPENING AND LABOUR INDUCTION IN LATE PREGNANCY: GENERIC PROTOCOL: (Hofmeyr GJ, Alfirevic Z, Kelly T, Kavanagh J, Thomas J, Brocklehurst P, Neilson JP) Protocol CD002074

ABRIDGED BACKGROUND: When a woman and her caregivers agree that labour induction is necessary (or desirable), the best method of induction needs to be chosen. The main problems experienced during induction of labour are an inability to achieve effective labour, or the production of excessively strong uterine contractions. The latter may cause both maternal and fetal distress, and both problems may lead to an increased risk of caesarean section. Excessive uterine activity, through inappropriate use of uterine stimulants, may occasionally lead to the very serious complication of uterine rupture (and fetal death).

There are several clinical factors which may influence the choice of induction method. These include parity, the condition of the cervix, membrane status and presence or absence of a uterine scar (usually from previous caesarean section). There are many methods of labour induction, that include administration of oxytocin, prostaglandins, prostaglandin analogues and smooth muscle stimulants such as herbs or castor oil, or mechanical methods such as digital stretching of the cervix and sweeping of the membranes, hygroscopic cervical dilators, extra-amniotic balloon catheters, artificial rupture of the membranes and nipple stimulation. Acupuncture and homeopathy have also been used.

OBJECTIVES: To determine, from the best available evidence, the effectiveness and safety of induction agents or procedures for third trimester cervical ripening and induction of labour (primary reviews); and to compare various methods for specific clinical categories of women (secondary reviews).

VAGINAL PROSTAGLANDIN (PGE2 AND PGF2A) FOR INDUCTION OF LABOUR AT TERM: increased the chance of vaginal birth within 24 hours; but PGE2 increased hyperstimulation. (Kelly AJ, Kavanagh J, Thomas J) CD003101

BACKGROUND: Prostaglandins have been used for induction of labour since the 1960s. Initial work focused on prostaglandin F2a as prostaglandin E2 was considered unsuitable for a number of reasons. With the development of alternative routes of administration, comparisons were made between various formulations of vaginal prostaglandins. This is one of a series of reviews of methods of cervical ripening and labour induction using standardised methodology.

OBJECTIVES: To determine the effects of vaginal prostaglandins E2 and F2a for third trimester cervical ripening or induction of labour in comparison with placebo/no treatment or other vaginal prostaglandins (except misoprostol).

METHODS: Standard PCG methods for labour induction reviews (see page xvii). Search date: May 2003.

MAIN RESULTS: In total, 101 studies were considered: 43 excluded and 57 (10039 women) included. One study is awaiting assessment.

Vaginal prostaglandin E2 compared with placebo or no treatment reduced the likelihood of vaginal delivery not being achieved within 24 hours (18% versus 99%, relative risk (RR) 0.19, 95% confidence interval (CI) 0.14 to 0.25, two trials, 384 women); there was no evidence of a difference between caesarean section rates although the risk of uterine hyperstimulation with fetal heart rate changes was increased (4.6% versus 0.51%, RR 4.14, 95% CI 1.93 to 8.90, 13 trials, 1203 women).

Comparison of vaginal prostaglandin F2a with placebo showed similar caesarean section rates but the cervical score was more likely to be improved (15% versus 60%, RR 0.25, 95% CI 0.13 to 0.49, five trials,

467 women) and the risk of oxytocin augmentation reduced (53.9% versus 89.1%, RR 0.60, 95% CI 0.43 to 0.84, 11 trials, 1265 women) with the use of vaginal PGF2a.

There were insufficient data to make meaningful conclusions for the comparison of vaginal PGE2 and PGF2a.

PGE2 tablet, gel and pessary appear to be as efficacious as each other. Lower dose regimens, as defined in the review, appear as efficacious as higher dose regimens.

AUTHORS' CONCLUSIONS: The primary aim of this review was to examine the efficacy of vaginal prostaglandin E2 and F2a. This is reflected by an increase in successful vaginal delivery rates in 24 hours, no increase in operative delivery rates and significant improvements in cervical favourability within 24 to 48 hours. Further research is needed to quantify the cost-analysis of induction of labour with vaginal prostaglandins, with special attention to different methods of administration.

☺ **INTRACERVICAL PROSTAGLANDINS FOR INDUCTION OF LABOUR:** less effective than intravaginal prostaglandins. (Boulvain M, Kelly A, Irion O) CD006971

BACKGROUND: Prostaglandins have been used for cervical ripening and induction of labour since the 1970s. The goal of the administration of prostaglandins in the process of induction of labour is to achieve cervical ripening before the onset of contractions. One of the routes of administration that was proposed is intracervical. Using this route, prostaglandins are less easy to administer and the need for exposing the cervix may cause discomfort to the woman.

OBJECTIVES: To determine the effects of intracervical prostaglandins for third trimester cervical ripening or induction of labour compared with placebo/no treatment and with vaginal prostaglandins (except misoprostol).

METHODS: Standard PCG methods for labour induction reviews (see page xvii). Search date: August 2007.

MAIN RESULTS: Fifty-six trials (7738 women) are included.

Intracervical PGE2 with placebo/no treatment: 28 trials, 3764 women
Four studies reported the number of women who did not achieve vaginal delivery within 24 hours, showing a decreased risk with PGE2 (relative risk (RR) 0.61; 95% confidence interval (CI) 0.47 to 0.79). There was a small, and statistically non-significant, reduction of the risk of

caesarean section when PGE2 was used (RR 0.88; 95% CI 0.77 to 1.00). The finding was statistically significant in a subgroup of women with intact membranes and unfavourable cervix only (RR 0.82; 95% CI 0.68 to 0.98). The risk of hyperstimulation with fetal heart rate (FHR) changes was not significantly increased (RR 1.21; 95% CI 0.72 to 2.05). However, the risk of hyperstimulation without FHR changes was significantly increased (RR 1.59; 95% CI 1.09 to 2.33).

Intracervical PGE2 with intravaginal PGE2: 29 trials, 3881 women
The risk of not achieving vaginal delivery within 24 hours was increased with intracervical PGE2 (RR 1.26; 95% CI 1.12 to 1.41). There was no change in the risk of caesarean section (RR 1.07; 95% CI 0.93 to 1.22). The risks of hyperstimulation with FHR changes (RR 0.76; 95% CI 0.39 to 1.49) and without FHR changes (RR 0.80; 95% CI 0.56 to 1.15) were non-significantly different with the two methods of PGE2 administration. Only one trial with small sample size reported on women's views, with no difference between groups.

Intracervical PGE2 low dose with intracervical PGE2 high dose: two trials, 102 women
The trials are too small to provide any useful information.

AUTHORS' CONCLUSIONS: Intracervical prostaglandins are effective compared to placebo, but appear inferior when compared to intravaginal prostaglandins.

☺ **INTRAVENOUS OXYTOCIN ALONE FOR CERVICAL RIPENING AND INDUCTION OF LABOUR:** increased the chance of vaginal birth within 24 hours; was generally less effective than prostaglandins; may have similar efficacy when membranes are ruptured. (Kelly AJ, Tan B) CD003246

BACKGROUND: Oxytocin is the commonest induction agent used worldwide. It has been used alone, in combination with amniotomy or following cervical ripening with other pharmacological or non-pharmacological methods. Prior to the introduction of prostaglandin agents oxytocin was used as a cervical ripening agent as well. In developed countries oxytocin alone is more commonly used in the presence of ruptured membranes, whether spontaneous or artificial. In developing countries where the incidence of HIV is high, delaying amniotomy in labour reduces vertical transmission rates and hence the use of oxytocin with intact membranes warrants further investigation.

This review will address the use of oxytocin alone for induction of labour. Amniotomy alone or oxytocin with amniotomy for induction of labour has been reviewed elsewhere in The Cochrane Library. Trials which consider concomitant administration of oxytocin and amniotomy will not be considered.

This is one of a series of reviews of methods of cervical ripening and labour induction using a standardised methodology.

OBJECTIVES: To determine the effects of oxytocin alone for third trimester cervical ripening or induction of labour in comparison with other methods of induction of labour or placebo/no treatment.

METHODS: Standard PCG methods for labour induction reviews (see page xvii). Search date: May 2001.

MAIN RESULTS: In total, 110 trials were considered; 52 have been excluded and 58 included examining a total of 11 129 women.

Comparing oxytocin alone with expectant management: Oxytocin alone reduced the rate of unsuccessful vaginal delivery within 24 hours when compared with expectant management (8.3% versus 54%, relative risk (RR) 0.16, 95% confidence interval (CI) 0.10 to 0.25) but the caesarean section rate was increased (10.4% versus 8.9%, RR 1.17, 95% CI 1.01 to 1.36). This increase in caesarean section rate was not apparent in the subgroup analyses. Women were less likely to be unsatisfied with induction rather than expectant management, in the one trial reporting this outcome (5.5% versus 13.7%, RR 0.43, 95% CI 0.33 to 0.56).

Comparing oxytocin alone with vaginal prostaglandins: Oxytocin alone was associated with an increase in unsuccessful vaginal delivery within 24 hours (52% versus 28%, RR 1.85, 95% CI 1.41 to 2.43), irrespective of membrane status, but there was no difference in caesarean section rates (11.4% versus 10%, RR 1.12, 95% CI 0.95 to 1.33).

Comparing oxytocin alone with intracervical prostaglandins: Oxytocin alone was associated with an increase in unsuccessful vaginal delivery within 24 hours when compared with intracervical PGE2 (51% versus 35%, RR 1.49, 95% CI 1.12 to 1.99). For all women with an unfavourable cervix regardless of membrane status, the caesarean section rates were increased (19.0% versus 13.1%, RR 1.42, 95% CI 1.11 to 1.82).

AUTHORS' CONCLUSIONS: Overall, comparison of oxytocin alone with either intravaginal or intracervical PGE2 reveals that the prostaglandin agents probably overall have more benefits than oxytocin alone. The amount of information relating to specific clinical subgroups is limited, especially with respect to women with intact membranes. Comparison of oxytocin alone to vaginal PGE2 in women with ruptured membranes reveals that both interventions are probably equally efficacious with each having some advantages and disadvantages over the others. With respect to current practice in women with ruptured membranes induction can be recommended by either method and in women with intact membranes there is insufficient information to make firm recommendations.

AMNIOTOMY ALONE FOR INDUCTION OF LABOUR: not enough data to provide reliable evidence. (Bricker L, Luckas M) CD002862

BACKGROUND: Amniotomy (deliberate rupture of the membranes) is a simple procedure which can be used alone for induction of labour if the membranes are accessible, thus avoiding the need for pharmacological intervention. However, the time interval from amniotomy to established labour may not be acceptable to clinicians and women, and in a number of cases labour may not ensue. This is one of a series of reviews of methods of cervical ripening and labour induction using standardised methodology.

OBJECTIVES: To determine the effects of amniotomy alone for third tri-mester labour induction in women with a live fetus.

METHODS: Standard PCG methods for labour induction reviews (see page xvii). Search date: January 2007.

MAIN RESULTS: Two trials, comprising 50 and 260 women, respec-tively were eligible for inclusion in this review. No conclusions could be drawn from comparisons of amniotomy alone versus no interven-tion, and amniotomy alone versus oxytocin alone (small trial, only one pre-specified outcome reported). No trials compared amniotomy alone with intracervical prostaglandins. One trial compared amniot-omy alone with a single dose of vaginal prostaglandins for women with a favourable cervix, and found a significant increase in the need for oxytocin augmentation in the amniotomy alone group (44% versus 15%; relative risk 2.85, 95% confidence interval 1.82 to 4.46). This should be viewed with caution as this was the result of a single-centre trial. Furthermore, secondary intervention occurred four hours after amniotomy, and this time interval may not have been appropriate.

AUTHORS' CONCLUSIONS: Data are lacking about the value of amniotomy alone for induction of labour. While there are now other modern methods available for induction of labour (pharmacological agents), there remain clinical scenarios where amniotomy alone may be desirable and appropriate, and this method is worthy of further research. This research should include evaluation of the appropriate time interval from amniotomy to secondary intervention, women and caregivers' satisfaction and economic analysis.

AMNIOTOMY PLUS INTRAVENOUS OXYTOCIN FOR INDUCTION OF LABOUR: not enough data to provide reliable evidence. (Howarth GR, Botha DJ) CD003250

BACKGROUND: Induction of labour is a common obstetric intervention. Amniotomy alone for induction of labour is reviewed separately and oxytocin alone for induction of labour is being prepared for inclusion in The Cochrane Library. This review will address the use of the combination of these two methods for induction of labour in the third trimester. This is one of a series of reviews of methods of cervical ripening and labour induction using standardised methodology.

OBJECTIVES: To determine, from the best available evidence, the efficacy and safety of amniotomy and intravenous oxytocin for third trimester induction of labour.

METHODS: Standard PCG methods for labour induction reviews (see page xvii). Search date: May 2001.

MAIN RESULTS: Seventeen trials involving 2566 women were included. Amniotomy and intravenous oxytocin were found to result in fewer women being undelivered vaginally at 24 hours than amniotomy alone (relative risk (RR) 0.03, 95% confidence intervals (CI) 0.001–0.49). This finding was based on the results of a single study of 100 women. As regards secondary results amniotomy and intravenous oxytocin resulted in significantly fewer instrumental vaginal deliveries than placebo (RR 0.18, CI 0.05–0.58). Amniotomy and intravenous oxytocin resulted in more postpartum haemorrhage than vaginal prostaglandins (RR 5.5, CI 1.26–24.07). Significantly more women were also dissatisfied with amniotomy and intravenous oxytocin when compared with vaginal prostaglandins (RR 53, CI 3.32–846.51).

AUTHORS' CONCLUSIONS: Data on the effectiveness and safety of amniotomy and intravenous oxytocin are lacking. No recommendations for clinical practice can be made on the basis of this review. Amniotomy and intravenous oxytocin is a combination of two methods of induction of labour and both methods are utilised in clinical practice. If their use is to be continued it is important to compare the effectiveness and safety of these methods, and to define under which clinical circumstances one may be preferable to another.

☺ **VAGINAL MISOPROSTOL FOR CERVICAL RIPENING AND INDUCTION OF LABOUR:** doses >25 mcg were more effective than dinoprostone but more uterine hyperstimulation; lower doses were similar to dinoprostone. (Hofmeyr GJ, Gülmezoglu AM) CD000941 (in RHL 11)

BACKGROUND: Misoprostol (Cytotec, Searle) is a prostaglandin E1 analogue widely used for off-label indications such as induction of abortion and of labour. This is one of a series of reviews of methods of cervical ripening and labour induction using standardised methodology.

OBJECTIVES: To determine the effects of vaginal misoprostol for third trimester cervical ripening or induction of labour.

METHODS: Standard PCG methods for labour induction reviews (see page xvii). Search date: February 2004.

MAIN RESULTS: Seventy trials have been included. Compared to placebo, misoprostol was associated with reduced failure to achieve vaginal delivery within 24 hours (relative risk (RR) 0.36, 95% confidence interval (CI) 0.19 to 0.68). Uterine hyperstimulation, without fetal heart rate changes, was increased (RR 11.66, 95% CI 2.78 to 49).

Compared with vaginal prostaglandin E2, intracervical prostaglandin E2 and oxytocin, vaginal misoprostol was associated with less epidural analgesia use, fewer failures to achieve vaginal delivery within 24 hours and more uterine hyperstimulation. Compared with vaginal or intracervical prostaglandin E2, oxytocin augmentation was less common with misoprostol and meconium-stained liquor more common.

Lower doses of misoprostol compared to higher doses were associated with more need for oxytocin augmentation and less uterine hyperstimulation, with and without fetal heart rate changes.

Information on women's views is conspicuously lacking.

AUTHORS' CONCLUSIONS: Vaginal misoprostol in doses above 25 mcg four-hourly was more effective than conventional methods of labour induction, but with more uterine hyperstimulation. Lower doses were similar to conventional methods in effectiveness and risks. The studies reviewed were not large enough to exclude the possibility of rare but serious adverse events, particularly uterine rupture, which has been reported anecdotally following misoprostol induction. The authors request information on cases of uterine rupture known to readers. Further research is needed to establish the ideal route of administration and dosage, and safety. Professional and governmental bodies should agree guidelines for the use of misoprostol, based on the best available evidence and local circumstances.

☺ **ORAL MISOPROSTOL FOR INDUCTION OF LABOUR:** was associated with fewer caesarean sections but more uterine hyperstimulation than vaginal dinoprostone; more meconium stained liquor than intravenous oxytocin; less uterine hyperstimulation and more meconium stained liquor than vaginal misoprostol. (Alfirevic Z, Weeks A) CD001338 (in RHL 11)

BACKGROUND: Misoprostol is a synthetic prostaglandin that can be given orally or vaginally. In most countries misoprostol has not been licensed for use in pregnancy, but its unlicensed use is common because misoprostol is cheap, stable at room temperature and effective in causing uterine contractions. Oral use of misoprostol may be convenient, but high doses could cause uterine hyperstimulation and uterine rupture which may be life-threatening for both mother and fetus.

OBJECTIVES: To assess the effectiveness and safety of oral misoprostol used for labour induction in women with a viable fetus in the third trimester of pregnancy.

METHODS: Standard PCG methods for labour induction reviews (see page xvii). Search date: January 2005.

MAIN RESULTS: 41 trials (8606 participants) were included. In four trials comparing oral misoprostol with placebo (474 participants), women using oral misoprostol were less likely to have long labours (relative risk (RR) 0.16, 95% confidence interval (CI) 0.05 to 0.49), needed less oxytocin (RR 0.32, 95% CI 0.24 to 0.43) and had a lower caesarean section rate (RR 0.62, 95% CI 0.40 to 0.96).

In nine trials comparing oral misoprostol with vaginal dinoprostone (2627 participants), women given oral misoprostol were less likely to need a caesarean section, but this reduction reached statistical significance only in the subgroup with intact membranes (RR 0.78, 95% CI 0.66 to 0.94). Uterine hyperstimulation was more common after oral misoprostol (RR 1.63, 95% CI 1.09 to 2.44) although this was not associated with any adverse fetal events.

Seven trials (1017 participants) compared oral misoprostol with intravenous oxytocin. The only difference between the groups was an increase in meconium-stained liquor in women with ruptured membranes following administration of oral misoprostol (RR 1.72, 95% CI 1.08 to 2.74).

16 trials (3645 participants) compared oral and vaginal misoprostol and found no difference in the primary outcomes. There was less uterine hyperstimulation without fetal heart rate changes in those given oral misoprostol (RR 0.37, 95% CI 0.23 to 0.59). Oral misoprostol was associated with increased need for oxytocin augmentation (RR 1.28, 95% CI 1.11 to 1.48) and more meconium-stained liquor (RR 1.27, 95% CI 1.01 to 1.60).

AUTHORS' CONCLUSIONS: Oral misoprostol appears to be more effective than placebo and at least as effective as vaginal dinoprostone. However, there remain questions about its safety because of a relatively high rate of uterine hyperstimulation and the lack of appropriate dose ranging studies. In countries where misoprostol remains unlicenced for the induction of labour, many practitioners will prefer the legal protection of using a licenced product like dinoprostone. There is no evidence that misoprostol given orally is inferior to the vaginal route and has lower rates of hyperstimulation. If misoprostol is used orally, the dose should not exceed 50 mcg.

> ☺ **MECHANICAL METHODS FOR INDUCTION OF LABOUR:** were less effective than prostaglandins; similar to misoprostol with less uterine hyperstimulation; showed less chance of caesarean section compared with oxytocin. (Boulvain M, Kelly A, Lohse C, Stan C, Irion O) CD001233

BACKGROUND: Mechanical methods were the first methods developed to ripen the cervix or to induce labour. Devices which were used include various types of catheters and laminaria tents, introduced into the cervical canal or into the extra-amniotic space. Mechanical methods were never completely abandoned, but were substituted by pharmacological methods during recent decades. Potential advantages of mechanical methods, compared with pharmacological methods, may include simplicity of preservation, lower cost and reduction of the side effects. However, special attention should be paid to contraindications (e.g. low-lying placenta), risk of infection and maternal discomfort when inserting these devices.

This is one of a series of reviews of methods of cervical ripening and labour induction using standardised methodology.

OBJECTIVES: To determine the effects of mechanical methods for third trimester cervical ripening or induction of labour in comparison with placebo/no treatment, prostaglandins (vaginal, intracervical, misoprostol) and oxytocin.

METHODS: Standard PCG methods for labour induction reviews (see page xvii). Search date: April 2001.

MAIN RESULTS: In total, 58 studies were considered; 45 studies have been included and 13 were excluded. Studies generally included women with unfavourable cervix and intact membranes.

Comparing mechanical methods with placebo/no treatment, only one study with 48 participants reported on vaginal delivery not achieved in 24 hours (69% with mechanical methods versus 77% with placebo/no treatment; relative risk (RR) 0.90; 95% confidence interval (CI): 0.64–1.26). Hyperstimulation with fetal heart rate changes was not reported. The risk of caesarean section, reported in six studies including 416 women, was similar between groups (34%; RR 1.00; 95% CI: 0.76–1.30). There were no reported cases of severe neonatal and maternal morbidity.

Comparing mechanical methods with vaginal PGE2, only one trial (109 women) reported on vaginal delivery not achieved in 24 hours (73% versus 42%; relative risk (RR) 1.74; 95% CI: 1.21–2.49). Compared with intracervical PGE2, only one trial (100 women) reported on vaginal delivery not achieved in 24 hours (68% versus 40%; relative risk (RR) 1.70; 95% CI: 1.15–2.51). Compared with misoprostol, the effectiveness of mechanical methods was similar (34% versus 30%; relative risk (RR) 1.15; 95% CI: 0.80–1.66). The use of mechanical method reduced the risk of hyperstimulation with fetal heart rate changes when compared with prostaglandins: vaginal PGE2 (0% versus 6%; RR 0.14; 95% CI: 0.04–0.53), intracervical PGE2 (0% versus 1%; RR 0.21; 95%

CI: 0.04–1.20) and misoprostol (4% versus 9%; RR 0.41; 95% CI: 0.20–0.87). There was no difference in the risk of caesarean section between mechanical methods and prostaglandins. Serious neonatal (three cases) and maternal morbidity (one case) were infrequently reported.

When compared with oxytocin, use of mechanical methods reduced the risk of caesarean section (four trials; 198 women; 17% versus 32%; RR 0.55; 95% CI: 0.33–0.91). The likelihood of vaginal delivery in 24 hours and of hyperstimulation with fetal heart rate changes was not reported. There were no reported cases of serious maternal morbidity and severe neonatal morbidity was not reported.

These results are similar whatever specific mechanical method was used, except with extra-amniotic infusion. When comparing extra-amniotic infusion with any prostaglandins, women were more likely to not achieve vaginal delivery within 24 hours (57% versus 42%; RR 1.33; 95% CI: 1.02–1.75) and the risk of caesarean section was increased (31% versus 22%; RR 1.48; 95% CI: 1.14–1.90), without a reduction of the risk of hyperstimulation.

AUTHORS' CONCLUSIONS: There is insufficient evidence to evaluate the effectiveness, in terms of likelihood of vaginal delivery in 24 hours, of mechanical methods compared with placebo/no treatment or with prostaglandins. The risk of hyperstimulation was reduced when compared with prostaglandins (intracervical, intravaginal or misoprostol). Compared to oxytocin in women with unfavourable cervix, mechanical methods reduce the risk of caesarean section. There is no evidence to support the use of extra-amniotic infusion.

MEMBRANE SWEEPING FOR INDUCTION OF LABOUR: reduced the need for formal labour induction; but was uncomfortable for women. (Boulvain M, Stan C, Irion O) CD000451

BACKGROUND: Sweeping of the membranes, also named stripping of the membranes, is a relatively simple technique usually performed without admission to hospital. During vaginal examination, the clinician's finger is introduced into the cervical os. Then, the inferior pole of the membranes is detached from the lower uterine segment by a circular movement of the examining finger. This intervention has the potential to initiate labour by increasing local production of prostaglandins and, thus, reduce pregnancy duration or pre-empt formal induction of labour with either oxytocin, prostaglandins or amniotomy. This is one of a series of reviews of methods of cervical ripening and labour induction using standardised methodology.

OBJECTIVES: To determine the effects of membrane sweeping for third trimester induction of labour.

METHODS: Standard PCG methods for labour induction reviews (see page xvii). Search date: July 2004.

MAIN RESULTS: 22 trials (2797 women) were included, 20 comparing sweeping of membranes with no treatment, three comparing sweeping with prostaglandins and one comparing sweeping with oxytocin (two studies reported more than one comparison). Risk of caesarean section was similar between groups (relative risk (RR) 0.90, 95% confidence interval (CI) 0.70 to 1.15). Sweeping of the membranes, performed as a general policy in women at term, was associated with reduced duration of pregnancy and reduced frequency of pregnancy continuing beyond 41 weeks (RR 0.59, 95% CI 0.46 to 0.74) and 42 weeks (RR 0.28, 95% CI 0.15 to 0.50). To avoid one formal induction of labour, sweeping of membranes must be performed in eight women (NNT = eight). There was no evidence of a difference in the risk of maternal or neonatal infection. Discomfort during vaginal examination and other adverse effects (bleeding, irregular contractions) were more frequently reported by women allocated to sweeping. Studies comparing sweeping with prostaglandin administration are of limited sample size and do not provide evidence of benefit.

AUTHORS' CONCLUSIONS: Routine use of sweeping of membranes from 38 weeks of pregnancy onwards does not seem to produce clinically important benefits. When used as a means for induction of labour, the reduction in the use of more formal methods of induction needs to be balanced against women's discomfort and other adverse effects.

EXTRA-AMNIOTIC PROSTAGLANDIN FOR INDUCTION OF LABOUR: not enough data to provide reliable evidence. (Hutton E, Mozurkewich E) CD003092

BACKGROUND: This is one of a series of reviews of methods of cervical ripening and labour induction using standardised methodology.

OBJECTIVES: To determine the effects of extra-amniotic prostaglandin for third trimester cervical ripening or induction of labour.

METHODS: Standard PCG methods for labour induction reviews (see page xvii). Search date: July 2001.

MAIN RESULTS: Oxytocin was used to initiate or augment labour significantly less frequently with extra-amniotic prostaglandins when compared to placebo (relative risk 0.50, 95% confidence interval 0.38–0.66). No other findings were significant in the comparisons that were made for this review, including when extra-amniotic prostaglandins were compared with other methods of cervical ripening or induction of labour. Although this could suggest that extra-amniotic prostaglandins are as effective as other agents, the findings are difficult to interpret because they are based on very small numbers and may lack the power to show a real difference.

AUTHORS' CONCLUSIONS: The studies in this review are limited by their small sample sizes which are in many cases further divided into multiple comparison groups. The analyses resulted in most comparisons showing no significant differences, with wide confidence intervals. Although extra-amniotic prostaglandins may be as effective as other modalities in initiating labour, there is little conclusive information from this review to guide clinical practice. An adequately powered randomised controlled trial would be useful to determine if the use of extra-amniotic prostaglandins would lower the rate of caesarean section. However, in the time since these studies were undertaken the use of extra-amniotic prostaglandins has largely been replaced by other modes of prostaglandin administration.

⊗ **INTRAVENOUS PROSTAGLANDIN FOR INDUCTION OF LABOUR:** showed more adverse effects than other methods. (Luckas M, Bricker L) CD002864

BACKGROUND: Intravenous prostaglandin E2 and F2 alpha can be used to induce labour, however their use is limited by unacceptable maternal side-effect profiles. This is one of a series of reviews of methods of cervical ripening and labour induction using standardised methodology.

OBJECTIVES: To determine the effects of intravenous prostaglandin for third trimester cervical ripening or induction of labour.

METHODS: Standard PCG methods for labour induction reviews (see page xvii). Search date: January 2004.

MAIN RESULTS: 13 trials (1165 women) were included in the review.

The use of intravenous prostaglandin was associated with higher rates of uterine hyperstimulation both with changes in the fetal heart rate (relative risk (RR) 6.76, 95% confidence interval (CI) 1.23 to 37.11) and without (RR 4.25, 95% CI 1.48 to 12.24) compared to oxytocin. Use of prostaglandin was also associated with significantly more maternal side-effects (gastrointestinal, thrombophlebitis and pyrexia, RR 3.75, 95% CI 2.46 to 5.70) than oxytocin. Prostaglandin was no more likely to result in vaginal delivery than oxytocin (RR 0.85, 95% CI 0.61 to 1.18).

No significant differences emerged from subgroup analysis or from the trials comparing combination oxytocin/prostaglandin F2 alpha and oxytocin or extra-amniotic versus intravenous prostaglandin E2.

AUTHORS' CONCLUSIONS: Intravenous prostaglandin is no more efficient than intravenous oxytocin for the induction of labour but its use is associated with higher rates of maternal side-effects and uterine hyperstimulation.

No conclusions can be drawn form the comparisons of combination of prostaglandin F2 alpha and oxytocin compared to oxytocin alone or extra-amniotic and intravenous prostaglandin E2.

☹ **ORAL PROSTAGLANDIN E2 FOR INDUCTION OF LABOUR:** had no clear advantages and more adverse effects, such as vomiting. (French L) CD003098

BACKGROUND: This is one of a series of reviews of methods of cervical ripening and labour induction using standardized methodology.

OBJECTIVES: To determine the effects of oral prostaglandin E2 for third trimester induction of labour.

METHODS: Standard PCG methods for labour induction reviews (see page xvii). Search date: January 2007.

MAIN RESULTS: There were 19 studies included in the review. Of these 15 included a comparison using either oral or intravenous oxytocin with or without amniotomy. The quality of studies reviewed was not high. Only seven studies had clearly described allocation concealment. Only two studies stated that providers or participants, or both, were blinded to treatment group.

For the outcome of vaginal delivery not achieved within 24 hours, in the composite comparison of oral PGE2 versus all oxytocin treatments (oral and intravenous, with and without amniotomy), there was a trend favoring oxytocin treatments (relative risk (RR) 1.97, 95% confidence interval (CI) 0.86 to 4.48). For the outcome of cesarean section, in the comparison of PGE2 versus no treatment or placebo, PGE2 was favored (RR 0.54, 95% CI 0.29 to 0.98). Otherwise, there were no significant differences between groups for this outcome.

Oral prostaglandin was associated with vomiting across all comparison groups.

AUTHORS' CONCLUSIONS: Oral prostaglandin consistently resulted in more frequent gastrointestinal side-effects, in particular vomiting, compared with the other treatments included in this review. There were no clear advantages to oral prostaglandin over other methods of induction of labour.

MIFEPRISTONE FOR INDUCTION OF LABOUR: not enough data to provide reliable evidence. (Neilson JP) CD002865

BACKGROUND: The steroid hormone, progesterone, inhibits contractions of the uterus. Antiprogestins (including mifepristone) have been developed to antagonise the action of progesterone, and these have a recognised role in medical termination of early or mid-pregnancy. Animal studies have suggested that mifepristone may also have a role in inducing labour in late pregnancy.

OBJECTIVES: To determine the effects of mifepristone for third trimester cervical ripening or induction of labour.

METHODS: Standard PCG methods for labour induction reviews (see page xvii). Search date: April 2001.

MAIN RESULTS: Seven trials, that recruited 594 women, are included. All trials compared mifepristone with placebo, except for one that compared mifepristone with no treatment. Compared to placebo, mifepristone treated women were less likely to have an unfavourable cervix at 48 hours (relative risk [RR] 0.36, 95% confidence intervals [CI] 0.2–0.63) or 96 hours (RR 0.39, 95% CI 0.23–0.66). Mifepristone treated women were more likely to have delivered within 48 and 96 hours of treatment than were placebo treated/no treatment women – 48 hours: RR 2.82, 95% CI 1.82–4.36; 96 hours: RR 3.40, 95% CI 1.96–5.92. Mifepristone treated women were less likely to undergo caesarean section (RR 0.71, 95% CI 0.53–0.95). There is little information about fetal outcome, although there was no evidence that neonatal hypoglycaemia might be more common after exposure to mifepristone. Similarly, there is little information about maternal side-effects although some nausea and vomiting was reported in one trial.

AUTHOR'S CONCLUSIONS: There is insufficient information available from clinical trials to support the use of mifepristone to induce labour. However, available data do show that mifepristone is better than placebo at ripening the cervix, and inducing labour. There is evidence of a possible reduction in the incidence of caesarean section following mifepristone treatment (compared to placebo) that would justify further trials. We found no trials that compared mifepristone with alternative methods of inducing labour, e.g. prostaglandins.

OESTROGENS ALONE OR WITH AMNIOTOMY FOR CERVICAL RIPENING OR INDUCTION OF LABOUR: not enough data to provide reliable evidence. (Thomas J, Kelly AJ, Kavanagh J) CD003393

BACKGROUND: Studies in sheep showed that there is a pre-labour rise in oestrogen and a decrease in progesterone; both of these changes stimulate prostaglandin production and may help initiate labour. Though oestrogen has been suggested as an effective cervical ripening or induction agent, research in humans has failed to demonstrate a similar physiological mechanism. The use of oestrogen as an induction agent is not currently common practice, and as such this systematic review should be regarded as an historical review.

This is one of a series of reviews of methods of cervical ripening and labour induction using a standardised methodology.

OBJECTIVES: To determine, from the best available evidence, the effectiveness and safety of oestrogens alone or with amniotomy for third trimester cervical ripening and induction of labour in comparison with other methods of induction of labour.

METHODS: Standard PCG methods for labour induction reviews (see page xvii). Search date: April 2001.

MAIN RESULTS: When comparing oestrogen with placebo there was no difference between the rate of caesarean section (7.1% versus 10.3%, relative risk (RR) 0.70, 95% confidence interval (CI) 0.30 to 1.62). There were no differences between rates of uterine hyperstimulation with or without fetal heart rate changes or instrumental vaginal delivery.

None of the studies reported the rates of either vaginal delivery not achieved in 24 hours, or cervix unfavourable/unchanged after 12–24 hours. There were insufficient data to make any meaningful conclusions when comparing oestrogen with vaginal PGE2, intracervical PGE2, oxytocin alone or extra amniotic PGF2a, as to whether oestrogen is effective in inducing labour.

AUTHORS' CONCLUSIONS: There were insufficient data to draw any conclusions regarding the efficacy of oestrogen as an induction agent.

⊗ **CORTICOSTEROIDS FOR CERVICAL RIPENING AND INDUCTION OF LABOUR:** are not supported by the limited data. (Kavanagh J, Kelly AJ, Thomas J) CD003100

BACKGROUND: The role of corticosteroids in the process of labour is not well understood. Animal studies have shown the importance of cortisol secretion by the fetal adrenal gland in initiating labour in sheep. Infusion of glucocorticosteroids into the fetus has also been shown to induce premature labour in sheep. Given these studies it has been postulated that corticosteroids will promote the induction of labour in women. This is one of a series of reviews of methods of cervical ripening and labour induction using standardised methodology.

OBJECTIVES: To determine the effects of corticosteroids for third trimester cervical ripening or induction of labour in comparison with other methods of cervical priming or induction of labour.

METHODS: Standard PCG methods for labour induction reviews (see page xvii). Search date: December 2005.

MAIN RESULTS: Only one small trial (66 women) was included. The primary outcome of vaginal birth within 24 hours was not reported. No benefit of intramuscular administration of corticosteroids with intravenous oxytocin was found when compared with oxytocin alone. However, given the small size of this trial this result should be interpreted cautiously.

AUTHORS' CONCLUSIONS: The effectiveness of corticosteroids for induction of labour is uncertain. This method of induction of labour is not commonly used and so further research in this area is probably unwarranted.

RELAXIN FOR CERVICAL RIPENING AND INDUCTION OF LABOUR: not enough data to provide reliable evidence. (Kelly AJ, Kavanagh J, Thomas J) CD003103

BACKGROUND: Relaxin is a protein hormone composed of two amino acid chains. The role played by relaxin in human pregnancy and parturition is unclear. Its use and involvement as a cervical ripening agent has been debated since the 1950s. Because the main source of human relaxin is the corpus luteum of pregnancy much of the early work on induction of labour has focused on porcine or bovine preparations. With the advent of DNA recombinant technology human relaxin has become available for evaluation. Relaxin is thought to have a promoting effect on cervical ripening. Due to a possible inhibitory effect on human myometrial activity, relaxin may not be associated with the concomitant increase in the rate of uterine hyperstimulation seen with other induction agents. This is one of a series of reviews of methods of cervical ripening and labour induction using a standardised methodology.

OBJECTIVES: To determine the effects of relaxin (purified porcine and recombinant human) for third trimester cervical ripening or induction of labour in comparison with other methods of induction.

METHODS: Standard PCG methods for labour induction reviews (see page xvii). Search date: May 2003.

MAIN RESULTS: Nine studies were considered; five have been excluded and four included examining a total of 267 women. There were no reported cases of uterine hyperstimulation with fetal heart rate (FHR) changes in any of the studies. There was no evidence of a difference between the rate of caesarean section in those women given relaxin compared with placebo (15.3% versus 14.2%; relative risk (RR) 0.79, 95% confidence interval (CI) 0.42 to 1.50, four trials, 257 women). There was a reduction in the risk of the cervix remaining unfavourable or unchanged with induction with relaxin (21.9% versus 49.3%; RR 0.45, 95% CI 0.28 to 0.72, three trials, 371 women). There were no reported cases of uterine hyperstimulation without FHR changes.

AUTHORS' CONCLUSIONS: The place of relaxin, either purified porcine or recombinant human, as an induction or cervical priming agent is unclear. Further trials are needed to estimate the true effect of relaxin within current clinical practice.

HYALURONIDASE FOR CERVICAL RIPENING AND INDUCTION OF LABOUR: reduced oxytocin augmentation and caesarean sections, but is invasive. (Kavanagh J, Kelly AJ, Thomas J) CD003097

BACKGROUND: Dilatation and effacement of the cervix are not only a result of uterine contractions, but are also dependent upon ripening processes within the cervix. The cervix is a fibrous organ composed principally of hyaluronic acid, collagen and proteoglycan. Hyaluronic acid increases markedly after the onset of labour. An increase in the level of hyaluronic acid is associated with an increase in tissue water content. Cervical ripening during labour is characterised by changes of the cervix and an increased water content. Cervical injection of hyaluronidase was postulated to increase cervical ripening. This is one of a series of reviews of methods of cervical ripening and labour induction using standardised methodology.

OBJECTIVES: To determine the effects of hyaluronidase for third trimester cervical ripening or induction of labour in comparison with other methods of induction of labour.

METHODS: Standard PCG methods for labour induction reviews (see page xvii). Search date: January 2006

MAIN RESULTS: One trial, with 168 women participating, was included in the review. When compared with placebo for cervical ripening intracervical injections of hyaluronidase resulted in women receiving significantly fewer caesarean sections (18% versus 49%, relative risk (RR) 0.37, 95% confidence interval (CI) 0.22 to 0.61), less need for oxytocin augmentation (10% versus 47%, RR 0.20, 95% CI 0.10 to 0.41) and increased cervical favourability after 24 hours (60% versus 98%, RR 0.62, 95% CI 0.52 to 0.74). No side-effects for mother or baby were reported in this trial.

AUTHORS' CONCLUSIONS: Intracervical injections of hyaluronidase for cervical ripening appear beneficial. However, this is not common practice. In addition it is an invasive procedure that women may find unacceptable in the presence of less invasive methods.

CASTOR OIL, BATH AND/OR ENEMA FOR CERVICAL PRIMING AND INDUCTION OF LABOUR: not enough data to provide reliable evidence. (Kelly AJ, Kavanagh J, Thomas J) CD003099

BACKGROUND: Castor oil, a potent cathartic, is derived from the bean of the castor plant. Anecdotal reports, which date back to ancient Egypt, have suggested the use of castor oil to stimulate labour. Castor oil has been widely used as a traditional method of initiating labour in midwifery practice. Its role in the initiation of labour is poorly understood and data examining its efficacy within a clinical trial are limited. This is one of a series of reviews of methods of cervical ripening and labour induction using standardised methodology.

OBJECTIVES: To determine the effects of castor oil or enemas for third trimester cervical ripening or induction of labour in comparison with other methods of cervical ripening or induction of labour.

METHODS: Standard PCG methods for labour induction reviews (see page xvii). Search date: May 2003.

MAIN RESULTS: In the one included study of 100 women, which compared a single dose of castor oil versus no treatment, no evidence of a difference was found between caesarean section rates (relative risk (RR) 2.31, 95% confidence interval (CI) 0.77 to 6.87). No data was presented on neonatal or maternal mortality or morbidity. There was no evidence of a difference between either the rate of meconium stained liquor (RR 0.77, 95% CI 0.25 to 2.36) or Apgar score less than seven at five minutes (RR 0.92, 95% CI 0.02 to 45.71) between the two groups. The number of participants was small, hence only large differences in outcomes could have been detected. All women who ingested castor oil felt nauseous (RR 97.08, 95% CI 6.16 to 1530.41).

AUTHORS' CONCLUSIONS: The only trial included in this review attempts to address the role of castor oil as an induction agent. The trial was small and of poor methodological quality. Further research is needed to attempt to quantify the efficacy of castor oil as an induction agent.

ACUPUNCTURE FOR INDUCTION OF LABOUR: not enough data to provide reliable evidence. (Smith CA, Crowther CA) CD002962

BACKGROUND: This is one of a series of reviews of methods of cervical ripening and labour induction using standardised methodology. The use of complementary therapies is increasing and some women look to complementary therapies during pregnancy and childbirth to be used alongside conventional medical practice. Acupuncture involves the insertion of very fine needles into specific points of the body. The limited observational studies to date suggest that acupuncture for induction of labour appears safe, has no known teratogenic effects and may be effective. The evidence regarding the clinical effectiveness of this technique is limited.

OBJECTIVES: To determine the effects of acupuncture for third trimester cervical ripening or induction of labour.

METHODS: Standard PCG methods for labour induction reviews (see page xvii). Search date: February 2003.

MAIN RESULTS: One trial of 56 women was included in the review. Data was not in a form that could be included in the meta-analysis.

AUTHORS' CONCLUSIONS: There is a need for well-designed randomised controlled trials to evaluate the role of acupuncture to induce labour and for trials to assess clinically meaningful outcomes.

BREAST STIMULATION FOR CERVICAL RIPENING AND INDUCTION OF LABOUR: increased the number of women in labour within 72 hours and reduced postpartum haemorrhage; more studies are needed to address safety. (Kavanagh J, Kelly AJ, Thomas J) CD003392

BACKGROUND: Breast stimulation has been suggested as a means of inducing labour. It is a non-medical intervention allowing women greater control over the induction process. This is one of a series of reviews of methods of cervical ripening and labour induction using a standardised methodology.

OBJECTIVES: To determine the effectiveness of breast stimulation for third trimester cervical ripening or induction of labour in comparison with placebo/no intervention or other methods of induction of labour.

METHODS: Standard PCG methods for labour induction reviews (see page xvii). Search date: June 2007.

MAIN RESULTS: Six trials (719 women) were included.

Analysis of trials comparing breast stimulation with no intervention found a significant reduction in the number of women not in labour at 72 hours (62.7% versus 93.6%, relative risk (RR) 0.67, 95% confidence interval (CI) 0.60 to 0.74). This result was not significant in women with an unfavourable cervix. A major reduction in the rate of postpartum haemorrhage was reported (0.7% versus 6%, RR 0.16, 95% CI 0.03 to 0.87). No significant difference was detected in the caesarean section rate (9% versus 10%, RR 0.90, 95% CI 0.38 to 2.12) or rates of meconium staining. There were no instances of uterine hyperstimulation. Three perinatal deaths were reported (1.8% versus 0%, RR 8.17, 95% CI 0.45 to 147.77).

When comparing breast stimulation with oxytocin alone the analysis found no difference in caesarean section rates (28% versus 47%, RR 0.60, 95% CI 0.31 to 1.18). No difference was detected in the number of women not in labour after 72 hours (58.8% versus 25%, RR 2.35, 95% CI 1.00 to 5.54) or rates of meconium staining. There were four perinatal deaths (17.6% versus 5%, RR 3.53, 95% CI 0.40 to 30.88).

AUTHORS' CONCLUSIONS: Breast stimulation appears beneficial in relation to the number of women not in labour after 72 hours, and reduced postpartum haemorrhage rates. Until safety issues have been fully evaluated it should not be used in high-risk women. Further research is required to evaluate its safety, and should seek data on postpartum haemorrhage rates, number of women not in labour at 72 hours and maternal satisfaction.

SEXUAL INTERCOURSE FOR CERVICAL RIPENING AND INDUCTION OF LABOUR: not enough data to provide reliable evidence. (Kavanagh J, Kelly AJ, Thomas J) CD003093

BACKGROUND: The role of prostaglandins for cervical ripening and induction of labour has been examined extensively. Human semen is the biological source that is presumed to contain the highest prostaglandin concentration. The role of sexual intercourse in the initiation of labour is uncertain. The action of sexual intercourse in stimulating labour is unclear; it may in part be due to the physical stimulation of the lower uterine segment, or endogenous release of oxytocin as a result of orgasm or from the direct action of prostaglandins in semen. Furthermore nipple stimulation may be part of the process of initiation. This is one of a series of reviews of methods of cervical ripening and labour induction using standardised methodology.

OBJECTIVES: To determine the effects of sexual intercourse for third trimester cervical ripening or induction of labour in comparison with other methods of induction.

METHODS: Standard PCG methods for labour induction reviews (see page xvii). Search date: June 2007.

MAIN RESULTS: There was one included study of 28 women which reported very limited data, from which no meaningful conclusions can be drawn.

AUTHORS' CONCLUSIONS: The role of sexual intercourse as a method of induction of labour is uncertain. This is an important issue to pregnant women and their partners. There is a need for well-designed randomised controlled trials to assess the impact of sexual intercourse on the onset of labour. Any future trials investigating sexual intercourse as a method of induction need to be of sufficient power to detect clinically relevant differences in standard outcomes.

HOMOEOPATHY FOR INDUCTION OF LABOUR: not enough data to provide reliable evidence. (Smith CA) CD003399

BACKGROUND: This is one of a series of reviews of cervical ripening and labour induction using standardised methodology. Homoeopathy involves the use, in dilution, of substances which cause symptoms in their undiluted form. A type of herb, 'caulophyllum', is one type of homoeopathic therapy that has been used to induce labour.

OBJECTIVES: To determine the effects of homoeopathy for third trimester cervical ripening or induction of labour.

METHODS: Standard PCG methods for labour induction reviews (see page xvii). Search date: May 2003.

MAIN RESULTS: Two trials involving 133 women were included in the review. The trials were placebo controlled and double blind, but the quality was not high. Insufficient information was available on the method of randomisation and the study lacked clinically meaningful outcomes. These trials demonstrated no differences in any primary or secondary outcome between the treatment and control group.

AUTHOR'S CONCLUSIONS: There is insufficient evidence to recommend the use of homoeopathy as a method of induction. It is likely that the demand for complementary medicine will continue and women will continue to consult a homoeopath during their pregnancy. Although caulophyllum is a commonly used homoeopathic therapy to induce labour, the treatment strategy used in the one trial in which it was evaluated may not reflect routine homoeopathy practice. Rigorous

evaluations of individualised homeopathic therapies for induction of labour are needed.

NITRIC OXIDE DONORS FOR CERVICAL RIPENING AND INDUCTION OF LABOUR: (Kelly AJ, Kavanagh J) Protocol [see page xviii] CD006901

ABRIDGED BACKGROUND: Nitric oxide is thought to be an essential mediator in the process of cervical ripening. There is increasing evidence that the use of nitric oxide donors (including isosorbide mononitrate, nitroglycerin and sodium nitroprusside) allows cervical ripening to occur in the absence of uterine contractions and this may be performed in an outpatient.

OBJECTIVES: To determine the effects of nitric oxide donors (isosorbide mononitrate, nitroglycerin and sodium nitroprusside) for third trimester cervical ripening or induction of labour, in comparison with placebo or no treatment or other treatments from a predefined hierarchy.

BUCCAL OR SUBLINGUAL MISOPROSTOL FOR CERVICAL RIPENING AND INDUCTION OF LABOUR: was at least as effective as the same dose orally; more studies are needed to establish the optimal dosage and risks. (Muzonzini G, Hofmeyr GJ) CD004221 (in RHL 11)

BACKGROUND: This is one of a series of reviews of cervical ripening and labour induction using standardised methodology. Misoprostol administered by the oral and sublingual routes has the advantage of rapid onset of action, while the sublingual and vaginal routes have the advantage of prolonged activity and greatest bioavailability.

OBJECTIVES: To determine the effectiveness and safety of misoprostol administered buccally or sublingually for third trimester cervical ripening and induction of labour.

METHODS: Standard PCG methods for labour induction reviews (see page xvii). Search date: December 2003.

MAIN RESULTS: Three studies (502 participants) compared buccal/sublingual misoprostol respectively with a vaginal regimen (200 µg versus 50 µg) and with oral administration (50 versus 50 µg and 50 versus 100 µg).

The buccal route was associated with a trend to fewer caesarean sections than with the vaginal route (18/73 versus 28/79; relative risk

(RR) 0.70; 95% confidence interval (CI) 0.42 to 1.15). There were no significant differences in any other outcomes.

When the same dosage was used sublingually versus orally, the sublingual route was associated with less failures to achieve vaginal delivery within 24 hours (12/50 versus 19/50; RR 0.63, 95% CI 0.34 to 1.16), reduced oxytocin augmentation (17/50 versus 23/50; RR 0.74, 95% CI 0.45 to 1.21) and reduced caesarean section (8/50 versus 15/50; RR 0.53, 95% CI 0.25 to 1.14), but the differences were not statistically significant.

When a smaller dose was used sublingually than orally, there were no differences in any of the outcomes.

AUTHORS' CONCLUSIONS: Based on only three small trials, sublingual misoprostol appears to be at least as effective as when the same dose is administered orally. There are inadequate data to comment on the relative complications and side-effects. Sublingual or buccal misoprostol should not enter clinical use until its safety and optimal dosage have been established by larger trials.

Nitric oxide for induction of labour

Hypnosis for induction of labour

No Cochrane reviews of these topics.

6.3 Techniques of labour induction – secondary reviews

These reviews will summarise data from the primary reviews relevant to women with specific clinical circumstances.

> **INDUCTION OF LABOUR IN SPECIFIC CLINICAL SITUATIONS: GENERIC PROTOCOL:** (Kelly A, Alfirevic Z, Hofmeyr GJ, Kavanagh J, Neilson JP, Thomas J) Protocol CD003398

ABRIDGED BACKGROUND: When deciding on the method of induction of labour certain clinical factors are considered. These include parity; the status of membranes, ruptured or intact; the status of the cervix, favourable or unfavourable; and any history of a previous caesarean section.

This generic protocol will form the basis of a series of secondary (clinical) reviews focusing on induction of labour in specific clinical situations arranged by potentially important clinical characteristics of the women (parity, favourability of cervix, state of membranes and previous caesarean section).

OBJECTIVES: To evaluate how parity, a history of a caesarean section, and membrane or cervical status may affect the performance of a variety of methods of third trimester cervical ripening or induction of labour when compared with each other and with placebo or no treatment.

CHAPTER 7: CARE DURING CHILDBIRTH

L abour and birth is in many ways the central focus of care for pregnant women. It is at once a time of unique emotional intensity for parents – anticipation, excitement, exhilaration, fear, pain or disappointment may be extreme – and a time of increased need for surveillance by caregivers. The timing of maternal deaths is clustered around the time of labour and the postpartum period. This includes deaths from hypertensive disorders, eclampsia, haemorrhage, uterine rupture, cardiac disease, AIDS, pulmonary embolism and complications of anaesthesia and surgery.

The intermittent interruption of maternal blood flow to the placenta during uterine contractions has no impact on the great majority of babies, but may compromise physiological function in babies without adequate reserve. Rare complications of labour such as placental abruption, uterine rupture, cord prolapse, shoulder dystocia and difficulty with breech delivery may be dangerous for the baby if interventions are not prompt. Prolonged obstructed labour presents dangers to both mothers and babies.

For these reasons, the World Health Organization has identified 'skilled attendance at birth' as the central theme in global attempts to reduce maternal deaths: the presence during labour and birth of a midwife or other caregiver with skills to identify complications and resources to provide or refer for further care when needed.

The context within which birth takes places varies considerably across societies and health systems, ranging from unattended births at home to patently excessive medical intervention. There is even a point of view which promotes avoiding labour altogether by routine elective caesarean section. Finding a balance between the need to ensure reasonable

A Cochrane Pocketbook: Pregnancy and Childbirth   G.J. Hofmeyr et al.
Copyright © 2008, Z. Alfiervic, C. A. Crowther, L. Duley, A. M. Gulmezoglu, G. ML. Gyte , E. D. Hodnett, G. J. Hofmeyr, J. P. Neilson

levels of safety, and excessive interventions, which may diminish the experience of childbirth for the family, and place the mother at increased risk from the immediate and long-term complications of interventions such as caesarean section, remains a matter of ongoing debate.

7.1 Place of birth

Choosing the appropriate place for birth may represent a compromise between considerations such as the emotional security, comfort, convenience, and preference of the parents, and perceived needs for medical surveillance. The relative benefits and risk of different settings are difficult to quantify. For a woman and her baby with no complications, the risk of an unexpected adverse event during a home birth may be smaller than risks specific to hospitalisation, such as hospital-acquired infections. For a woman with pregnancy complications, the balance of benefit and risk may be in the other direction. Other options include home-like birth units within a hospital, or free-standing birth units.

> **HOME VERSUS HOSPITAL BIRTH:** not enough data to provide reliable evidence. (Olsen O, Jewell MD) CD000352

BACKGROUND: A meta-analysis of observational studies has suggested that planned home birth may be safe and with less interventions than planned hospital birth.

OBJECTIVES: To assess the effects of planned home birth compared to hospital birth on the rates of interventions, complications and morbidity as determined in randomized trials.

METHODS: Standard PCG methods (see page xvii). Search date: April 2006.

MAIN RESULTS: One study involving 11 women was included. The trial was of reasonable quality, but was too small to be able to draw conclusions.

AUTHORS' CONCLUSIONS: There is no strong evidence to favour either planned hospital birth or planned home birth for low-risk pregnant women.

> ☺**HOME-LIKE VERSUS CONVENTIONAL INSTITUTIONAL SETTINGS FOR BIRTH:** were associated with fewer medical interventions; greater satisfaction and breastfeeding success; but a trend to higher perinatal mortality. (Hodnett ED, Downe S, Edwards N, Walsh D) CD000012

BACKGROUND: Home-like birth settings have been established in or near conventional labour wards for the care of pregnant women who prefer and require little or no medical intervention during labour and birth.

OBJECTIVES: Primary: to assess the effects of care in a home-like birth environment compared to care in a conventional labour ward. Secondary: to determine if the effects of birth settings are influenced by staffing or organizational models or geographical location of the birth centre.

METHODS: Standard PCG methods (see page xvii). Search date: May 2004.

MAIN RESULTS: Six trials involving 8677 women were included. No trials of freestanding birth centres were found. Between 29% and 67% of women allocated to home-like settings were transferred to standard care before or during labour. Allocation to a home-like setting significantly increased the likelihood of: no intrapartum analgesia/anaesthesia (four trials; n = 6703; relative risk (RR) 1.19, 95% confidence interval (CI) 1.01 to 1.40), spontaneous vaginal birth (five trials; n = 8529; RR 1.03, 95% CI 1.01 to 1.06), vaginal/perineal tears (four trials; n = 8415; RR 1.08, 95% CI 1.03 to 1.13), preference for the same setting the next time (one trial; n = 1230; RR 1.81, 95% CI 1.65 to 1.98), satisfaction with intrapartum care (one trial; n = 2844; RR 1.14, 95% CI 1.07 to 1.21), and breastfeeding initiation (two trials; n = 1431; RR 1.05, 95% CI 1.02 to 1.09) and continuation to six to eight weeks (two trials; n = 1431; RR 1.06, 95% CI 1.02 to 1.10). Allocation to a home-like setting decreased the likelihood of episiotomy (five trials; n = 8529; RR 0.85, 95% CI 0.74 to 0.99). There was a trend towards higher perinatal mortality in the home-like setting (five trials; n = 8529; RR 1.83, 95% CI 0.99 to 3.38). No firm conclusions could be drawn regarding the effects of staffing or organizational models.

AUTHORS' CONCLUSIONS: When compared to conventional institutional settings, home-like settings for childbirth are associated with modest benefits, including reduced medical interventions and increased maternal satisfaction. Caregivers and clients should be vigilant for signs of complications.

7.2   Routine care during labour

During the last century, routines for care of women during labour evolved, largely without objective evidence of effectiveness. In recent years, many of the routines have been challenged and found to be ineffective or harmful. One of the most extensively studied routines is the practice of excluding from the labour ward supportive companions of the woman (see below). To view a motivational video on the value of childbirth companions, particularly in low-resource settings, see the video presentation 'Childbirth companions: Every woman's choice': WHO Reproductive Health Library, **www.rhlibrary.com**.

> **ANTENATAL EDUCATION FOR SELF-DIAGNOSIS OF THE ONSET OF ACTIVE LABOUR AT TERM:** not enough data to provide reliable evidence. (Lauzon L, Hodnett E) CD000935

BACKGROUND: A specific programme designed to teach women to recognise active labour may be beneficial through potentially decreasing the incidence of early admission to hospital, increasing women's confidence, feelings of control and empowerment, and decreasing their anxiety.

OBJECTIVES: To assess the effects of teaching pregnant women specific criteria for self-diagnosis of active labour onset in term pregnancy.

METHODS: Standard PCG methods (see page xvii). Search date: October 2007.

MAIN RESULTS: One study involving 245 women was included. Method of randomisation was unclear and 15% of the sample was lost to follow-up in this trial. A specific antenatal education programme was associated with a reduction in the mean number of visits to the labour suite before the onset of labour (weighted mean difference -0.29, 95% confidence interval to -0.47 to -0.11). It is unclear whether this resulted in fewer women being sent home because they were not in labour.

AUTHORS' CONCLUSIONS: There is not enough evidence to evaluate the use of a specific set of criteria for self-diagnosis of active labour.

> ☺ **LABOUR ASSESSMENT PROGRAMMES TO DELAY ADMISSION TO LABOUR WARDS:** reduced the time spent in labour ward, use of oxytocin and analgesia; improved women's sense of control. (Lauzon L, Hodnett E) CD000936

BACKGROUND: The aim of labour assessment programmes is to delay hospital admission until labour is in the active phase, and thereby to prevent unnecessary interventions in women who are not in established labour.

OBJECTIVES: To assess the effects of labour assessment programmes that aim to delay hospital admission until labour is in the active phase.

METHODS: Standard PCG methods (see page xvii). Search date: January 2004.

MAIN RESULTS: One study of 209 women was included. The trial was of excellent quality. Women who were randomised to the labour assessment unit spent less time in the labour ward (weighted mean difference −5.20 hours, 95% confidence interval −7.06 to −3.34), were less likely to receive intrapartum oxytocics (odds ratio 0.45, 95% confidence interval 0.25 to 0.80) and analgesia (odds ratio 0.36, 95% confidence interval 0.16 to 0.78) than women who were admitted directly to the labour ward. Women in the labour assessment group reported higher levels of control during labour (weighted mean difference 16.00, 95% confidence interval 7.52 to 24.48). There is insufficient evidence to assess effects on rate of caesarean section and other important measures of maternal and neonatal outcome.

AUTHORS' CONCLUSIONS: Labour assessment programmes, which aim to delay hospital admission until active labour, may benefit women with term pregnancies.

☺ **CONTINUOUS SUPPORT FOR WOMEN DURING CHILDBIRTH:** reduced labour duration, use of analgesia and operative births; increased satisfaction. (Hodnett ED, Gates S, Hofmeyr GJ, Sakala C) CD003766 (in RHL 11)

BACKGROUND: Historically, women have been attended and supported by other women during labour. However, in recent decades in hospitals worldwide, continuous support during labour has become the exception rather than the routine. Concerns about the consequent dehumanization of women's birth experiences have led to calls for a return to continuous support by women for women during labour.

OBJECTIVES: Primary: to assess the effects, on mothers and their babies, of continuous, one-to-one intrapartum support compared with usual care. Secondary: to determine whether the effects of continuous support are influenced by: (1) routine practices and policies in the birth environment that may affect a woman's autonomy, freedom of movement and ability to cope with labour; (2) whether the caregiver is a member of the staff of the institution; and (3) whether the continuous support begins early or later in labour.

METHODS: Standard PCG methods (see page xvii). Search date: February 2007.

MAIN RESULTS: 16 trials involving 13 391 women met inclusion criteria and provided usable outcome data. Primary comparison: women who had continuous intrapartum support were likely to have a slightly shorter labour, were more likely to have a spontaneous vaginal birth and less likely to have intrapartum analgesia or to report dissatisfaction with their childbirth experiences. Subgroup analyses: in general, continuous intrapartum support was associated with greater benefits when the provider was not a member of the hospital staff, when it began early in labour and in settings in which epidural analgesia was not routinely available.

AUTHORS' CONCLUSIONS: All women should have support throughout labour and birth.

> **ENEMAS DURING LABOUR:** the evidence does not support the routine use of enemas. (Reveiz L, Gaitṫn HG, Cuervo LG) CD000330

BACKGROUND: The use of enemas during labour usually reflects the preference of the attending healthcare provider. However, enemas may cause discomfort for women and increase the costs of delivery.

OBJECTIVES: To assess the effects of enemas applied during the first stage of labour on infection rates in mothers and newborns, duration of labour, perineal wound dehiscence in the mother, perineal pain and faecal soiling.

METHODS: Standard PCG methods (see page xvii). Search date: March 2007.

MAIN RESULTS: Three RCTs (1765 women) met the inclusion criteria. Meta-analysis revealed no significant differences for infection rates in puerperal women (2 RCTs; 594 women; relative risk (RR) 0.66, 95% CI 0.42 to 1.04) or newborn children (1 RCT; 370 newborns; RR 1.12, 95% CI 0.76 to 1.67) after one month of follow up. No significant differences were found in the incidence of lower or upper respiratory tract infections. One trial described labour to be significantly shorter with enema versus no enema (1 RCT, 1027 women; 409.4 minutes versus 459.8

minutes; weighted mean difference (WMD) −50,40 CI 95% −75.68 to −25.12; P < 0.001), but another, adjusted for parity, did not confirm this (median 515 minutes with enemas versus 585 minutes without enemas, P = 0.24). Two trials found no significant differences in neonatal umbilical infection (2 RCTs; 592 newborns; RR 3.16 95% CI 0.50 to 19.82). The one trial that researched women's views found no significant differences in satisfaction between groups.

AUTHORS' CONCLUSIONS: The evidence provided by the three included RCTs shows that enemas do not have a significant effect on infection rates such as perineal wound infection or other neonatal infections and women's satisfaction. This evidence does not support the routine use of enemas during labour; therefore, such practice should be discouraged.

MATERNAL POSITIONS AND MOBILITY DURING FIRST STAGE LABOUR: (Lewis L, Webster J, Carter A, McVeigh C, Devenish-Meares P) Protocol [see page xviii] CD003934

ABRIDGED BACKGROUND: In cultures not influenced by Western society, women progress through the first stage of labour in upright positions and change position as they wish with no evidence of harmful effects to either the mother or the fetus. It is more common for women in the developed world to labour in bed. However, when these women are encouraged, they will choose a number of different positions as the first stage progresses. Numerous studies have shown that a supine position in labour may have adverse physiological effects on the condition of the woman and her fetus and the progression of labour. Moving about can increase a woman's sense of control in labour by providing a self regulated distraction from the challenge of labour.

OBJECTIVES: The purpose of this review is to assess the effects of different upright and recumbent positions and mobilisation for women in the first stage of labour on length of labour, type of delivery and other important maternal, fetal and neonatal outcomes.

This primary objective is:

- To compare the effects of upright (defined as walking and upright non walking, e.g. sitting, standing, kneeling, squatting and all fours) positions with recumbent positions (supine, semi recumbent and lateral) assumed by women in the first stage of labour on maternal, fetal and neonatal outcomes.

The secondary objectives are:

- To compare the effects of semi recumbent and supine positions with lateral positions assumed by women in the first stage of labour on maternal, fetal and neonatal outcomes.
- To compare the effects of walking with upright non walking positions (sitting, standing, kneeling, squatting, all fours) assumed by women in the first stage of labour on maternal, fetal and neonatal outcomes.
- To compare the effects of walking with recumbent positions (supine, semi recumbent and lateral) assumed by women in the first stage of labour on maternal, fetal and neonatal outcomes.
- To compare allowing women to assume the position/s they choose with recumbent positions (supine, semi recumbent and lateral) assumed by women in the first stage of labour on maternal, fetal and neonatal outcomes.

IMMERSION IN WATER IN PREGNANCY, LABOUR AND BIRTH: reduced pain and analgesia use in the first stage of labour; more research on second stage immersion is needed. (Cluett E R, Nikodem VC, McCandlish RE, Burns EE) CD000111

BACKGROUND: Enthusiasts for immersion in water during labour and birth have advocated its use to increase maternal relaxation, reduce analgesia requirements and promote a midwifery model of supportive care. Sceptics are concerned that there may be greater harm to women and/or babies, for example, a perceived risk associated with neonatal inhalation of water and maternal/neonatal infection.

OBJECTIVES: To assess the evidence from randomised controlled trials about the effects of immersion in water during pregnancy, labour or birth on maternal, fetal, neonatal and caregiver outcomes.

METHODS: Standard PCG methods (see page xvii). Search date: September 2003.

MAIN RESULTS: Eight trials are included (2939 women). No trials were identified that evaluated immersion versus no immersion during pregnancy, considered different types of baths/pools or considered the management of third stage of labour. There was a statistically significant reduction in the use of epidural/spinal/paracervical analgesia/anaesthesia amongst women allocated to water immersion water during the first stage of labour compared to those not allocated to water immersion (odds ratio (OR) 0.84, 95% confidence interval (CI) 0.71 to 0.99, four trials). There was no significant difference in vaginal operative deliveries (OR 0.83, 95% CI 0.66 to 1.05, six trials) or caesarean sections (OR 1.33, 95% CI 0.92 to 1.91). Women who used water immersion during the first stage of labour reported statistically significantly less pain than those not labouring in water (40/59 versus 55/61) (OR 0.23, 95% CI 0.08 to 0.63, one trial). There were no significant differences in incidence of an Apgar score less than seven at five minutes (OR 1.59, 95% CI 0.63 to 4.01), neonatal unit admissions (OR 1.05, 95% CI 0.68 to 1.61) or neonatal infection rates (OR 2.01, 95% CI 0.50 to 8.07).

AUTHORS' CONCLUSIONS: There is evidence that water immersion during the first stage of labour reduces the use of analgesia and reported maternal pain, without adverse outcomes on labour duration, operative delivery or neonatal outcomes. The effects of immersion in water during pregnancy or in the third stage are unclear. One trial explores birth in water, but is too small to determine the outcomes for women or neonates.

EFFECT OF PARTOGRAM USE ON OUTCOMES FOR WOMEN IN SPONTANEOUS LABOUR AT TERM: (Lavender T, O'Brien P, Hart A)
Protocol [*see* page xviii] CD005461

ABRIDGED BACKGROUND: The partogram (or partograph) is a simple, inexpensive tool to provide a continuous pictorial overview of labour. The partogram is a pre-printed form, usually in paper version, on which midwives and obstetricians record labour observations. Most partograms have three distinct sections where observations are entered on maternal condition, fetal condition and labour progress; this last section assists in the detection of prolonged labour. The partogram has been heralded as one of the most important advances in modern obstetric care; however, this was prior to any rigorous evaluation.

OBJECTIVES: Objective 1: The primary objective is to determine the effect of use of the partogram on perinatal and maternal morbidity and mortality.

Objective 2: To determine the effect of partogram design on perinatal and maternal morbidity and mortality.

INTERVENTIONS FOR KETOSIS DURING LABOUR: (Toohill J, Soong B, Flenady V) Protocol [*see* page xviii] CD004230

ABRIDGED BACKGROUND: Ketone bodies are molecules which transport fat-derived energy from the liver to other organs and are normally oxidised to carbon dioxide, water and usable energy by peripheral tissue. However, when placed under more severe conditions, for example starvation and excessive exercise, peripheral metabolic processes cannot cope and ketones accumulate in the blood. This state is known as ketosis and usually becomes evident by the presence of ketone bodies in the urine (ketonuria).

In labour, ketosis is not an uncommon occurrence due to the increased physical stress and is often compounded by reduced oral intake. The clinical importance of detecting ketosis in labour is not clear.

OBJECTIVES: The primary objectives of the review are:

1. To assess the effects on maternal, fetal and neonatal outcomes of intravenous fluids with or without additional oral intake (fluids and food) administered to women in labour for the treatment of ketosis compared with no intervention defined as no oral intake, ice chips only, or oral intake on demand.
2. To assess the effects on maternal, fetal and neonatal outcomes of additional oral intake alone (fluids and food) for women in labour in the treatment of ketosis compared with no intervention defined as no oral intake, ice chips only, or oral intake on demand.
3. To assess the effects on maternal, fetal and neonatal outcomes of different types of intravenous fluids with or without additional oral intake (fluids and food) administered to women in labour for the treatment of ketosis.

A secondary objective of the review is to determine whether the effects on the primary outcome measures of spontaneous vaginal delivery, maternal satisfaction with labour care, maternal adverse effects, and neonatal admission to intensive care nursery are influenced by different types of oral and intravenous fluids as follows:

(i) intravenous therapy solutions, i.e. glucose solutions, balanced salt solutions (i.e. Hartmanns), normal saline;
(ii) high carbohydrate oral fluids.

RESTRICTING ORAL FLUID AND FOOD INTAKE DURING LABOUR: (Singata M, Tranmer JE) Protocol [see page xviii] CD003930

ABRIDGED BACKGROUND: Restricting oral food and fluid intake of women in active labour in hospitals is a strongly held obstetric tradition. The rationale for withholding food and fluid during labour is to decrease the risk of maternal morbidity and mortality from Mendelson's syndrome if a general anaesthetic is required, as fasting will ensure small gastric volumes. Recent reviews suggest that there is no evidence to support this belief.

Intravenous therapy instead of oral hydration is common practice during labour. The value and safety of routine intravenous fluid therapy has been questioned.

Despite these risks, and lack of evidence of benefit, routine restriction of foods and fluids in labour has persisted.

OBJECTIVES: To determine the benefits and risks of oral food or fluid restriction during labour, with or without intravenous hydration.

⊗ **ROUTINE PERINEAL SHAVING ON ADMISSION IN LABOUR:** was associated with more bacterial colonisation and no benefits. (Basevi V, Lavender T) CD001236

BACKGROUND: Pubic or perineal shaving is a procedure performed before birth in order to lessen the risk of infection if there is a spontaneous perineal tear or if an episiotomy is performed.

OBJECTIVES: To assess the effects of routine perineal shaving on admission in labour on maternal and neonatal outcomes, according to the best available evidence.

METHODS: Standard PCG methods (see page xvii). Search date: November 2003.

MAIN RESULTS: Only two trials fulfilled the prespecified criteria. In the earlier trial, 389 women were alternately allocated to receive either skin preparation and perineal shaving (control) or clipping of vulval hair only (experimental). In the second trial, which included 150 participants, perineal shaving was compared with the cutting of long hairs for procedures only. The primary outcome for both trials was maternal febrile morbidity. No differences were found (combined odds ratio (OR) 1.26, 95% confidence interval (CI) 0.75 to 2.12).

In the smaller trial, fewer women who had not been shaved had Gram-negative bacterial colonisation compared with women who had been shaved (OR 0.43, 95% CI 0.20 to 0.92).

AUTHORS' CONCLUSIONS: There is insufficient evidence to recommend perineal shaving for women on admission in labour.

CAESAREAN SECTION FOR NON-MEDICAL REASONS AT TERM: no randomised trials to provide reliable evidence; systematic review of observational studies and qualitative data needed. (Lavender T, Hofmeyr GJ, Neilson JP, Kingdon C, Gyte GML) CD004660

BACKGROUND: Caesarean section rates are progressively rising in many parts of the world. One suggested reason is increasing requests by women for caesarean section in the absence of clear medical indications, such as placenta praevia, HIV infection, contracted pelvis and, arguably, breech presentation or previous caesarean section. The reported benefits of planned caesarean section include greater safety for the baby, less pelvic floor trauma for the mother, avoidance of labour pain and convenience. The potential disadvantages, from observational studies, include increased risk of major morbidity or mortality for the mother, adverse psychological sequelae and problems in subsequent pregnancies, including uterine scar rupture and greater risk of stillbirth and neonatal morbidity. An unbiased assessment of advantages and disadvantages would assist discussion of what has become a contentious issue in modern obstetrics.

OBJECTIVES: To assess, from randomised trials, the effects on perinatal and maternal morbidity and mortality, and on maternal psychological morbidity, of planned caesarean delivery versus planned vaginal birth in women with no clear clinical indication for caesarean section.

METHODS: Standard PCG methods (see page xvii). Search date: December 2005.

We identified no studies that met the inclusion criteria.

MAIN RESULTS: There were no included trials.

AUTHORS' CONCLUSIONS: There is no evidence from randomised controlled trials upon which to base any practice recommendations regarding planned caesarean section for non-medical reasons at term. In the absence of trial data, there is an urgent need for a systematic review of observational studies and a synthesis of qualitative data to better assess the short- and long-term effects of caesarean section and vaginal birth.

PACKAGE OF CARE FOR ACTIVE MANAGEMENT IN LABOUR FOR REDUCING CAESAREAN SECTION RATES IN LOW-RISK WOMEN: (Brown H, Paranjothy S, Thomas J) Protocol [see page xviii] CD004907

ABRIDGED BACKGROUND: Since the 1960s active management of labour has been proposed as an effective way in which to decrease caesarean section rates by reducing the proportion of women with 'failure to progress'. Active management of labour refers to a labour ward protocol for low-risk women that includes one-to-one support in labour, routine amniotomy (artificial rupture of the amniotic membranes) and the use of the intravenous drug oxytocin. Other components of active management include strict criteria for the diagnosis of labour, abnormal progress in labour and fetal compromise and peer review of assisted deliveries (daily retrospective and critical review of the reasons why assisted deliveries were carried out). Possible disadvantages of active management are related to the need for more interventions during labour, more invasive monitoring leading to a more medicalised birth process in which women have less control and hence lower levels of satisfaction.

OBJECTIVES: To determine whether a predefined package of interventions during childbirth such as 'active management of labour' can reduce the caesarean section rate in low-risk women and improve women's satisfaction.

⊗ **ROUTINE PROPHYLACTIC DRUGS IN NORMAL LABOUR FOR REDUCING GASTRIC ASPIRATION AND ITS EFFECTS:** had no clear benefits. (Gyte GML, Richens Y) CD005298

BACKGROUND: Women in normal labour may sometimes go on to have general anaesthesia if labour becomes abnormal, for example if a caesarean section is required. General anaesthesia carries a very small risk of regurgitation and inhalation of stomach contents into the lungs. This can cause inflammation, particularly if the fluid is acidic, and can lead to severe morbidity and very occasionally mortality. Labour hormones increase the risk of gastric aspiration or Mendelson's syndrome, though the exact incidence is unknown. The routine administration of acid prophylaxis drugs to all women in normal labour is commonly practiced worldwide, to reduce gastric aspiration by reducing the volume and acidity of stomach contents.

OBJECTIVES: To assess the effectiveness of routine prophylaxis drugs for women in normal labour to reduce gastric aspiration and its effects.

METHODS: Standard PCG methods (see page xvii). Search date: December 2005.

MAIN RESULTS: Three trials were included, involving 2465 women, assessing the effects of antacids, H_2 receptor antagonists and dopamine antagonists. There were no trials on proton-pump inhibitors. None of the trials were of good quality, and none assessed the incidence of gastric aspiration, Mendelson's syndrome or their consequences. All the studies assessed vomiting, and there was limited evidence that vomiting may be reduced by antacids (relative risk (RR) 0.46, 95% confidence interval (CI) 0.27 to 0.77, n = 578, one trial) or by dopamine antagonists given alongside pethidine (RR 0.40, 95% CI 0.23 to 0.68, n = 584, one trial). Comparisons between different drugs showed no significant differences, though the number of participants was small. There was no evidence that H_2 receptor antagonists improved outcomes compared with antacids, though only one trial addressed this issue.

AUTHORS' CONCLUSIONS: There is no good evidence to support the routine administration of acid prophylaxis drugs in normal labour to prevent gastric aspiration and its consequences. Giving such drugs to women, once a decision to give general anaesthesia is made, is assessed in another Cochrane review.

7.2.1 Normal birth – second stage

7.2.2 Episiotomy

In 1920, writing in the first volume of the *American Journal of Obstetrics and Gynecology*, De Lee advocated that all first-time mothers and most women having a second or subsequent baby should labour under twilight sedation and be delivered under general anaesthesia with prophylactic forceps and routine episiotomy. Cogent reasons were given for prophylactic episiotomy which influenced obstetric practice for the next 60 years. Only in the 1980s did randomised trials begin to indicate how misleading these concepts had been.

> ☹ **EPISIOTOMY FOR VAGINAL BIRTH:** a liberal episiotomy policy increased perineal trauma, suturing and complications; reduced anterior vaginal trauma. (Carroli G, Belizan J) CD000081 (in RHL 11)

BACKGROUND: Episiotomy is done to prevent severe perineal tears, but its routine use has been questioned. The relative effects of midline compared with midlateral episiotomy are unclear.

OBJECTIVES: To assess the effects of restrictive use of episiotomy compared with routine episiotomy during vaginal birth.

METHODS: Standard PCG methods (see page xvii).

MAIN RESULTS: Six studies were included. In the routine episiotomy group, 72.7% (1752/2409) of women had episiotomies, while the rate in the restrictive episiotomy group was 27.6% (673/2441). Compared with routine use, restrictive episiotomy involved less posterior perineal trauma (relative risk 0.88, 95% confidence interval 0.84 to 0.92), less suturing (relative risk 0.74, 95% confidence interval 0.71 to 0.77) and fewer healing complications (relative risk 0.69, 95% confidence interval 0.56 to 0.85). Restrictive episiotomy was associated with more anterior perineal trauma (relative risk 1.79, 95% 1.55 to 2.07). There was no difference in severe vaginal or perineal trauma (relative risk 1.11, 95% confidence interval 0.83 to 1.50), dyspareunia (relative risk 1.02, 95% confidence interval 0.90 to 1.16), urinary incontinence (relative risk 0.98, 95% confidence interval 0.79 to 1.20) or several pain measures. Results for restrictive versus routine mediolateral versus midline episiotomy were similar to the overall comparison.

AUTHORS' CONCLUSIONS: Restrictive episiotomy policies appear to have a number of benefits compared to routine episiotomy policies. There is less posterior perineal trauma, less suturing and fewer complications, no difference for most pain measures and severe vaginal or perineal trauma, but there was an increased risk of anterior perineal trauma with restrictive episiotomy.

POSITION IN THE SECOND STAGE OF LABOUR FOR WOMEN
WITHOUT EPIDURAL ANAESTHESIA: upright or lateral postures
reduced the duration of second stage, assisted deliveries, episiotomy, severe pain and abnormal fetal heart rate patterns; perineal
tears and blood loss were increased. (Gupta JK, Hofmeyr GJ, Smyth
R) CD002006 (in RHL 11)

BACKGROUND: For centuries, there has been controversy around
whether being upright (sitting, birthing stools, chairs, squatting) or lying
down have advantages for women delivering their babies.

OBJECTIVES: To assess the benefits and risks of the use of different positions during the second stage of labour (i.e. from full dilatation of the
cervix).

METHODS: Standard PCG methods (see page xvii). Search date:
September 2005.

MAIN RESULTS: Results should be interpreted with caution as the
methodological quality of the 20 included trials (6135 participants)
was variable. Use of any upright or lateral position, compared with
supine or lithotomy positions, was associated with: reduced duration of second stage of labour (nine trials: mean 4.28 minutes, 95%
confidence interval (CI) 2.93 to 5.63 minutes) – this was largely
due to a considerable reduction in women allocated to the use
of the birth cushion; a small reduction in assisted deliveries
(19 trials: relative risk (RR) 0.80, 95% CI 0.69 to 0.92); a reduction
in episiotomies (12 trials: RR 0.83, 95% CI 0.75 to 0.92); an increase
in second degree perineal tears (11 trials: RR 1.23, 95% CI 1.09 to
1.39); increased estimated blood loss greater than 500 ml (11 trials:
RR 1.63, 95% CI 1.29 to 2.05); reduced reporting of severe pain
during second stage of labour (one trial: RR 0.73, 95% CI 0.60 to
0.90); fewer abnormal fetal heart rate patterns (one trial: RR 0.31,
95% CI 0.08 to 0.98).

AUTHORS' CONCLUSIONS: The tentative findings of this review suggest several possible benefits for upright posture, with the possibility
of increased risk of blood loss greater than 500 ml. Women should be
encouraged to give birth in the position they find most comfortable.
Until such time as the benefits and risks of various delivery positions
are estimated with greater certainty, when methodologically stringent

trials' data are available, women should be allowed to make informed choices about the birth positions they might wish to assume for delivery of their babies.

PERINEAL TECHNIQUES DURING THE SECOND STAGE OF LABOUR FOR REDUCING PERINEAL TRAUMA: (Aasheim V, Nilsen ABV, Lukasse M, Reinar LM) Protocol [see page xviii] CD006672

ABRIDGED BACKGROUND: Most vaginal births are associated with some form of trauma to the genital tract. Perineal trauma can occur spontaneously or result from a surgical incision of the perineum, called episiotomy. It is uncertain which role exercise, demographic factors and nutrition in the years before and during pregnancy play in the occurrence of perineal trauma. Nulliparity, a large baby (both weight and head circumference), a prolonged second stage and malposition increase the risk for perineal trauma. Perineal management techniques termed as guiding or support techniques are believed to reduce perineal trauma.

OBJECTIVES: The objective of this review is to assess the effect of perineal techniques during the second stage of labour on the incidence of perineal trauma.

FUNDAL PRESSURE FOR SHORTENING THE SECOND STAGE OF LABOUR: (Verheijen E, Raven JH, Hofmeyr GJH) Protocol [see page xviii] CD006067

ABRIDGED BACKGROUND: Fundal pressure during the second stage of a vaginal delivery is a controversial manoeuvre. The obstetric technique involves application of manual pressure to the uppermost part of the uterus directed towards the birth canal in an attempt to shorten the second stage. Fundal pressure has also been applied using an inflatable girdle. The practice varies greatly between countries. While in many low- and middle-income countries the manoeuvre appears to be routine practice during delivery, in some, mainly English speaking, Western countries, it is seen as an obsolete procedure. Several anecdotal reports suggest that fundal pressure is associated with maternal and fetal complications, for example, uterine rupture, fetal fractures and brain damage. On the other hand, if fundal pressure could prevent instrumental delivery, the risk of a third-degree tear as a result of the instrument used would also be decreased.

OBJECTIVES: To determine if fundal pressure is effective in shortening the second stage of labour and reducing assisted vaginal deliveries or caesarean sections.

To explore maternal and fetal adverse effects related to fundal pressure.

7.2.3   Normal birth – third stage

The sense of relief and joy which accompanies the birth of a healthy child should not distract caregivers from the need for vigilance in the third stage of labour. For women without ready access to medical care, death from haemorrhage after childbirth often occurs too quickly and unpredictably to allow time for referral to a health facility. Creative methods are needed to improve global access to routine preventive measures known to be effective. Techniques of third stage management are demonstrated in the video presentation 'Active management of the third stage of labour': WHO reproductive Health Library, **www. rhlibrary.com.**

☺ **ACTIVE VERSUS EXPECTANT MANAGEMENT IN THE THIRD STAGE OF LABOUR:** reduced third stage labour duration and haemorrhage; side effects were increased when ergometrine was used. (Prendiville WJ, Elbourne D, McDonald S) CD000007 (in RHL 11)

BACKGROUND: Expectant management of the third stage of labour involves allowing the placenta to deliver spontaneously or aiding by gravity or nipple stimulation. Active management involves administration of a prophylactic oxytocic before delivery of the placenta, and usually early cord clamping and cutting, and controlled cord traction of the umbilical cord.

OBJECTIVES: To assess the effects of active versus expectant management on blood loss, post partum haemorrhage and other maternal and perinatal complications of the third stage of labour.

METHODS: Standard PCG methods (see page xvii). Search date: 2000.

MAIN RESULTS: Five studies were included. Four of the trials were of good quality. Compared to expectant management, active management (in the setting of a maternity hospital) was associated with the following reduced risks: maternal blood loss (weighted mean difference −79.33 millilitres, 95% confidence interval −94.29 to −64.37); post partum haemorrhage of more than 500 millilitres (relative risk

0.38, 95% confidence interval 0.32 to 0.46); prolonged third stage of labour (weighted mean difference −9.77 minutes, 95% confidence interval −10.00 to −9.53). Active management was associated with an increased risk of maternal nausea (relative risk 1.83, 95% confidence interval 1.51 to 2.23), vomiting and raised blood pressure (probably due to the use of ergometrine). No advantages or disadvantages were apparent for the baby.

AUTHORS' CONCLUSIONS: Routine 'active management' is superior to 'expectant management' in terms of blood loss, post partum haemorrhage and other serious complications of the third stage of labour. Active management is, however, associated with an increased risk of unpleasant side effects (e.g. nausea and vomiting), and hypertension, where ergometrine is used. Active management should be the routine management of choice for women expecting to deliver a baby by vaginal delivery in a maternity hospital. The implications are less clear for other settings including domiciliary practice (in developing and industrialised countries).

☺ **PROPHYLACTIC OXYTOCIN FOR THE THIRD STAGE OF LABOUR:** reduced postpartum haemorrhage; compared with ergot alkaloids reduced manual removal of the placenta. (Cotter A, Ness A, Tolosa J) CD001808 (in RHL 11)

BACKGROUND: Complications of the third stage of labour are a significant cause of maternal mortality worldwide.

OBJECTIVES: To examine the effect of oxytocin given prophylactically in the third stage of labour on maternal and neonatal outcomes.

METHODS: Standard PCG methods (see page xvii). Search date: December 2004.

MAIN RESULTS: 14 trials are included.

In seven trials involving over 3000 women, prophylactic oxytocin showed benefits of reduced blood loss (relative risk (RR) for blood loss greater than 500 ml 0.50; 95% confidence interval (CI) 0.43 to 0.59) and need for therapeutic oxytocics (RR 0.50; 95% CI 0.39 to 0.64) compared to no uterotonics.

In six trials involving over 2800 women, there was little evidence of differential effects for oxytocin versus ergot alkaloids, except that oxytocin was associated with fewer manual removals of the placenta

(RR 0.57; 95% CI 0.41 to 0.79), and with the suggestion of less raised blood pressure (RR 0.53; 95% CI 0.19 to 1.52) than with ergot alkaloids.

In five trials involving over 2800 women, there was little evidence of a synergistic effect of adding oxytocin to ergometrine versus ergometrine alone.

AUTHORS' CONCLUSIONS: Oxytocin appears to be beneficial for the prevention of postpartum haemorrhage. However, there is insufficient information about other outcomes and side-effects hence it is difficult to be confident about the trade-offs for these benefits. There seems little evidence in favour of ergot alkaloids alone compared to either oxytocin alone or to ergometrine–oxytocin, but the data are sparse. More trials are needed in domiciliary deliveries in developing countries, which shoulder most of the burden of third stage complications.

☺ **PROPHYLACTIC ERGOMETRINE–OXYTOCIN VERSUS OXYTOCIN FOR THE THIRD STAGE OF LABOUR:** reduced blood loss but increased side effects. (McDonald S, Abbott JM, Higgins SP) CD000201 (in RHL 11)

BACKGROUND: The routine prophylactic administration of a uterotonic agent is an integral part of active management of the third stage of labour, helping to prevent postpartum haemorrhage (PPH). The two most widely used uterotonic agents are: ergometrine–oxytocin (Syntometrine®) (a combination of oxytocin five international units (iu) and ergometrine 0.5 mg) and oxytocin (Syntocinon®).

OBJECTIVES: To compare the effects of ergometrine–oxytocin with oxytocin in reducing the risk of PPH (blood loss of at least 500 ml) and other maternal and neonatal outcomes.

METHODS: Standard PCG methods (see page xvii). Search date: April 2007.

MAIN RESULTS: Six trials were included (9332 women). Compared with oxytocin, ergometrine–oxytocin was associated with a small reduction in the risk of PPH using the definition of PPH of blood loss of at least 500 ml (odds ratio 0.82, 95% confidence interval 0.71 to 0.95). This advantage was found for both a dose of 5 iu oxytocin and a dose of 10 iu oxytocin, but was greater for the lower dose. There was no difference detected between the groups using either 5 or 10 iu for the stricter definition of PPH of blood loss at least 1000 ml. Adverse effects of vomiting, nausea and hypertension were more likely to be associated with the use of ergometrine–oxytocin. When heterogeneity between trials was taken into account there were no statistically significant differences found for the other maternal or neonatal outcomes.

AUTHORS' CONCLUSIONS: The use of ergometrine–oxytocin as part of the routine active management of the third stage of labour appears to be associated with a small but statistically significant reduction in the risk of PPH when compared to oxytocin for blood loss of 500 ml or more. No statistically significant difference was observed between the groups for blood loss of 1000 ml or more. A statistically significant difference was observed in the presence of maternal side-effects, including elevation of diastolic blood pressure, vomiting and nausea, associated with ergometrine–oxytocin use compared to oxytocin use. Thus, the advantage of a reduction in the risk of PPH, between 500 and 1000 ml blood loss, needs to be weighed against the adverse side-effects associated with the use of ergometrine–oxytocin.

☺ **PROPHYLACTIC USE OF ERGOT ALKALOIDS IN THE THIRD STAGE OF LABOUR:** reduced blood loss but increased vomiting, blood pressure and pain. (Liabsuetrakul T, Choobun T, Peeyananjarassri K, Islam QM) CD005456

BACKGROUND: Previous research has shown that the prophylactic use of uterotonic agents in the third stage of labour reduces postpartum blood loss and moderate to severe postpartum haemorrhage. This is one of a series of systematic reviews assessing the effects of prophylactic use of uterotonic drugs – here, prophylactic ergot alkaloids compared with no uterotonic agents, and different regimens of administration of ergot alkaloids.

OBJECTIVES: To determine the effectiveness and safety of prophylactic use of ergot alkaloids in the third stage of labour compared with no uterotonic agents, as well as with different routes or timing of administration for prevention of postpartum haemorrhage.

METHODS: Standard PCG methods (see page xvii). Search date: December 2006.

MAIN RESULTS: We included six studies comparing ergot alkaloids with no uterotonic agents, with a total of 1996 women in ergot alkaloids group and 1945 women in placebo or no treatment group. The use of injected ergot alkaloids in the third stage of labour significantly decreased mean blood loss (weighted mean difference −83.03 ml, 95% confidence interval (CI) −99.39 to −66.66 ml) and postpartum haemorrhage of at least 500 ml (relative risk (RR) 0.38, 95% CI 0.21 to 0.69). The risk of retained placenta or manual removal of the placenta, or both, was inconsistent. Ergot alkaloids increased the risk of vomiting (RR 11.81, 95% CI 1.78 to 78.28), elevation of blood pressure (RR 2.60, 95% CI 1.03 to 6.57) and pain after birth requiring analgesia (RR 2.53, 95% CI 1.34 to 4.78). One study compared oral ergometrine with placebo and showed no significant benefit of ergometrine over placebo. No maternal adverse effects were reported. There were no included trials that compared different administration regimens of ergot alkaloids.

AUTHORS' CONCLUSIONS: Prophylactic intramuscular or intravenous injections of ergot alkaloids are effective in reducing blood loss and postpartum haemorrhage, but adverse effects include vomiting, elevation of blood pressure and pain after birth requiring analgesia, particularly with the intravenous route of administration.

PROSTAGLANDINS FOR PREVENTING POSTPARTUM HAEMORRHAGE: misoprostol may reduce postpartum haemorrhage when other uterotonics are not available, but was less effective than conventional uterotonics. (Gülmezoglu AM, Forna F, Villar J, Hofmeyr GJ) CD000494 (in RHL 11)

BACKGROUND: Prostaglandins have mainly been used for postpartum haemorrhage (PPH) when other measures fail. Misoprostol, a new and inexpensive prostaglandin E1 analogue, has been suggested as an alternative for routine management of the third stage of labour.

OBJECTIVES: To assess the effects of prophylactic prostaglandin use in the third stage of labour.

METHODS: Standard PCG methods (see page xvii). Search date: February 2007.

MAIN RESULTS: 37 misoprostol and nine intramuscular prostaglandin trials (42 621 women) were included. Oral (seven trials, 2849 women) or sublingual misoprostol (relative risk (RR) 0.66; 95% confidence interval (CI) 0.45 to 0.98; one trial, 661 women) compared to placebo may be effective in reducing severe PPH and blood transfusion (RR 0.31; 95% CI 0.10 to 0.94; five oral misoprostol trials, 3519 women).

The severe PPH analysis of oral misoprostol trials was not totalled due to significant heterogeneity.

Compared to conventional injectable uterotonics, oral misoprostol was associated with higher risk of severe PPH (RR 1.32; 95% CI 1.16 to 1.51; 16 trials, 29 042 women) and use of additional uterotonics but with fewer blood transfusions (RR 0.81; 95% CI 0.64 to 1.02; 15 trials, 27 858 women). Additional uterotonic data were not totalled due to heterogeneity. Misoprostol use is associated with significant increases in shivering and a temperature of 38°C.

There are scarce data comparing injectable prostaglandins with the conventional injectable uterotonics on severe PPH and the use of additional uterotonics, the primary outcomes of this review

AUTHORS' CONCLUSIONS: Misoprostol orally or sublingually at a dose of 600 mcg shows promising results when compared to placebo in reducing blood loss after delivery. The margin of benefit may be affected by whether other components of management of the third stage of labour are used or not. As side-effects are dose-related, research should be directed towards establishing the lowest effective dose for routine use, and the optimal route of administration. Neither intramuscular prostaglandins nor misoprostol are preferable to conventional injectable uterotonics as part of the management of the third stage of labour, especially for low-risk women.

OXYTOCIN AGONISTS FOR PREVENTING POSTPARTUM HAEMORRHAGE: not enough data to provide reliable evidence. (Su LL, Chong YS, Samuel M) CD005457

BACKGROUND: Postpartum haemorrhage (PPH) is one of the major contributors to maternal mortality and morbidity worldwide. Active management of the third stage of labour has been proven to be effective in the prevention of PPH. Syntometrine is more effective than oxytocin but is associated with more side-effects. Carbetocin, a long-acting oxytocin agonist, appears to be a promising agent for the prevention of PPH.

OBJECTIVES: To determine if the use of oxytocin agonist is as effective as conventional uterotonic agents for the prevention of PPH, and assess the best routes of administration and optimal doses of oxytocin agonist.

METHODS: Standard PCG methods (see page xvii). Search date: September 2006.

MAIN RESULTS: Four studies (1037 women) were included in the review (three studies on caesarean delivery and one on vaginal delivery). The risk of PPH was similar in both oxytocin and carbetocin arms for participants who underwent caesarean delivery as well as participants, with risk factor(s) for PPH, who underwent vaginal delivery. Use of carbetocin resulted in a statistically significant reduction in the need for therapeutic uterotonic agent (relative risk (RR) 0.44, 95% confidence interval (CI) 0.25 to 0.78) compared to oxytocin for those who underwent caesarean section, but not for vaginal delivery. Carbetocin is also associated with a reduced need for uterine massage in both caesarean and vaginal deliveries (RR 0.38, 95% CI 0.18 to 0.80; RR 0.70, 95% CI 0.51 to 0.94) respectively. However, this outcome measure was only documented in one study on caesarean delivery and in the only study on vaginal delivery. Pooled data from the trials did not reveal any statistically significant differences in terms of the adverse effects between carbetocin and oxytocin.

AUTHORS' CONCLUSIONS: There is insufficient evidence that 100 micrograms of intravenous carbetocin is as effective as oxytocin to prevent PPH. In comparison to oxytocin, carbetocin was associated with reduced need for additional uterotonic agents, and uterine massage. There was limited comparative evidence on adverse events.

CORD TRACTION VERSUS FUNDAL PRESSURE FOR THE THIRD STAGE OF LABOUR: no data to provide reliable evidence. (Peña-Martí G, Comunián-Carrasco G) CD005462

BACKGROUND: There are two basic interventions to help to deliver the placenta as part of the active management of the third stage of labour: (1) fundal pressure, and (2) controlled traction on the umbilical cord. Both of these methods may, in addition, have adverse outcomes. Fundal pressure may interrupt the process of placental detachment and cause pain, haemorrhage or uterine inversion, and controlled cord traction, if undertaken before placental separation or without prior administration of a uterotonic drug, may have similar adverse effects. The obstetric clinical practice on this issue is not standardised.

OBJECTIVES: To determine the efficacy of fundal pressure versus controlled cord traction as part of the active management of the third stage of labour.

METHODS: Standard PCG methods (see page xvii). Search date: June 2007

MAIN RESULTS: The search strategies yielded five studies for consideration of inclusion. However, none of these studies fulfilled the requirements for inclusion in this review.

AUTHORS' CONCLUSIONS: We identified no randomised controlled trials comparing the efficacy of fundal pressure versus controlled cord traction as part of the active management of the third stage of labour. Hence controlled cord traction, after awaiting signs of placental separation, should remain the third component of the active management of third stage of labour, and follow the routine administration of a uterotonic drug and cord clamping.

EFFECT OF TIMING OF UMBILICAL CORD CLAMPING OF TERM INFANTS ON MATERNAL AND NEONATAL OUTCOMES: (McDonald SJ, Abbott JM) Protocol [*see* page xviii] CD004074

ABRIDGED BACKGROUND: There are two contrasting approaches to managing the third stage of labour, active management and expectant or physiological management.

In an active management strategy the umbilical cord is usually clamped shortly following birth of the infant. Delaying clamping allows time for a transfer of the fetal blood in the placenta to the infant at the time of birth; placental transfusion. The suggested neonatal benefits associated with this increased placental transfusion with delayed cord clamping include higher haematocrit and haemoglobin levels, additional iron stores and less anaemia later in infancy, higher red blood cell flow to vital organs, better cardiopulmonary adaptation and increased duration of early breastfeeding.

It has also been argued that the increased placental transfusion can be a disadvantage, causing an excess of red blood cells (polycythaemia), and/or an abnormal increase in the volume of circulating fluid in the body. There is some concern that such increases in blood volume and the amount of red blood cells could result in overload of the heart and respiratory difficulties.

OBJECTIVES: The objective of this review is to determine the maternal and neonatal effects of different strategies for the timing of umbilical cord clamping of term infants during the third stage of labour.

> **TIMING OF PROPHYLACTIC OXYTOCICS FOR THE THIRD STAGE OF LABOUR AFTER VAGINAL BIRTH:** (Soltani H, Dickinson) Protocol [see page xviii] CD006173

ABRIDGED BACKGROUND: The delivery of the placenta after childbirth can be a critical stage in relation to maternal and neonatal well-being. The routine prophylactic use of oxytocics such as oxytocin or combined oxytocin/ergometrine (syntometrine) has been shown to reduce the risk of postpartum haemorrhage (PPH). The timing of the administration of oxytocic drugs, however, varies greatly among practitioners. The main recommended approach in the active management is to administer relevant drugs at the delivery of the anterior shoulder. This, however, can make the process complicated in many busy maternity units and increases the demand for having more than one healthcare professional present at the time of birth. In the practical setting, many clinicians use oxytocics immediately after the birth of the baby. There are others who administer the oxytocic drugs at the crowning of the head or even after the delivery of the placenta. The timing of oxytocic drugs can potentially impact on the blood perfusion to the baby and on the amount of maternal blood loss at the time of delivery.

OBJECTIVES: To assess the specific effect of the timing of administration of prophylactic oxytocics as part of the active management on the progress of the third stage of labour.

> **UMBILICAL VEIN INJECTION FOR THE ROUTINE MANAGEMENT OF THIRD STAGE OF LABOUR:** (Nardin JM, Carroli G, Weeks AD, Mori R) Protocol [see page xviii] CD006176

ABRIDGED BACKGROUND: Among the different causes of maternal death, haemorrhage alone is responsible for at least 25% of these deaths, with the majority due to postpartum haemorrhage (PPH). Umbilical (or intraumbilical) vein injection (UVI, IUVI) for the *treatment* of retained placenta was first described by Mojon and Asdrubali in 1826.

Routine umbilical vein injection has been suggested as an alternative way of managing the third stage of labour, as it directs the treatment to the placental bed and uterine wall, resulting in an earlier uterine contraction and placental separation. It also allows higher doses to be used, and a reduction of systemic side-effects. Balanced against this is a need for training in the technique and a possible higher cost of materials.

OBJECTIVES: The objective of this review is to compare, from the best available evidence, the effects of umbilical vein injection of a saline solution alone or with any uterotonic drug versus an alternative solution with or without any other uterotonic agent or expectant management or any other method for routine management of the third stage of labour, on maternal and perinatal outcomes. We will only consider management of third stage of labour when the umbilical vein injection is administered within 15 minutes after the delivery of the baby.

Additional subgroup analyses for the main outcomes will be based on the following characteristics:

1) total volume administered;
2) volume of oxytocin administered;
3) method of injection (catheter, syringe, milked, etc).

UTERINE MASSAGE FOR PREVENTING POSTPARTUM HAEMOR-RHAGE: (Hofmeyr GJ, Abdel-Aleem H) Protocol [*see* page xviii] CD006431

ABRIDGED BACKGROUND: Postpartum haemorrhage (PPH) (bleeding from the genital tract after childbirth) is a major cause of maternal mortality and disability, particularly in under-resourced areas. Uterine atony, when the uterus fails to contract after delivery, is the most important cause of primary PPH. Uterine massage involves placing a hand on the woman's lower abdomen and stimulating the uterus by repetitive massaging or squeezing movements. Massage is thought to stimulate uterine contraction, possibly through stimulation of local prostaglandin release and thus to reduce haemorrhage. However, it is not done routinely after delivery in a systematic way. If shown to be effective, it would have important advantages as it is inexpensive and requires no access to medication or other specialized services, and could be used in any location in which women give birth. Disadvantages include the use of staff time, and discomfort caused to women. However, there is very little empirical research to evaluate the effectiveness of this method.

OBJECTIVES: To determine the effectiveness of uterine massage after birth and before and/or after delivery of the placenta to reduce postpartum blood loss and associated morbidity and mortality.

⊗ **EARLY VERSUS DELAYED UMBILICAL CORD CLAMPING IN PRETERM INFANTS:** increased neonatal blood transfusions and intraventricular haemorrhage. (Rabe H, Reynolds G, Diaz-Rossello J) CD003248 (in RHL 11)

BACKGROUND: Optimal timing for clamping of the umbilical cord at birth is unclear. Early clamping allows for immediate resuscitation of the newborn. Delaying clamping may facilitate transfusion of blood between the placenta and the baby.

OBJECTIVES: To delineate the short- and long-term effects for infants born at less than 37 completed weeks' gestation, and their mothers, of early compared to delayed clamping of the umbilical cord at birth.

METHODS: Standard PCG methods (see page xvii). Search date: February 2004. Randomized controlled trials comparing early with delayed (30 seconds or more) clamping of the umbilical cord for infants born before 37 completed weeks' gestation.

MAIN RESULTS: Seven studies (297 infants) were eligible for inclusion. The maximum delay in cord clamping was 120 seconds. Delayed cord clamping was associated with fewer transfusions for anaemia (three trials, 111 infants; relative risk (RR) 2.01, 95% CI 1.24 to 3.27) or low blood pressure (two trials, 58 infants; RR 2.58, 95% CI 1.17 to 5.67) and less intraventricular haemorrhage (five trials, 225 infants; RR 1.74, 95% CI 1.08 to 2.81) than early clamping.

AUTHORS' CONCLUSIONS: Delaying cord clamping by 30 to 120 seconds, rather than early clamping, seems to be associated with less need for transfusion and less intraventricular haemorrhage. There are no clear differences in other outcomes.

☺ **PLACENTAL CORD DRAINAGE AFTER SPONTANEOUS VAGINAL DELIVERY AS PART OF THE MANAGEMENT OF THE THIRD STAGE OF LABOUR:** reduced the duration of the third stage of labour. (Soltani H, Dickinson F, Symonds I) CD004665

BACKGROUND: Cord drainage in the third stage of labour involves unclamping the previously clamped and separated umbilical cord and allowing the blood from the placenta to drain freely into an appropriate receptacle. Currently there are no systematic reviews of the effects of placental cord drainage on the management of the third stage of labour.

OBJECTIVES: To assess the specific effects of placental cord drainage on the third stage of labour, with or without the prophylactic use of oxytocics.

METHODS: Standard PCG methods (see page xvii). Search date: July 2005.

MAIN RESULTS: Two studies met our inclusion criteria in terms of quality and relevance. Cord drainage could impact the third stage of labour as the results show a statistically significant reduction in the length of third stage of labour (one trial, n = 147, weighted mean difference (minutes) −5.46, 95% confidence interval (CI) −8.02 to −2.90). In the incidence of retained placenta at 30 minutes after birth (one trial, n = 477, relative risk 0.28, 95% CI 0.10 to 0.73) a significant difference was found, but this should be interpreted with caution due to potential intervention bias.

AUTHORS' CONCLUSIONS: It is difficult to draw conclusions from such a small number of studies, especially where the review outcomes were presented in a variety of formats. However, there does appear to be some potential benefit from the use of placental cord drainage in terms of reducing the length of the third stage of labour. More research is required to investigate the impact of cord drainage on the management of the third stage of labour.

TOPICAL UMBILICAL CORD CARE AT BIRTH: had no clear benefits in high income settings; there was insufficient evidence from low-income settings. (Zupan J, Garner P, Omari AAA) CD001057 (in RHL 11)

BACKGROUND: Umbilical cord infection caused many neonatal deaths before aseptic techniques were used.

OBJECTIVES: To assess the effects of topical cord care in preventing cord infection, illness and death.

METHODS: Standard PCG methods (see page xvii). Search date: September 2003.

MAIN RESULTS: 21 studies (8959 participants) were included, the majority of which were from high-income countries. No systemic infections or deaths were observed in any of the studies reviewed. No difference was demonstrated between cords treated with antiseptics compared with dry cord care or placebo. There was a trend to reduced colonization with antibiotics compared to topical antiseptics and no treatment. Antiseptics prolonged the time to cord separation. Use of antiseptics was associated with a reduction in maternal concern about the cord.

AUTHORS' CONCLUSIONS: Good trials in low-income settings are warranted. In high-income settings, there is limited research which has not shown an advantage of antibiotics or antiseptics over simply keeping the cord clean. Quality of evidence is low.

7.3 Pain during labour

Approaches and attitudes to the pain of labour vary greatly between both caregivers and individual women. Some women see the pain of labour as part of a natural process and are motivated to cope with this pain without 'artificial' help; others prefer medical methods of analgesia.

7.3.1 Non-pharmacological methods of pain relief in labour

In the last century, several philosophies of pain control evolved, such as strategies to break the cycle of fear/tension/pain; relaxation techniques; visualisation techniques; and psychoprophylaxis. Methods shown to reduce the perception of pain covered elsewhere in this book include companionship (page 255); immersion in water (page 258); and upright posture (page 257).

COMPLEMENTARY AND ALTERNATIVE THERAPIES FOR PAIN MANAGEMENT IN LABOUR: labour pain appeared reduced by acupuncture and hypnotherapy; not by aromatherapy, music or audio-analgesia. (Smith CA, Collins CT, Cyna AM, Crowther CA) CD003521

BACKGROUND: Many women would like to avoid pharmacological or invasive methods of pain management in labour and this may contribute towards the popularity of complementary methods of pain management. This review examined currently available evidence supporting the use of alternative and complementary therapies for pain management in labour.

OBJECTIVES: To examine the effectiveness of complementary and alternative therapies for pain management in labour on maternal and perinatal morbidity.

METHODS: Standard PCG methods (see page xvii). Search date: February 2006.

MAIN RESULTS: Fourteen trials were included in the review with data reporting on 1537 women using different modalities of pain management; 1448 women were included in the meta-analysis. Three trials involved acupuncture (n = 496), one audio-analgesia (n = 24), two trials acupressure (n = 172), one aromatherapy (n = 22), five trials hypnosis (n = 729), one trial of massage (n = 60), and relaxation (n = 34). The trials of acupuncture showed a decreased need for pain relief (relative risk (RR) 0.70, 95% confidence interval (CI) 0.49 to 1.00, two trials 288 women). Women taught self-hypnosis had decreased requirements for pharmacological analgesia (RR 0.53, 95% CI 0.36 to 0.79, five trials 749 women) including epidural analgesia (RR 0.30, 95% CI 0.22 to 0.40) and were more satisfied with their pain management in labour compared with controls (RR 2.33, 95% CI 1.15 to 4.71, one trial). No differences were seen for women receiving aromatherapy, or audio-analgesia.

AUTHORS' CONCLUSIONS: Acupuncture and hypnosis may be beneficial for the management of pain during labour; however, the number of women studied has been small. Few other complementary therapies have been subjected to proper scientific study.

TRANSCUTANEOUS ELECTRICAL NERVE STIMULATION FOR PAIN RELIEF IN LABOUR: (Johnston RV, Burrows E, Merrin MIJ, Burrows R) Protocol [see page xviii] CD003578

ABRIDGED BACKGROUND: Transcutaneous electrical nerve stimulation (TENS) is a non-invasive technique that applies non-painful low-voltage electrical stimulation via cutaneous electrodes to treat pain arising from several conditions including surgical pain, back pain, arthritis, neuropathic pain, menstrual pain and labour. As TENS is non-invasive, there may be expected to be few adverse events associated with its use and an advantage may be that the woman in labour has some control over the intensity and frequency of the stimulations used.

OBJECTIVES: To determine the effectiveness and safety of TENS in reducing labour pain.

BIOFEEDBACK FOR PAIN DURING LABOUR: (Barragan Loayza IM, Gonzales F) Protocol [see page xviii] CD006168

ABRIDGED BACKGROUND: Pain experienced by pregnant women during labour is caused by contractions of the uterus, dilatation of the cervix and, at the end of the first stage and during the second stage of labour, by vaginal and pelvic floor dilatation to accommodate the baby. Pain, however, is not simply a consequence of the physiological process of delivery. Instead, pain during labour is a result of a complex and subjective interaction of multiple factors (psychological, social, physiological and spiritual), which are related to the personal interpretation each woman may give to the feelings and physical stimuli they experience during labour and delivery. Biofeedback or biological feedback encompasses a therapeutic technique by which individuals receive training to improve their health and wellbeing through signals coming from their own bodies (temperature, heart rate, muscular tension, etc). The underlying principle is that changes in thoughts and emotions may result in changes in body functioning. It consists of an alternative treatment that aims to gain control over physiological responses with the aid of electronic instruments, under the supervision of experts in biofeedback technique. Participants are trained to be able to modify a body function by trial and error using continuous feedback by means of what is known as a 'directed learning process'.

OBJECTIVES: To examine the effectiveness of the use of biofeedback in prenatal lessons for managing pain during labour.

7.3.2 *Pharmacological methods of pain relief in labour*

'We are having the baby and we shall have the chloroform' Queen Victoria, 1853. In Bennion E. *Antique Medical instruments*. Berkeley, California: University of California Press, 1979: 15.

☻ **EPIDURAL VERSUS NON-EPIDURAL OR NO ANALGESIA IN LABOUR:** improved pain relief; but increased instrumental births. (Anim-Somuah M, Smyth R, Howell C) CD000331

BACKGROUND: Epidural analgesia is a central nerve block technique achieved by injection of a local anaesthetic close to the nerves that transmits pain and is widely used as a form of pain relief in labour. However, there are concerns regarding unintended adverse effects on the mother and infant.

OBJECTIVES: To assess the effects of all modalities of epidural analgesia (including combined spinal-epidural) on the mother and the baby, when compared with non-epidural or no pain relief during labour.

METHODS: Standard PCG methods (see page xvii). Search date: June 2005.

MAIN RESULTS: 21 studies involving 6664 women were included; all but one study compared epidural analgesia with opiates. For technical reasons, data on women's perception of pain relief in labour could only be included from one study which found epidural analgesia to offer better pain relief than non-epidural analgesia (weighted mean difference (WMD) −2.60, 95% confidence interval (CI) −3.82 to −1.38, one trial, 105 women). However, epidural analgesia was associated with an increased risk of instrumental vaginal birth (relative risk (RR) 1.38, 95% CI 1.24 to 1.53, 17 trials, 6162 women). There was no evidence of a significant difference in the risk of caesarean delivery (RR 1.07, 95% CI 0.93 to 1.23, 20 trials, 6534 women), long-term backache (RR 1.00, 95% CI 0.89 to 1.12, two trials, 814 women), low neonatal Apgar scores at five minutes (RR 0.70, 95% CI 0.44 to 1.10, 14 trials, 5363 women) and maternal satisfaction with pain relief (RR 1.18 95% CI 0.92 to 1.50, five trials, 1940 women). No studies reported on rare but potentially serious adverse effects of epidural analgesia.

AUTHORS' CONCLUSIONS: Epidural analgesia appears to be effective in reducing pain during labour. However, women who use this form of pain relief are at increased risk of having an instrumental delivery. Epidural analgesia had no statistically significant impact on the risk of caesarean section, maternal satisfaction with pain relief and long-term backache and did not appear to have an immediate effect on neonatal status as determined by Apgar scores. Further research may be helpful to evaluate rare but potentially severe adverse effects of epidural analgesia on women in labour and long-term neonatal outcomes.

☺ **COMBINED SPINAL-EPIDURAL VERSUS EPIDURAL ANALGE-SIA IN LABOUR:** produced quicker effect and more pruritis; no difference in maternal satisfaction. (Simmons SW, Cyna AM, Dennis AT, Hughes D) CD003401

BACKGROUND: Traditional epidural techniques have been associated with prolonged labour, use of oxytocin augmentation, and increased incidence of instrumental vaginal delivery. The combined spinal-epidural (CSE) technique has been introduced in an attempt to reduce these adverse effects. CSE is believed to improve maternal mobility during labour and provide more rapid onset of analgesia than epidural analgesia, which could contribute to increased maternal satisfaction.

OBJECTIVES: To assess the relative effects of CSE versus epidural analgesia during labour.

METHODS: Standard PCG methods (see page xvii). Search date: December 2006.

MAIN RESULTS: 19 trials (2658 women) met our inclusion criteria. 26 outcomes in two sets of comparisons involving CSE versus traditional epidurals and CSE versus low-dose epidural techniques were analysed. Of the CSE versus traditional epidural analyses only three outcomes showed a difference. CSE was more favourable in relation to need for rescue analgesia and urinary retention, but associated with more pruritus.

For CSE versus low-dose epidurals, four outcomes were statistically significant. CSE had a faster onset of effective analgesia from time of injection but was associated with more pruritus. CSE was also associated with a clinically non-significant lower umbilical arterial pH.

No differences between CSE and epidural were seen for maternal satisfaction, mobilisation in labour, modes of birth, incidence of post dural puncture headache or blood patch and maternal hypotension. It was not possible to draw any conclusions with respect to maternal respiratory depression, maternal sedation and need for labour augmentation.

AUTHORS' CONCLUSIONS: There appears to be little basis for offering CSE over epidurals in labour, with no difference in overall maternal satisfaction despite a slightly faster onset with CSE and less pruritus with epidurals. There is no difference in ability to mobilise, obstetric

outcome or neonatal outcome. However, the significantly higher incidence of urinary retention and rescue interventions with traditional techniques would favour the use of low-dose epidurals. It is not possible to draw any meaningful conclusions regarding rare complications such as nerve injury and meningitis.

⊗ **DISCONTINUATION OF EPIDURAL ANALGESIA LATE IN LABOUR FOR REDUCING THE ADVERSE DELIVERY OUTCOMES ASSOCIATED WITH EPIDURAL ANALGESIA:** increased the rate of inadequate pain relief without clear benefits. (Torvaldsen S, Roberts CL, Bell JC, Raynes-Greenow CH) CD004457

BACKGROUND: Although epidural analgesia provides the most effective labour analgesia, it is associated with some adverse obstetric consequences, including an increased risk of instrumental delivery. Many centres discontinue epidural analgesia late in labour to improve a woman's ability to push and reduce the rate of instrumental delivery.

OBJECTIVES: To assess the impact of discontinuing epidural analgesia late in labour on:

 i) rates of instrumental deliveries and other delivery outcomes; and
ii) analgesia and satisfaction with labour care.

METHODS: Standard PCG methods (see page xvii). Search date: October 2007.

MAIN RESULTS: We identified six studies, of which five were included (462 participants). Three of these were high quality studies whilst the other two were judged to be of lower quality because placebo was not used and the method of randomisation not described. All studies used different epidural analgesia protocols (type of drug, dosage or method of administration). Overall, the reduction in instrumental delivery rate was not statistically significant (23% versus 28%, RR 0.84, 95% confidence interval (CI) 0.61 to 1.15) nor was there any statistically significant difference in rates of other delivery outcomes. The only statistically significant result was an increase in inadequate pain relief when the epidural was stopped (22% versus 6%, RR 3.68, 95% CI 1.99 to 6.80).

AUTHORS' CONCLUSIONS: There is insufficient evidence to support the hypothesis that discontinuing epidural analgesia late in labour

reduces the rate of instrumental delivery. There is evidence that it increases the rate of inadequate pain relief in the second stage of labour. The practice of discontinuing epidurals is widespread and the size of the reduction in instrumental delivery rate could be clinically important; therefore, we recommend a larger study than those included in this review be undertaken to determine whether this effect is real or has occurred by chance, and to provide stronger evidence about the safety aspects.

PROPHYLACTIC INTRAVENOUS PRELOADING FOR REGIONAL ANALGESIA IN LABOUR: reduced hypotension and fetal heart rate abnormalities for high-dose epidurals, not for low-dose or combined spinal-epidurals. (Hofmeyr GJ, Cyna AM, Middleton P) CD000175

BACKGROUND: Reduced uterine blood flow from maternal hypotension may contribute to fetal heart rate changes which are common following regional analgesia (epidural or spinal or combined spinal-epidural (CSE)) during labour. Intravenous fluid preloading may help to reduce maternal hypotension but using lower doses of local anaesthetic, and opioid only blocks, may reduce the need for preloading.

OBJECTIVES: To assess the effects of prophylactic intravenous fluid preloading before regional analgesia during labour on maternal and fetal well-being.

METHODS: Standard PCG methods (see page xvii). Search date: February 2004.

MAIN RESULTS: Six studies are included (473 participants). In one epidural trial using high-dose local anaesthetic, preloading with intravenous fluids was shown to counteract the hypotension which frequently follows traditional epidural analgesia (relative risk (RR) 0.07, 95% confidence interval (CI) 0.01 to 0.53; 102 women). This trial was also associated with a reduction in fetal heart rate abnormalities (RR 0.36, 95% CI 0.16 to 0.83; 102 women); no differences were detected in other perinatal and maternal outcomes for this trial and another high-dose epidural trial. In the two epidural low-dose anaesthetic trials, no significant difference in maternal hypotension was found (RR 0.73, 95% CI 0.36 to 1.48; 260 women), although they were underpowered to detect less than a very large effect. No significant differences were seen between groups in these trials for fetal heart rate abnormalities (RR 0.64, 95% CI 0.39 to 1.05; 233 women).

In the two CSE trials, no differences were reported between preloading and no preloading groups. In the spinal/opioid trial the RR for hypotension was 0.89 (95% CI 0.43 to 1.83; 40 women) and was 0.70, (95% CI 0.36 to 1.37; 32 women) for fetal heart rate abnormalities. In the opioid only study (30 women), there were no instances of hypotension or fetal heart rate abnormalities in either group.

AUTHORS' CONCLUSIONS: Preloading prior to traditional high-dose local anaesthetic blocks may have some beneficial fetal and maternal effects in healthy women. Low-dose epidural and CSE analgesia techniques may reduce the need for preloading. The studies reviewed were too small to show whether preloading is beneficial for women having regional analgesia during labour using the lower-dose local anaesthetics or opioids. Further investigation of low-dose epidural or CSE (including opioid only) blocks, and the risks and benefits of intravenous preloading for women with pregnancy complications, is required.

7.4   Slow progress during labour

The duration of the latent phase of labour, and whether or when to intervene, is poorly defined, in part because of difficulty in pinpointing the time of onset of labour. The active phase of rapid cervical dilation is more clearly defined. Progress may be assessed by plotting cervical dilation in cm and descent of the head in fifths above the pelvic brim, against time in hours on a labour graph (partogram). When progress is slow, this may be a sign of ineffective uterine contractions or that the baby is possibly too big for the pelvis (fetopelvic disproportion).

7.4.1   Ineffective uterine contractions

Uterine contractions may be 'augmented' by rupturing the amniotic membranes (if HIV infection has been excluded) or by administering uteritonics (drugs that stimulate contractions of the uterus) such as oxytocin. For women having a second or subsequent baby there is reason for caution, as slow progress is less likely to be due to inadequate uterine activity, and rupture of the uterus is more common.

> **AMNIOTOMY FOR SHORTENING SPONTANEOUS LABOUR:** did not improve labour outcomes. (Smyth RMD, Alldred SK, Markham C) CD006167

BACKGROUND: Intentional artificial rupture of the amniotic membranes during labour, sometimes called amniotomy or 'breaking of the waters', is one of the most commonly performed procedures in modern obstetric and midwifery practice. The primary aim of amniotomy is to speed up contractions and, therefore, shorten the length of labour. However, there are concerns regarding unintended adverse effects on the woman and baby.

OBJECTIVES: To determine the effectiveness and safety of amniotomy alone for (1) routinely shortening all labours that start spontaneously, and (2) shortening labours that have started spontaneously, but have become prolonged.

METHODS: Standard PCG methods (see page xvii). Search date: March 2007.

MAIN RESULTS: We have included 14 studies in this review, involving 4893 women. There was no evidence of any statistical difference in length of first stage of labour (weighted mean difference −20.43 minutes, 95% confidence interval (CI) −95.93 to 55.06), maternal satisfaction with childbirth experience (standardised mean difference 0.27, 95% CI −0.49 to 1.04) or low Apgar score less than seven at five minutes (RR 0.55, 95% CI 0.29 to 1.05). Amniotomy was associated with an increased risk of delivery by caesarean section compared to women in the control group, although the difference was not statistically significant (RR 1.26, 95% CI 0.98 to 1.62).

There was no consistency between papers regarding the timing of amniotomy during labour in terms of cervical dilatation.

AUTHORS' CONCLUSIONS: On the basis of the findings of this review, we cannot recommend that amniotomy should be introduced routinely as part of standard labour management and care. We do recommend that the evidence presented in this review should be made available to women offered an amniotomy and may be useful as a foundation for discussion and any resulting decisions made between women and their caregivers.

EARLY AMNIOTOMY AND EARLY OXYTOCIN FOR DELAY IN FIRST STAGE SPONTANEOUS LABOR COMPARED WITH ROUTINE CARE: (Wei SQ, Wo BL, Xu HR, Roy C, Turcot L, Fraser WD). Protocol [see page xviii] CD006794

ABRIDGED BACKGROUND: Caesarean section rates are over 20% in many developed countries. The main diagnosis contributing to this increase is dystocia or prolonged labor. The Active Management of Labor is a clinical protocol that was designed to facilitate the organization of obstetrical care in a busy labor ward. Active Management includes: selective admission to the labor ward; selective use of electronic fetal monitoring; early intervention with amniotomy and oxytocin for delay in labor progress; routine use of a simplified 1cm/hr partogram to guide clinical decision making; and continuous professional support. As dystocia is primarily a problem of women who are in their first labor, Active Management focuses on nulliparous women. To date, there is no consensus with respect to the timing of amniotomy and oxytocin administration in the presence of a labor delay. Early intervention is not without its risks. Uterine hyperstimulation and fetal heart rate abnormalities may result from oxytocin and amniotomy.

OBJECTIVES: 1) To estimate the effects of early augmentation with amniotomy plus oxytocin on the cesarean birth rate and on indicators of maternal and neonatal morbidity, in women whose labor is abnormally delayed. 2) To evaluate the effects of routine early augmentation with amniotomy plus oxytocin on the cesarean birth rate and on indicators of maternal and neonatal morbidity.

USE OF INTRA-UTERINE PRESSURE CATHETER (IUPC) VERSUS EXTERNAL TOCODYNAMOMETRY (TOCO) DURING LABOUR FOR REDUCING ADVERSE OUTCOMES: (Bakker JJH, Janssen PF, Mol BWJ, Papatsonis D, van Lith JMM, van der Post JAM) Protocol [see page xviii] CD006947

ABRIDGED BACKGROUND: During induction, or augmentation, of labour in pregnant women with intravenous oxytocin, uterine activity can be monitored by external tocodynamometry (TOCO) or by the use of an intra-uterine pressure catheter (IUPC). Reducing the risk of hyperstimulation and thus fetal hypoxia by accurate measurement of contractions could lead to a reduction in fetal and maternal morbidity. Some argue that the use of an IUPC might facilitate the clinical diagnosis of uterine rupture because one might expect that the pressure inside the uterine cavity lowers when the uterine wall is ruptured. The value of IUPC is questioned by the possibility of infrequent but potentially hazardous risks.

OBJECTIVES: To evaluate the effectiveness of an intra-uterine pressure catheter when intravenous oxytocin is used for induction or augmentation of labour compared with the effect of using external tocodynamometry.

7.4.2   Diagnosis of fetopelvic disproportion

In previous decades, considerable attention was paid to efforts to diagnose fetopelvic disproportion before labour. Screening methods included the mother's height and shoe size, and diagnostic methods included assessment of the size of the mother's pelvis and the baby, either clinically or with X-rays, ultrasound, computed tomography or magnetic resonance imaging. However, static measurements are unable to account for the dynamics of labour, including the efficiency of uterine contractions and the orientation and moulding of the baby's head. In practice, fetopelvic disproportion is suspected when slow progress of labour is accompanied by the development of caput succedaneum and moulding of the baby's head, or there is blood in the urine.

The definition of slow progress of the second stage of labour is controversial. Traditionally, the second stage was regarded as prolonged after 60 minutes in first time mothers and 30 minutes in multiparous women. More recently longer durations of second stage have been allowed provided fetal heart rate monitoring is reassuring, particularly in women with epidural analgesia.

⊗ **PELVIMETRY FOR FETAL CEPHALIC PRESENTATIONS AT OR NEAR TERM:** x-ray pelvimetry increased caesarean section rates. (Pattinson RC, Farrell E) CD000161

BACKGROUND: Pelvimetry assesses the size of a woman's pelvis aiming to predict whether she will be able to deliver or not. This can be done by clinical examination or by conventional x-rays, computerised tomography scanning, or magnetic resonance imaging.
OBJECTIVES: To assess the effects of pelvimetry (performed antenatally, intrapartum or postpartum) on the method of delivery, and on perinatal mortality and morbidity, and on maternal morbidity.
METHODS: Standard PCG methods (see page xvii). Search date: June 2007.

MAIN RESULTS: Four trials of over 1000 women were included. All used x-ray pelvimetry to assess the pelvis. The trials were generally not of good quality. Women undergoing x-ray pelvimetry were more likely to be delivered by caesarean section (odds ratio 2.17, 95% confidence interval 1.63 to 2.88). No significant impact was detected on perinatal outcome.

AUTHORS' CONCLUSIONS: There is not enough evidence to support the use of x-ray pelvimetry in women whose fetuses have a cephalic presentation.

7.4.3 Management of fetopelvic disproportion

When progress of the presenting part of the baby is delayed, this can usually be overcome with forceps or vacuum extraction (see page xvii), or caesarean section. On the other hand, obstruction of a partly born baby, such as in shoulder dystocia or entrapped aftercoming head during breech birth, may be catastrophic.

Strategies to assist delivery include, encouragement, support and positioning of the mother, and episiotomy (see page 264). Fundal pressure (the Kristellar manoeuvre) is both widely used and condemned as dangerous.

In low-resource settings without safe caesarean section facilities, the only option for management of fetopelvic disproportion may be symphysiotomy, or if the baby has died a destructive procedure such as craniotomy. For obstructed aftercoming head in a breech birth, symphysiotomy may be life-saving.

> **SYMPHYSIOTOMY FOR FETO-PELVIC DISPROPORTION:** (Hofmeyr GJ, Shweni PM) Protocol [*see* page xviii] CD005299

ABRIDGED BACKGROUND: Symphysiotomy is an operation in which fibres of the symphysis pubis are divided with a scalpel using local analgesic infiltration. This allows the pubic bones to separate, creating more space in the pelvis for the birth of the baby.

Symphysiotomy has come to be regarded as an unacceptable operation because of perceptions that complications for the mother are prohibitive, and the view that it is a 'second-class' operation used only in women from poor communities. Emotions and sensitivity to political correctness make it difficult to reach an objective evaluation of the benefits and risks of symphysiotomy.

When caesarean section is not available or unsafe, symphysiotomy may be life-saving for both mother and baby. Complications of the procedure have been reduced by improved operative techniques (such as partial rather than complete symphysiotomy) and postoperative care (early mobilisation).

The main indications for symphysiotomy are cephalo-pelvic disproportion with cephalic presentation and arrested aftercoming head of the breech. Symphysiotomy may be lifesaving for women too ill to survive caesarean section following neglected labour.

The contention that symphysiotomy is an unacceptable operation has seldom been based on the views of clients. A Nigerian survey of pregnant women's views in a region where symphysiotomy has been practised for many years and is well known among women found that 63% of women given the choice would prefer symphysiotomy to caesarean section.

OBJECTIVES: To determine, from the best available evidence, the relative benefits and risks of symphysiotomy in defined clinical situations, compared with alternative management; and the relative benefits and risks of alternative symphysiotomy techniques.

7.5   Shoulder dystocia

With increasing weight, the size of a baby's shoulders increases relative to the size of the head. Birth of a baby's head, usually with chubby cheeks, where the head is drawn back immovably against the mother's perineum and no further descent takes place, signifies shoulder dystocia. Quick, co-ordinated and skilful interventions are needed to achieve safe birth of the baby. Efforts may include hyperflexion of the mother's hips (McRobert's manouver); getting the mother to kneel (Gaskin manoeuvre); suprapubic pressure; posterior traction on the baby's head; delivery of the posterior arm; rotation of the posterior shoulder to anterior (Wood's method); delivery of the anterior shoulder, fracture of the clavicle or cephalic replacement with tocolysis and caesarean section (Zavanelli's method).

INTRAPARTUM INTERVENTIONS FOR PREVENTING SHOULDER DYSTOCIA: not enough data to provide reliable evidence. (Athukorala C, Middleton P, Crowther CA) CD005543

BACKGROUND: The early management of shoulder dystocia involves the administration of various manoeuvres which aim to relieve the dystocia by manipulating the fetal shoulders and increasing the functional size of the maternal pelvis.

OBJECTIVES: To assess the effects of prophylactic manoeuvres in preventing shoulder dystocia.

METHODS: Standard PCG methods (see page xvii). Search date: June 2006.

SELECTION CRITERIA: Randomised controlled trials comparing the prophylactic implementation of manoeuvres and maternal positioning with routine or standard care.

DATA COLLECTION AND ANALYSIS: Two review authors independently applied exclusion criteria, assessed trial quality and extracted data.

MAIN RESULTS: Two trials were included; one comparing the McRobert's manoeuvre and suprapubic pressure with no prophylactic manoeuvres in 185 women likely to give birth to a large baby and one trial comparing the use of the McRobert's manoeuvre versus lithotomy positioning in 40 women. We decided not to pool the results of the two trials. One study reported fifteen cases of shoulder dystocia in the therapeutic (control) group compared to five in the prophylactic group (relative risk (RR) 0.44, 95% confidence interval (CI) 0.17 to 1.14) and the other study reported one episode of shoulder dystocia in both prophylactic and lithotomy groups. In the first study, there were significantly more caesarean sections in the prophylactic group and when these were included in the results significantly fewer instances of shoulder dystocia were seen in the prophylactic group (RR 0.33, 95% CI 0.12 to 0.86). In this study, 13 women in the control group required therapeutic manoeuvres after delivery of the fetal head compared to three in the treatment group (RR 0.31, 95% CI 0.09 to 1.02).

One study reported no birth injuries or low Apgar scores recorded. In the other study, one infant in the control group had a brachial plexus injury (RR 0.44, 95% CI 0.02 to 10.61), and one infant had a five-minute Apgar score less than seven (RR 0.44, 95% CI 0.02 to 10.61).

AUTHORS' CONCLUSIONS: There are no clear findings to support or refute the use of prophylactic manoeuvres to prevent shoulder dystocia, although one study showed an increased rate of caesareans in the prophylactic group. Both included studies failed to address important maternal outcomes such as maternal injury, psychological outcomes and satisfaction with birth. Due to the low incidence of shoulder dystocia, trials with larger sample sizes investigating the use of such manoeuvres are required.

7.6   Abnormal presentations and positions of the baby

At the time of birth, most babies have actively assumed the position of 'best fit' in the uterine cavity: a longitudinal lie, vertex presentation and occipito-anterior position. Other orientations are less favourable: transverse or oblique lie, breech, brow, face or compound presentation, occipito-lateral or occipito-posterior position. They warrant investigation for possible causes such as abnormalities of the uterus, placenta praevia, increased or decreased volume of amniotic fluid, multiple pregnancy, and anomalies or inactivity of the baby. Several methods are used to correct the baby's position.

The most extensively evaluated technique for correcting malpresentations is external cephalic version for breech presentation (see below). For details of the procedure, see the video presentation 'External cephalic version: why and how': WHO Reproductive Health Library, www.rhllibrary.com.

CEPHALIC VERSION BY POSTURAL MANAGEMENT FOR BREECH PRESENTATION: not enough data to provide reliable evidence. (Hofmeyr GJ, Kulier R) CD000051 (in RHL 11)

BACKGROUND: Babies with breech presentation (bottom first) are at increased risk of complications during birth, and are often delivered by caesarean section. The chance of breech presentation persisting at the time of delivery, and the risk of caesarean section, can be reduced by external cephalic version (ECV – turning the baby by manual manipulation through the mother's abdomen). It is also possible that maternal posture may influence fetal position. Many postural techniques have been used to promote cephalic version.

OBJECTIVES: To assess the effects of postural management of breech presentation on measures of pregnancy outcome. Procedures in which the mother rests with her pelvis elevated were evaluated. These include the knee-chest position, and a supine position with the pelvis elevated with a wedge-shaped cushion.

METHODS: Standard PCG methods (see page xvii). Search date: September 2001.

MAIN RESULTS: Five studies involving a total of 392 women were included. No effect of postural management on the rate of non-cephalic births was detected, either for the sub-group in which no external cephalic version was attempted, or for the group overall (relative risk 0.95, 95% confidence interval 0.81 to 1.11). No differences were detected for caesarean sections or Apgar scores below seven at one minute.

AUTHORS' CONCLUSIONS: There is insufficient evidence from well-controlled trials to support the use of postural management for breech presentation. The numbers of women studied to date remain relatively small. Further research is needed.

EXTERNAL CEPHALIC VERSION FOR BREECH PRESENTATION BEFORE TERM: further trials are needed to confirm possible benefits of commencing ECV attempts before term. (Hutton EK, Hofmeyr GJ) CD000084 (in RHL 11)

BACKGROUND: External cephalic version (ECV) of the breech fetus at term (after 37 weeks) has been shown to be effective in reducing the number of breech presentations and caesarean sections, but the rates of success are relatively low. This review examines studies initiating ECV prior to term (before 37 weeks' gestation).

OBJECTIVES: To assess the effectiveness of a policy of beginning ECV before term (before 37 weeks' gestation) for breech presentation on fetal presentation at birth, method of delivery, and the rate of preterm birth, perinatal morbidity, stillbirth or neonatal mortality.

METHODS: Standard PCG methods (see page xvii). Search date: April 2005.

MAIN RESULTS: Three studies are included. One study reported on ECV that was undertaken and completed before 37 weeks' gestation compared to no ECV. No difference was found in the rate of non-cephalic presentation at birth. One study reported on a policy of ECV that was initiated before term (33 weeks) and up until 40 weeks' gestation and which could be repeated up until delivery compared to no ECV. This study showed a decrease in the rate of non-cephalic presentation at birth (relative risk 0.59, 95% confidence interval 0.45 to 0.77). One study reported on ECV started at between 34 to 35 weeks' gestation compared to beginning at 37 to 38 weeks' gestation. Although findings were not statistically significant, a 9.5% decrease in the rate of non-cephalic presentation at birth and a 7% decrease in the caesarean section rate were reported when ECV was started early.

AUTHORS' CONCLUSIONS: Compared with no ECV attempt, ECV commenced before term reduces non-cephalic births. Compared with ECV at term, beginning ECV at between 34 to 35 weeks may have some benefit in terms of decreasing the rate of non-cephalic presentation, and caesarean section. Further trials are needed to confirm this finding and to rule out increased rates of preterm birth, or other adverse perinatal outcomes. A large pragmatic trial is ongoing (www.utoronto.ca/miru/eecv2).

☺ **EXTERNAL CEPHALIC VERSION FOR BREECH PRESENTATION AT TERM:** reduced breech births and caesarean sections. (Hofmeyr GJ, Kulier R) CD000083 (in RHL 11)

BACKGROUND: Management of breech presentation is controversial, particularly in regard to manipulation of the position of the fetus by external cephalic version (ECV). ECV may reduce the number of breech presentations and caesarean sections, but there also have been reports of complications with the procedure.

OBJECTIVES: To assess the effects of ECV at or near term on measures of pregnancy outcome. Methods of facilitating ECV, and ECV before term, are reviewed separately.

METHODS: Standard PCG methods (see page xvii). Search date: April 2005.

MAIN RESULTS: Five studies were included. The pooled data from these studies show a statistically significant and clinically meaningful reduction in non-cephalic birth (five trials, 433 women; relative risk (RR) 0.38, 95% confidence interval (CI) 0.18 to 0.80) and caesarean section (five trials, 433 women; RR 0.55, 95% CI 0.33 to 0.91) when ECV was attempted. There were no significant differences in the incidence of

Apgar score ratings below seven at one minute (two trials, 108 women; RR 0.95, 95% 0.47 to 1.89) or five minutes (four trials, 368 women; RR 0.76, 95% 0.32 to 1.77), low umbilical artery pH levels (one trial, 52 women; RR 0.65, 95% 0.17 to 2.44), neonatal admission (one trial, 52 women; RR 0.36, 95% 0.04 to 3.24), perinatal death (five trials, 433 women; RR 0.51, 95% 0.05 to 5.54), or time from enrolment to delivery (2 trials, 256 women; weighted mean difference −0.25 days, 95% −2.81 to 2.31).

AUTHORS' CONCLUSIONS: Attempting cephalic version at term reduces the chance of non-cephalic births and caesarean section. There is not enough evidence from randomised trials to assess complications of external cephalic version at term. Large observational studies suggest that complications are rare.

CEPHALIC VERSION BY MOXIBUSTION FOR BREECH PRESENTATION: not enough data to provide reliable evidence. (Coyle ME, Smith CA, Peat B) CD003928

BACKGROUND: Moxibustion (a type of Chinese medicine which involves burning a herb close to the skin) to the acupuncture point Bladder 67 (BL67) (Chinese name *Zhiyin*), located at the tip of the fifth toe, has been proposed as a way of correcting breech presentation. As caesarean section is often suggested for breech babies due to the potential difficulties during labour, it is preferable to turn the baby before labour starts.

OBJECTIVES: To examine the effectiveness and safety of moxibustion on changing the presentation of an unborn baby in the breech position, the need for external cephalic version (ECV), mode of birth and perinatal morbidity and mortality for breech presentation.

METHODS: Standard PCG methods (see page xvii). Search date: August 2004.

The outcome measures were baby's presentation at birth, need for external cephalic version, mode of birth, perinatal morbidity and mortality, maternal complications and maternal satisfaction, and adverse events.

MAIN RESULTS: Three trials involving a total of 597 women were included. Due to differences in interventions and sample size it was not appropriate to perform a meta-analysis for the main outcome. Only one trial reported on other outcome measures relevant to this review. Moxibustion reduced the need for ECV (relative risk (RR) 0.47, 95% confidence interval (CI) 0.33 to 0.66) and resulted in decreased use of oxytocin before or during labour for women who had vaginal deliveries (RR 0.28, 95% CI 0.13 to 0.60).

AUTHORS' CONCLUSIONS: There is insufficient evidence to support the use of moxibustion to correct a breech presentation. Moxibustion may be beneficial in reducing the need for ECV, and decreasing the use of oxytocin, however there is a need for well-designed randomised controlled trials to evaluate moxibustion for breech presentation which report on clinically relevant outcomes as well as the safety of the intervention.

☺ **INTERVENTIONS TO HELP EXTERNAL CEPHALIC VERSION FOR BREECH PRESENTATION AT TERM:** ECV was facilitated by beta-stimulants and possibly epidural analgesia. (Hofmeyr GJ, Gyte G) CD000184 (in RHL 11)

BACKGROUND: Breech presentation places a fetus at increased risk. The outcome for the baby is improved by planned caesarean section compared with current medical practice for planned vaginal birth. External cephalic version (turning the fetus to the vertex position by external manipulation) attempts to reduce the chances of breech presentation at birth, and thus reduce the adverse effects of caesarean section, but is not always successful. Tocolytic drugs to relax the uterus, as well as other methods, have been used in an attempt to facilitate external cephalic version at term.

OBJECTIVES: To assess the effects of routine tocolysis, fetal acoustic stimulation, epidural or spinal analgesia and transabdominal amnioinfusion for external cephalic version at term on successful version and measures of pregnancy outcome.

METHODS: Standard PCG methods (see page xvii). Search date: March 2004.

MAIN RESULTS: 16 studies were included. Routine tocolysis with beta-stimulants was associated with fewer failures of external cephalic version (six trials, 617 women, relative risk (RR) 0.74, 95% confidence interval (CI) 0.64 to 0.87). The reduction in non-cephalic presentations at birth was not statistically significant. Caesarean sections were reduced (three trials, 444 women, RR 0.85, 95% CI 0.72

to 0.99). In four small trials, sublingual nitroglycerine was associated with significant side-effects, and was not found to be effective. Fetal acoustic stimulation in midline fetal spine positions was associated with fewer failures of external cephalic version at term (one trial, 26 women, RR 0.17, 95% CI 0.05 to 0.60). External cephalic version failure, non-cephalic births and caesarean sections were reduced in two trials with epidural but not in three with spinal analgesia. We postulate that large volume preloading with epidural may have increased the amniotic fluid volume. No randomised trials of transabdominal amnioinfusion for external cephalic version at term were located.

AUTHORS' CONCLUSIONS: Although the methodological quality of the trials was not ideal, routine tocolysis appears to increase the success rate of external cephalic version at term. There is not enough evidence to evaluate the use of fetal acoustic stimulation in midline fetal spine positions, nor of epidural or spinal analgesia.

HANDS AND KNEES POSTURE IN LATE PREGNANCY OR LABOUR FOR FETAL MALPOSITION (LATERAL OR POSTERIOR): in late pregnancy, no substantive benefits were found; in labour, hands and knees posture reduced backache. (Hunter S, Hofmeyr GJ, Kulier R) CD001063

BACKGROUND: Lateral and posterior position of the baby's head (the back of the baby's head facing to the mother's side or back) may be associated with more painful, prolonged or obstructed labour and difficult delivery. It is possible that certain positions adopted by the mother may influence the baby's position.

OBJECTIVES: To assess the effects of adopting a hands and knees maternal posture in late pregnancy or during labour when the presenting part of the fetus is in a lateral or posterior position compared with no intervention.

METHODS: Standard PCG methods (see page xvii). Search date: July 2007.

MAIN RESULTS: Three trials (2794 women) were included. In one trial (100 women), four different postures (four groups of 20 women) were combined for comparison with the control group of 20 women. Lateral or posterior position of the presenting part of the fetus was less likely to persist following 10 minutes in the hands and knees position compared to a sitting position (one trial, 100 women, relative risk (RR)

0.26, 95% confidence interval (CI) 0.18 to 0.38). In a second trial (2547 women), advice to assume the hands and knees posture for 10 minutes twice daily in the last weeks of pregnancy had no effect on the baby's position at delivery or any of the other pregnancy outcomes measured. The third trial studied the use of hands and knees position in labour and involved 147 labouring women at 37 or more weeks' gestation. Occipito-posterior position of the baby was confirmed by ultrasound. Seventy women, who were randomised in the intervention group, assumed hands and knees positioning for a period of at least 30 minutes, compared to 77 women in the control group who did not assume hands and knees positioning in labour. The reduction in occipito-posterior or -transverse positions at delivery and operative deliveries was not statistically significant. There was a significant reduction in back pain.

AUTHORS' CONCLUSIONS: Use of hands and knees position for 10 minutes twice daily to correct occipito-posterior position of the fetus in late pregnancy cannot be recommended as an intervention. This is not to suggest that women should not adopt this position if they find it comfortable. The use of position in labour was associated with reduced backache. Further trials are needed to assess the effects on other labour outcomes.

7.6.1 Breech birth

Several techniques for vaginal breech births have been developed over time, but their relative effectiveness has not been assessed systematically. Factors considered favourable for vaginal breech birth include a baby of average size with flexed neck and hips, and good progress of labour. Flexed hips create a large presenting part comprising both body and thighs (frank breech) or lower limbs as well (complete breech). Undelayed, spontaneous delivery of the flexed breech indicates that fetopelvic disproportion is most unlikely.

The trend to preference for caesarean section in recent years has restricted the opportunities for practical training in the techniques of breech birth. Increasingly, simulated training and video demonstrations are used (see video: 'Vaginal breech delivery and symphysiotomy', WHO Reproductive Health Library www.rhlibrary.com).

☺ **PLANNED CAESAREAN SECTION FOR TERM BREECH DELIV-ERY:** improved short-term outcomes for babies; increased maternal morbidity. (Hofmeyr GJ, Hannah ME) CD000166 (in RHL 11)

BACKGROUND: Poor outcomes after breech birth might be the result of underlying conditions causing breech presentation or to factors associated with the delivery.

OBJECTIVES: To assess the effects of planned caesarean section for singleton breech presentation at term on measures of pregnancy outcome.

METHODS: Standard PCG methods (see page xvii). Search date: October 2004.

MAIN RESULTS: Three trials (2396 participants) were included in the review.

Caesarean delivery occurred in 550/1227 (45%) of those women allocated to a vaginal delivery protocol. Perinatal or neonatal death (excluding fatal anomalies) or serious neonatal morbidity was reduced with planned caesarean section (relative risk (RR) 0.33, 95% confidence interval (CI) 0.19 to 0.56). This reduction was less for countries with high national perinatal mortality rates. Perinatal or neonatal death (excluding fatal anomalies) was also reduced with planned caesarean section (RR 0.29, 95% CI 0.10 to 0.86). The proportional reductions were similar for countries with low and high national perinatal mortality rates. Planned caesarean section was associated with modestly increased short-term maternal morbidity (RR 1.29, 95% CI 1.03 to 1.61). At three months after delivery, women allocated to the planned caesarean section group reported less urinary incontinence (RR 0.62, 95% CI 0.41 to 0.93); more abdominal pain (RR 1.89, 95% CI 1.29 to 2. 79); and less perineal pain (RR 0.32, 95% CI 0.18 to 0.58).

At two years, there were no differences in the combined outcome 'death or neurodevelopmental delay'. Maternal outcomes at two years were also similar.

AUTHORS' CONCLUSIONS: Planned caesarean section compared with planned vaginal birth reduced perinatal or neonatal death or serious neonatal morbidity, at the expense of somewhat increased maternal morbidity. The option of external cephalic version is dealt with in separate reviews. The data from this review cannot be generalised to

settings where caesarean section is not readily available, or to methods of breech delivery that differ materially from the clinical delivery protocols used in the trials reviewed. The review will help to inform individualised decision-making regarding breech delivery. Research on strategies to improve the safety of breech delivery is needed.

> **EXPEDITED VERSUS CONSERVATIVE APPROACHES FOR VAGINAL DELIVERY IN BREECH PRESENTATION:** no randomised trials to provide reliable evidence. (Hofmeyr GJ, Kulier R) CD000082

BACKGROUND: In a vaginal breech birth there may be benefit from rapid delivery of the baby to prevent progressive acidosis. However, this needs to be weighed against the potential trauma of a quick delivery.
OBJECTIVES: To assess the effects of expedited vaginal delivery (breech delivery from umbilicus to delivery of the head within one contraction) on perinatal outcomes.
METHODS: Standard PCG methods (see page xvii). Search date: June 2007.
MAIN RESULTS: No studies were included.

AUTHORS' CONCLUSIONS: There is not enough evidence to evaluate the effects of expedited vaginal breech delivery.

7.7   Babies with compromised condition during labour

7.7.1   Diagnosis

During labour contractions, the pressure inside the uterus and intervillous space increases, and prevents blood flow from the mother's circulation through the placenta. Between contractions, the blood flow resumes. Normally, this intermittent interruption of flow has no noticeable effect on the baby. However, if the baby's condition is compromised, placental function is poor or periods of relaxation between uterine contractions are inadequate, the baby may become hypoxic (short of oxygen). The baby may compensate by a redistribution of blood flow away from non-essential organs, with overall increased peripheral resistance and slowing of the heart rate. Recovery of the heart rate after the contraction is then not immediate, as recovery of the baby's oxygenation takes a while. These 'late' decelerations may be heard by listening to the baby's heart rate before, during and after a contraction, or recording it with a cardiotocograph. Further deterioration of the baby's condition may depress the central nervous system and thus blunt the variability of the heart rate and the accelerative response to movements or stimuli.

During labour, clinical or electronic assessment of the baby's heart rate pattern is used to assess the baby's wellbeing. These methods tend to overdiagnose fetal compromise, so it is important to establish whether the benefits of accurately detected compromise outweigh the harms from false diagnoses of compromise. Other techniques have been developed to try to improve the specificity of fetal heart rate testing (see below).

☺ **CONTINUOUS CARDIOTOCOGRAPHY (CTG) AS A FORM OF ELECTRONIC FETAL MONITORING (EFM) FOR FETAL ASSESSMENT DURING LABOUR:** reduced neonatal seizures but not cerebral palsy; increased caesarean sections and operative vaginal births; no effect on perinatal mortality. (Alfirevic Z, Devane D, Gyte GML) CD006066 (in RHL 11)

BACKGROUND: Cardiotocography (sometimes known as electronic fetal monitoring) records changes in the fetal heart rate and their temporal relationship to uterine contractions. The aim is to identify babies who may be short of oxygen (hypoxic), so additional assessments of fetal well-being may be used, or the baby delivered by caesarean section or instrumental vaginal birth.

OBJECTIVES: To evaluate the effectiveness of continuous cardiotocography during labour.

METHODS: Standard PCG methods (see page xvii). Search date: March 2006.

MAIN RESULTS: 12 trials were included (over 37 000 women); only two were high quality. Compared to intermittent auscultation, continuous cardiotocography showed no significant difference in overall perinatal death rate (relative risk (RR) 0.85, 95% confidence interval (CI) 0.59 to 1.23, n = 33 513, 11 trials), but was associated with a halving of neonatal seizures (RR 0.50, 95% CI 0.31 to 0.80, n = 32 386, nine trials) although no significant difference was detected in cerebral palsy (RR 1.74, 95% CI 0.97 to 3.11, n = 13 252, two trials). There was a significant increase in caesarean sections associated with continuous cardiotocography (RR 1.66, 95% CI 1.30 to 2.13, n =18761, 10 trials). Women were also more likely to have an instrumental vaginal birth (RR 1.16, 95% CI 1.01 to 1.32, n = 18151, nine trials). Data for subgroups of low-risk, high-risk, preterm pregnancies and high quality trials were consistent with overall results. Access to fetal blood sampling did not appear to influence the difference in neonatal seizures or any other prespecified outcome.

AUTHORS' CONCLUSIONS: Continuous cardiotocography during labour is associated with a reduction in neonatal seizures, but no significant differences in cerebral palsy, infant mortality or other standard measures of neonatal well-being. However, continuous cardiotocography was associated with an increase in caesarean sections and instrumental vaginal births. The real challenge is how best to convey this uncertainty to women to enable them to make an informed choice without compromising the normality of labour.

☺ FETAL ELECTROCARDIOGRAM (ECG) FOR FETAL MONITOR-ING DURING LABOUR: reduced scalp sampling, neonatal encephalopathy and operative delivery; is more invasive than cardiotocography alone. (Neilson JP) CD000116

BACKGROUND: Hypoxaemia during labour can alter the shape of the fetal electrocardiogram (ECG) waveform, notably the relation of the PR to RR intervals, and elevation or depression of the ST segment. Technical systems have therefore been developed to monitor the fetal ECG during labour as an adjunct to continuous electronic fetal heart rate monitoring with the aim of improving fetal outcome and minimising unnecessary obstetric interference.

OBJECTIVES: To compare the effects of analysis of fetal ECG waveforms during labour with alternative methods of fetal monitoring.

METHODS: Standard PCG methods (see page xvii). Search date: April 2006.

MAIN RESULTS: Four trials including a total of 9829 women were included. In comparison to continuous electronic fetal heart rate monitoring alone, the use of adjunctive ST waveform analysis (three trials, 8872 women) was associated with fewer babies with severe metabolic acidosis at birth (cord pH less than 7.05 and base deficit greater than 12 mmol/l) (relative risk (RR) 0.64, 95% confidence interval (CI) 0.41

to 1.00, data from 8108 babies), fewer babies with neonatal enceph-alopathy (three trials, RR 0.33, 95% CI 0.11 to 0.95) although the absolute number of babies with encephalopathy was low (n = 17), fewer fetal scalp samples during labour (three trials, RR 0.76, 95% CI 0.67 to 0.86) and fewer operative vaginal deliveries (three trials, RR 0.87, 95% CI 0.78 to 0.96). There was no statistically significant difference in caesarean section (three trials, RR 0.97, 95% CI 0.84 to 1.11), Apgar score less than seven at five minutes (three trials, RR 0.80, 95% CI 0.56 to 1.14) or admissions to special care unit (three trials, RR 0.90, 95% CI 0.75 to 1.08). Apart from a trend towards fewer operative deliveries (one trial, RR 0.87, 95% CI 0.76 to 1.01), there was little evidence that monitoring by PR interval analysis con-veyed any benefit.

AUTHOR'S CONCLUSIONS: These findings provide some support for the use of fetal ST waveform analysis when a decision has been made to undertake continuous electronic fetal heart rate monitoring dur-ing labour. However, the advantages need to be considered along with the disadvantages of needing to use an internal scalp electrode, after membrane rupture, for ECG waveform recordings.

> ⊗ **FETAL PULSE OXIMETRY FOR FETAL ASSESSMENT IN LABOUR:** has not been shown to improve substantive outcomes. (East CE, Chan FY, Colditz PB, Begg LM) CD004075

BACKGROUND: Pulse oximetry could contribute to the evaluation of fetal well-being during labour.
OBJECTIVES: To compare the effectiveness and safety of fetal pulse oxi-metry with conventional surveillance techniques.
METHODS: Standard PCG methods (see page xvii). Search date: November 2006.
MAIN RESULTS: Five published trials comparing fetal pulse oximetry and CTG with CTG alone (or when fetal pulse oximetry values were blinded) were included. The published trials, with some unpublished data, reported on a total of 7424 pregnancies. Differing entry criteria necessitated separate analyses, rather than meta-analysis of all trials.

Four trials reported no significant differences in the overall caesarean section rate between those monitored with fetal oximetry and those not monitored with fetal pulse oximetry or for whom the fetal pulse oximetry results were masked. Neonatal seizures and hypoxic ischaemic encephalopathy were rare. No studies reported details of assessment of long-term disability.

There was a statistically significant decrease in caesarean section for non-reassuring fetal status in the fetal pulse oximetry plus CTG group compared to the CTG group in two analyses: (i) gestation from 36 weeks with fetal blood sample (fetal blood sampling) not required prior to study entry (relative risk (RR) 0.68, 95% confidence interval (CI) 0.47 to 0.99); and (ii) when fetal blood sampling was required prior to study entry (RR 0.03, 95% CI 0.00 to 0.44). There was no statistically significant difference in caesarean section for dystocia when fetal pulse oximetry (fetal pulse oximetry) was added to CTG monitoring, compared with CTG monitoring alone, although the incidence rates varied between the trials.

AUTHORS' CONCLUSIONS: The data provide limited support for the use of fetal pulse oximetry when used in the presence of a nonreassuring CTG, to reduce caesarean section for non-reassuring fetal status. The addition of fetal pulse oximetry does not reduce overall caesarean section rates. A better method to evaluate fetal well-being in labour is required.

NEAR-INFRARED SPECTROSCOPY FOR FETAL ASSESSMENT DURING LABOUR: no randomised trials to provide reliable evidence. (Mozurkewich E, Wolf FM) CD002254

BACKGROUND: Over the past four decades, continuous electronic fetal monitoring (EFM) has been increasingly employed to detect fetal acidaemia in labour, with a view toward prevention of hypoxic ischaemic encephalopathy, permanent neurologic injury and death. Although very sensitive, this technology has low specificity and a high false positive rate. This false positive rate has resulted in operative intervention on behalf of many fetuses who were not in fact in danger of neurologic injury or death. Near-infrared spectroscopy has been developed to directly measure fetal cerebral oxygenation, with a view toward identification of those fetuses truly at risk.

OBJECTIVES: To determine the effects of the use of near-infrared spectroscopy to assess fetal condition during labour on maternal and perinatal outcomes.

METHODS: Standard PCG methods (see page xvii). Search date: April 2007.

MAIN RESULTS: No randomised trials were identified. Thus no studies were included.

AUTHORS' CONCLUSIONS: There is currently insufficient evidence to assess the efficacy of fetal surveillance by near-infrared spectroscopy.

VIBROACOUSTIC STIMULATION FOR FETAL ASSESSMENT IN LABOUR IN THE PRESENCE OF A NON-REASSURING FETAL HEART RATE TRACE: no randomised trials to provide reliable evidence. (East CE, Smyth R, Leader LR, Henshall NE, Colditz PB, Tan KH) CD004664

BACKGROUND: Fetal vibroacoustic stimulation is a simple, non-invasive technique where a device is placed on the maternal abdomen over the region of the fetal head and sound is emitted at a predetermined level for several seconds. It is hypothesised that the resultant startle reflex in the fetus and subsequent fetal heart rate acceleration or transient tachycardia following vibroacoustic stimulation provide reassurance of fetal well-being. This technique has been proposed as a tool to assess fetal well-being in the presence of a non-reassuring cardiotocographic trace during the first and second stages of labour.

OBJECTIVES: To evaluate the clinical effectiveness and safety of vibroacoustic stimulation in the assessment of fetal well-being during labour compared with mock or no stimulation for women with a singleton pregnancy exhibiting a non-reassuring fetal heart rate pattern.

METHODS: Standard PCG methods (see page xvii). Search date: September 2004.

MAIN RESULTS: The search strategies yielded six studies for consideration of inclusion. However, none of these studies fulfilled the requirements for inclusion in this review.

AUTHORS' CONCLUSIONS: There are currently no randomised controlled trials that address the safety and efficacy of vibroacoustic stimulation used to assess fetal well-being in labour in the presence of a non-reassuring cardiotocographic trace. Although vibroacoustic stimulation has been proposed as a simple, non-invasive tool for assessment of fetal well-being, there is insufficient evidence from

randomised trials on which to base recommendations for use of vibroacoustic stimulation in the evaluation of fetal well-being in labour in the presence of a non-reassuring cardiotocographic trace.

CARDIOTOCOGRAPHY VERSUS INTERMITTENT AUSCULTATION OF FETAL HEART ON ADMISSION TO LABOUR WARD FOR ASSESSMENT OF FETAL WELLBEING: (Devane D, Lalor J, Daly S, McGuire W) Protocol [see page xviii] CD005122

ABRIDGED BACKGROUND: The fetal heart rate undergoes constant changes as it responds to the intrauterine environment and to other stimuli such as uterine contractions. These changes in the fetal heart rate can be monitored to assess the wellbeing of the fetus during pregnancy and labour.

The two most common methods of monitoring the fetal heart rate are by intermittent auscultation and by an electronic fetal monitoring (EFM) machine that produces a paper printout called a cardiotocograph (CTG). The admission cardiotocograph is a commonly used screening test consisting of a short, usually 20 minutes, recording of the fetal heart rate and uterine activity performed on the mother's admission to the labour ward. Although the admission CTG remains in widespread use, several issues remain controversial and under discussion. These include whether the admission CTG (a) should be routinely offered to all women without risk factors for intrapartum hypoxia; (b) whether the admission CTG is effective at predicting those fetuses who will subsequently develop intrapartum hypoxia; and (c) the effect of the admission CTG on neonatal mortality and on maternal and neonatal morbidity.

OBJECTIVES: To compare the effects of admission cardiotocography with intermittent auscultation of the fetal heart rate on maternal and infant outcomes for pregnant women without risk factors on their admission to the labour ward.

INTRAPARTUM FETAL SCALP LACTATE SAMPLING FOR FETAL ASSESSMENT IN THE PRESENCE OF A NON-REASSURING FETAL HEART RATE TRACE: (East CE, Leader LR, Colditz PB, Henshall NE) Protocol [see page xviii] CD006174

ABRIDGED BACKGROUND: *Standard methods of assessment of fetal wellbeing during labour:*

Cardiotocography (CTG), often referred to as electronic fetal monitoring (EFM), records the fetal heart rate and uterine contractions to paper or computer, or both. It was introduced in the 1960s with the aim of improving neonatal outcomes by improving intrapartum fetal surveillance. The differences in individual fetal responses to a decrease in oxygen (and therefore differences in heart rate changes) mean that the positive predictive value of CTG for adverse outcome is low and the negative predictive value high, although this is improving with computerised interpretation of CTGs. This means that a normal CTG usually indicates reassuring fetal status, while a non-reassuring CTG does not necessarily equate with 'fetal distress'. These features, combined with marked inter-observer variation in CTG interpretation by midwives and doctors, result in variable but inappropriately high operative delivery rates for non-reassuring fetal status in many hospitals.

The addition of fetal scalp blood sampling (FBS) for pH estimation to standard EFM may reduce the caesarean section rate, although the odds of having a caesarean birth are still increased compared to intermittent auscultation of the fetal heart

Fetal lactate testing equipment requiring a much smaller blood volume (as little as 5 microlitres) has recently become available.

OBJECTIVES: To evaluate the effectiveness and risks of fetal scalp lactate sampling in the assessment of fetal wellbeing during labour, compared with no testing or alternative additional testing (pH, fetal pulse oximetry, etc) for women exhibiting a non-reassuring cardiotocograph trace.

A secondary objective of the review is to determine whether effectiveness and risks of intrapartum fetal scalp lactate sampling are influenced by the following:

1) stage of labour;
2) gestation less than 37, greater than or equal to 37 completed weeks;
3) additional tests performed to confirm the presence or absence of fetal acidaemia during labour.

7.7.2 Preventing compromise of the baby's condition during labour

Apart from avoiding interventions which may compromise the baby's condition such as hyperstimulation of the uterus and the supine position, specific measures have been developed to prevent such compromise.

⊗ **PROPHYLACTIC VERSUS THERAPEUTIC AMNIOINFUSION FOR OLIGOHYDRAMNIOS IN LABOUR:** did not improve outcomes, and was associated with increased fever. (Hofmeyr GJ) CD000176

BACKGROUND: Amnioinfusion aims to relieve umbilical cord compression during labour by infusing a liquid into the uterine cavity.

OBJECTIVES: To assess the effects of prophylactic amnioinfusion for oligohydramnios compared with therapeutic amnioinfusion only if fetal heart rate decelerations or thick meconium-staining of the liquor occur.

METHODS: Standard PCG methods (see page xvii). Search date: October 2001.

MAIN RESULTS: Two studies of 285 women were included. No differences were found in the rate of caesarean section (relative risk 0.98, 95% confidence interval 0.58 to 1.66) or forceps delivery. There were no differences in Apgar scores, cord arterial pH, oxytocin augmentation, meconium aspiration, neonatal pneumonia or postpartum endometritis. Prophylactic amnioinfusion was associated with increased intrapartum fever (relative risk 3.48, 95% confidence interval 1.21 to 10.05).

AUTHOR'S CONCLUSIONS: There appears to be no advantage of prophylactic amnioinfusion over therapeutic amnioinfusion carried out only when fetal heart rate decelerations or thick meconium-staining of the liquor occur.

⊗ **TOCOLYSIS FOR PREVENTING FETAL DISTRESS IN SECOND STAGE OF LABOUR:** increased forceps deliveries without showing benefits. (Hofmeyr GJ, Kulier R) CD000037

BACKGROUND: Prophylactic tocolysis with betamimetics and other agents has become widespread as a treatment for fetal distress. Uterine relaxation may improve placental blood flow and therefore fetal oxygenation. However, there may also be adverse maternal cardiovascular effects.

OBJECTIVES: To assess the effects of prophylactic betamimetic therapy during the second stage of labour on perinatal outcome.

METHODS: Standard PCG methods (see page xvii). Search date: October 2004.

MAIN RESULTS: One study involving 100 women was included. Compared to placebo, prophylactic betamimetic therapy was associated with an increase in forceps deliveries (relative risk 1.83, 95% confidence interval 1.02 to 3.29). There were no clear effects on postpartum haemorrhage, neonatal irritability, feeding slowness, umbilical arterial pH values or Apgar scores at two minutes.

AUTHORS' CONCLUSIONS: There is no evidence to support the prophylactic use of betamimetics during the second stage of labour.

7.7.3 Treatment of babies with evidence of compromised condition

Possible methods used to improve the baby's condition during labour include positioning the mother on her side, stopping uterine stimulants, administering oxygen to the mother, providing pain relief, administering tocolytics to reduce contractions of the uterus, and amnioinfusion to relieve umbilical cord compression or dilute meconium.

> **TOCOLYTICS FOR SUSPECTED INTRAPARTUM FETAL DISTRESS:** reduced fetal heart rate abnormalities; more evidence is needed on substantive outcomes. (Kulier R, Hofmeyr GJ) CD000035

BACKGROUND: Prophylactic tocolysis with betamimetics and other agents has become widespread as a treatment for fetal distress. Uterine relaxation may improve placental blood flow and therefore fetal oxygenation. However there may also be adverse maternal cardiovascular effects.

OBJECTIVES: To assess the effects of tocolytic therapy for suspected fetal distress on fetal, maternal and perinatal outcomes.

METHODS: Standard PCG methods (see page xvii). Search date: May 2006.

MAIN RESULTS: Three studies were included. Compared with no treatment, there were fewer failed improvements in fetal heart rate abnormalities with tocolytic therapy (relative risk 0.26, 95% 0.13 to 0.53). Betamimetic therapy compared with magnesium sulphate showed a non-significant trend towards reduced uterine activity (relative risk 0.07, 95% confidence interval 0.00 to 1.10).

AUTHORS' CONCLUSIONS: Betamimetic therapy appears to be able to reduce the number of fetal heart rate abnormalities and perhaps reduce uterine activity. However there is not enough evidence based on clinically important outcomes to evaluate the use of betamimetics for suspected fetal distress.

MATERNAL OXYGEN ADMINISTRATION FOR FETAL DISTRESS: has not been evaluated; prophylactic oxygen administration may be harmful. (Fawole B, Hofmeyr GJ) CD000136

BACKGROUND: Maternal oxygen administration has been used in an attempt to lessen fetal distress by increasing the available oxygen from the mother. This has been used for suspected fetal distress during labour, and prophylactically during the second stage of labour on the assumption that the second stage is a time of high risk for fetal distress.

OBJECTIVES: The objective of this review was to assess the effects of maternal oxygenation for fetal distress during labour and to assess the effects of prophylactic oxygen therapy during the second stage of labour on perinatal outcome.

METHODS: Standard PCG methods (see page xvii). Search date: June 2007

MAIN RESULTS: We located no trials addressing maternal oxygen therapy for fetal distress. We included two trials which addressed prophylactic oxygen administration during labour. Abnormal cord blood pH values (less than 7.2) were recorded significantly more frequently in the oxygenation group than the control group (RR 3.51, 95% CI 1.34 to 9.19). There were no other statistically significant differences between the groups. There were conflicting conclusions on the effect of the duration of oxygen administration on umbilical artery pH values between the two trials.

AUTHORS' CONCLUSIONS:

Implications for practice

There is not enough evidence to support the use of prophylactic oxygen therapy for women in labour, nor to evaluate its effectiveness for fetal distress.

Implications for research

In view of the widespread use of oxygen administration during labour and the possibility that it may be ineffective or harmful, there is an urgent need for randomized trials to assess its effects.

☺ **AMNIOINFUSION FOR POTENTIAL OR SUSPECTED UMBILI-CAL CORD COMPRESSION IN LABOUR:** improved short term perinatal outcomes; the possibility of rare adverse events cannot be excluded. (Hofmeyr GJ) CD000013 (in RHL 11)

BACKGROUND: Amnioinfusion aims to prevent or relieve umbilical cord compression or amniotic fluid infection during labour by infusing a solution into the uterine cavity.

OBJECTIVES: To assess the effects of amnioinfusion on maternal and perinatal outcome for potential or suspected umbilical cord compression or potential amnionitis.

METHODS: Standard PCG methods (see page xvii). Search date: November 2004.

MAIN RESULTS: 14 studies were included, most with fewer than 200 participants. Transcervical amnioinfusion for potential or suspected umbilical cord compression was associated with the following reductions: fetal heart rate decelerations (four studies, 227 women: relative risk (RR) 0.54; 95% confidence interval (CI) 0.43 to 0.68); caesarean section overall (nine studies, 953 women: RR 0.52; CI 0.40 to 0.69); Apgar score less than seven at five minutes (seven studies, 828 women: RR 0.54; CI 0.30 to 0.97); low cord arterial pH (six studies, 660 women: RR 0.45; CI 0.31 to 0.64); neonatal hospital stay greater than three days (one study, 305 women: RR 0.40; CI 0.26 to 0.62); postpartum endometritis (five studies, 619 women: RR 0.45; CI 0.25 to 0.81); maternal hospital stay greater than three days (two studies, 465 women: RR 0.41; CI 0.27 to 0.63). Transabdominal amnioinfusion showed similar trends, though numbers studied were small. Transcervical amnioinfusion to prevent infection in women with membranes ruptured for more than six hours was associated with a reduction in puerperal infection (one study, 68 women: RR 0.50; CI 0.26 to 0.97).

AUTHOR'S CONCLUSIONS: Amnioinfusion appears useful to reduce the occurrence of variable fetal heart rate decelerations, improve short-term measures of neonatal outcome and lower the use of caesarean section, mainly for 'fetal distress' diagnosed by fetal heart rate monitoring alone. However, most of the included studies were small, and there were methodological shortcomings. In one trial puerperal infection was reduced. The trials reviewed are too small to address

the possibility of rare but serious maternal adverse effects of amnio-infusion. More research is needed to confirm the findings and assess longer-term measures of fetal outcome and the impact on caesarean section when the diagnosis of fetal distress is more stringent.

> **AMNIOINFUSION FOR MECONIUM-STAINED LIQUOR IN LA-BOUR:** improved perinatal outcomes in settings with limited peripartum surveillance; not enough data to provide reliable evidence for settings with adequate peripartum surveillance. (Hofmeyr GJ) CD000014 (in RHL 11)

BACKGROUND: Amnioinfusion aims to prevent or relieve umbilical cord compression during labour by infusing a solution into the uterine cavity. It is also thought to dilute meconium when present in the amniotic fluid and so reduce the risk of meconium aspiration. However, it may be that the mechanism of effect is that it corrects oligohydramnios (reduced amniotic fluid), for which thick meconium staining is a marker.

OBJECTIVES: To assess the effects of amnioinfusion for meconium-stained liquor on perinatal outcome.

METHODS: Standard PCG methods (see page xvii). Search date: October 2001.

MAIN RESULTS: 12 studies, most involving small numbers of participants, were included. Under standard perinatal surveillance, amnioinfusion was associated with a reduction in the following: heavy meconium staining of the liquor (relative risk 0.03, 95% confidence interval 0.01 to 0.15); variable fetal heart rate deceleration (relative risk 0.65, 95% confidence interval 0.49 to 0.88); and reduced caesarean section overall (relative risk 0.82, 95% confidence interval 0.69 to 0.97). No perinatal deaths were reported. Under limited perinatal surveillance, amnioinfusion was associated with a reduction in the following: meconium aspiration syndrome (relative risk 0.24, 95% confidence interval 0.12 to 0.48); neonatal hypoxic ischaemic encephalopathy (relative risk 0.07, 95% confidence interval 0.01 to 0.56) and neonatal ventilation or intensive care unit admission (relative risk 0.56, 95% confidence interval 0.39 to 0.79); there was a trend towards reduced perinatal mortality (relative risk 0.34, 95% confidence interval 0.11 to 1.06).

AUTHOR'S CONCLUSIONS: Amnioinfusion is associated with improvements in perinatal outcome, particularly in settings where facilities for perinatal surveillance are limited. The trials reviewed are too small to address the possibility of rare but serious maternal adverse effects of amnioinfusion.

> **OPERATIVE VERSUS CONSERVATIVE MANAGEMENT FOR 'FETAL DISTRESS' IN LABOUR:** not enough data to provide reliable evidence. (Hofmeyr GJ, Kulier R) CD001065

BACKGROUND: Suspected fetal distress usually results in expedited delivery of a baby (often operatively). The potential harm to a mother and baby from operative delivery may not always be justified especially when fetal distress may be misdiagnosed. Even with a correct diagnosis it is not clear whether an operative or conservative approach is better.
OBJECTIVES: To assess the effects of operative management for fetal distress on maternal and perinatal morbidity.
METHODS: Standard PCG methods (see page xvii). Search date: March 2006.
MAIN RESULTS: One study of 350 women was included. This trial was carried out in 1959. There was no difference in perinatal mortality (relative risk 1.18, 95% confidence interval 0.56 to 2.48).

AUTHORS' CONCLUSIONS: There have been no contemporary trials of operative versus conservative management of suspected fetal distress. In settings without modern obstetric facilities, a policy of operative delivery in the event of meconium-stained liquor or fetal heart rate changes has not been shown to reduce perinatal mortality.

> **PIRACETAM FOR FETAL DISTRESS IN LABOUR:** not enough data to provide reliable evidence. (Hofmeyr GJ, Kulier R) CD001064

BACKGROUND: Piracetam is thought to promote the metabolism of brain cells when they are hypoxic. It has been used to prevent adverse effects of fetal distress.
OBJECTIVES: To assess the effects of piracetam for suspected fetal distress in labour on method of delivery and perinatal morbidity.
METHODS: Standard PCG methods (see page xvii). Search date: October 2004.
MAIN RESULTS: One study of 96 women was included. Piracetam compared with placebo was associated with a trend to reduced need for caesarean section (relative risk 0.57, 95% confidence interval

0.32 to 1.03). There were no statistically significant differences in relative risk between the piracetam and placebo group for neonatal morbidity (measured by neonatal respiratory distress) or Apgar score.

AUTHORS' CONCLUSIONS: There is not enough evidence to evaluate the use of piracetam for fetal distress in labour.

ENDOTRACHEAL INTUBATION AT BIRTH FOR PREVENTING MORBIDITY AND MORTALITY IN VIGOROUS, MECONIUM-STAINED INFANTS BORN AT TERM: no evidence of benefit (Halliday HL, Sweet D) CD000500 (in RHL 11). (Cochrane Neonatal Group)

BACKGROUND: On the basis of evidence from non-randomised studies, it has been recommended that all babies born through thick meconium should have their tracheas intubated so that suctioning of their airways can be performed. The aim is to reduce the incidence and severity of meconium aspiration syndrome. However, for term babies who are vigorous at birth endotracheal intubation may be both difficult and unnecessary.

OBJECTIVES: To determine if endotracheal intubation and suction of the airways at birth in vigorous term meconium-stained babies is more beneficial than routine resuscitation including aspiration of the oro-pharynx.

SEARCH STRATEGY: The search was made from the Oxford Database of Perinatal Trials, Cochrane Controlled Trials Register (The Cochrane Library, Issue 3, 2002), MEDLINE from 1966 to September 2002 and information obtained from knowledgeable practising neonatologists.

SELECTION CRITERIA: Randomised trials which compared a policy of routine vs no (or selective) use of endotracheal intubation and aspiration in the immediate management of vigorous term meconium-stained babies at birth.

DATA COLLECTION AND ANALYSIS: Data regarding clinical outcomes including mortality, meconium aspiration syndrome, other respiratory conditions, pneumothorax, need for oxygen supplementation, stridor, convulsions and hypoxic-ischaemic encephalopathy (HIE) were abstracted and analysed using Revman 4.1.

MAIN RESULTS: Four randomised controlled trials of endotracheal intubation at birth in vigorous term meconium-stained babies were identified. Meta-analysis of these trials does not support routine use of endotracheal intubation at birth in vigorous meconium-stained babies to reduce mortality, meconium aspiration syndrome, other respiratory symptoms or disorders, pneumothorax, oxygen need, stridor, HIE and convulsions. However, the event rate of many of these outcomes is low in the reported trials making reliable estimates of treatment effect impossible.

AUTHORS' CONCLUSIONS: Routine endotracheal intubation at birth in vigorous term meconium-stained babies has not been shown to be superior to routine resuscitation including oro-pharyngeal suction. This procedure cannot be recommended for vigorous infants until more research is available.

7.8   Cord prolapse

Presentation of the umbilical cord below the baby's presenting part with intact membranes, or prolapse once the membranes rupture, may be suspected because of variable decelerations of the baby's heart rate, or felt during a vaginal examination; or the prolapsed cord may protrude from the vagina. The baby's heart rate is checked clinically or electronically (absence of cord pulsation is an unreliable sign). Strategies intended to reduce compression of the cord while preparing to deliver the baby include replacement of the cord in the vagina; lateral or knee-chest positioning; tocolysis; digitally elevating the presenting part; and filling the bladder with fluid.

There are no Cochrane reviews of this topic.

7.9   Perineal trauma

During childbirth the perineum undergoes considerable stretching, which may be accompanied by bruising, tears and episiotomy wounds. Perineal pain is common in the days after childbirth, and may persist for years, particularly pain associated with sexual intercourse. Damage to the anal sphincter may result in incontinence of flatus and/or faeces. Avoidance of perineal trauma is one of the arguments advanced in favour of elective caesarean section.

Strategies originally devised to reduce perineal trauma include episiotomy (page 264), antenatal perineal massage, alternative birth postures, manual support for the perineum during the birth and birth in water.

Whether lacerations are sutured, and the methods of suturing, may also have a bearing on the long-term outcome of these injuries.

7.9.1   Preventing perineal trauma

☺ ANTENATAL PERINEAL MASSAGE FOR REDUCING PERINEAL TRAUMA: was effective for reducing perineal trauma in primiparous women; for multiparous women perineal pain was reduced at three months. (Beckmann MM, Garrett AJ) CD005123

BACKGROUND: Perineal trauma following vaginal birth can be associated with significant short- and long-term morbidity. Antenatal perineal massage has been proposed as one method of decreasing the incidence of perineal trauma.

OBJECTIVES: To assess the effect of antenatal perineal massage on the incidence of perineal trauma at birth and subsequent morbidity.

METHODS: Standard PCG methods (see page xvii). Search date: January 2005.

MAIN RESULTS: Three trials (2434 women) comparing digital perineal massage with control were included. All were of good quality. Antenatal perineal massage was associated with an overall reduction in the incidence of trauma requiring suturing (three trials, 2417 women, relative risk (RR) 0.91 (95% confidence interval (CI) 0.86 to 0.96), number needed to treat (NNT) 16 (10 to 39)). This reduction was statistically significant for women without previous vaginal birth only (three trials, 1925 women, RR 0.90 (95% CI 0.84 to 0.96), NNT 14 (9 to 35)). Women who practised perineal massage were less likely to have an episiotomy (three trials, 2417 women, RR 0.85 (95% CI 0.75 to 0.97), NNT 23 (13 to 111)). Again this reduction was statistically significant for women without previous vaginal birth only (three trials, 1925 women, RR 0.85 (95% CI 0.74 to 0.97), NNT 20 (11 to 110)). No differences were seen in the incidence of first or second degree perineal tears or third/fourth degree perineal trauma. Only women who have previously birthed vaginally reported a statistically significant reduction in the incidence of pain at three months' postpartum (one trial, 376 women, RR 0.68 (95% CI 0.50 to 0.91) NNT 13 (7 to 60)). No significant differences were observed in the incidence of instrumental deliveries, sexual satisfaction, or incontinence of urine, faeces or flatus for any women who practised perineal massage compared with those who did not massage.

AUTHORS' CONCLUSIONS: Antenatal perineal massage reduces the likelihood of perineal trauma (mainly episiotomies) and the reporting of ongoing perineal pain and is generally well accepted by women. As such, women should be made aware of the likely benefit of perineal massage and provided with information on how to massage.

7.9.2   Repair of perineal trauma

Considering the long-term discomfort which may follow perineal trauma, attention to optimising the quality of surgical repair is of importance.

ABSORBABLE SYNTHETIC VERSUS CATGUT SUTURE MATERIAL FOR PERINEAL REPAIR: reduced pain and suture dehiscence; needed removal more often. (Kettle C, Johanson RB) CD000006

BACKGROUND: Approximately 70% of women will experience some degree of perineal trauma following vaginal delivery and will require stitches. This may result in perineal pain and superficial dyspareunia.
OBJECTIVES: To assess the effects of absorbable synthetic suture material as compared with catgut on the amount of short and long term pain experienced by mothers following perineal repair.
METHODS: Standard PCG methods (see page xvii). Search date: 1999.
MAIN RESULTS: Eight trials were included. Compared with catgut, the polyglycolic acid and polyglactin groups were associated with less pain in the first three days (odds ratio 0.62, 95% confidence interval 0.54 to 0.71). There was also less need for analgesia (odds ratio 0.63, 95% confidence interval 0.52 to 0.77) and less suture dehiscence (odds ratio 0.45, 95% confidence interval 0.29 to 0.70). There was no significant difference in long term pain (odds ratio 0.81, 95% confidence interval 0.61 to 1.08). Removal of suture material was significantly more common in the polyglycolic acid and polyglactin groups (odds ratio 2.01, 95% confidence interval 1.56 to 2.58). There was no difference in the amount of dyspareunia experienced by women.

AUTHORS' CONCLUSIONS: Absorbable synthetic suture material (in the form of polyglycolic acid and polyglactin sutures) for perineal repair following childbirth appears to decrease women's experience of short term pain. The length of time taken for the synthetic material

to be absorbed is of concern. A trial addressing the use of polyglactin has recently been completed and this has been included in this updated review.

> ☺ **CONTINUOUS VERSUS INTERRUPTED SUTURES FOR PERINEAL REPAIR:** reduced short term pain, particularly when used for all layers. (Kettle C, Hills RK, Ismail KMK) CD000947

BACKGROUND: Millions of women worldwide undergo perineal suturing after childbirth and the type of repair may have an impact on pain and healing. For more than 70 years, researchers have been suggesting that continuous non-locking suture techniques for repair of the vagina, perineal muscles and skin are associated with less perineal pain than traditional interrupted methods.

OBJECTIVES: To assess the effects of continuous versus interrupted absorbable sutures for repair of episiotomy and second degree perineal tears following childbirth.

METHODS: Standard PCG methods (see page xvii). Search date: June 2007.

MAIN RESULTS: Seven studies, involving 3822 women at point of entry, from four countries, have been included. The trials were heterogeneous in respect of operator skill and training. Meta-analysis showed that continuous suture techniques compared with interrupted sutures for perineal closure (all layers or perineal skin only) are associated with less pain for up to 10 days' postpartum (relative risk (RR) 0.70, 95% confidence interval 0.64 to 0.76). Subgroup analysis showed that there is a greater reduction in pain when continuous suturing techniques are used for all layers (RR 0.65, 95% CI 0.60 to 0.71). There was an overall reduction in analgesia use associated with the continuous subcutaneous technique versus interrupted stitches for repair of perineal skin (RR 0.70, 95% CI 0.58 to 0.84). Subgroup analysis showed some evidence of reduction in dyspareunia experienced by participants in the groups that had continuous suturing for all layers (RR 0.83, 95% CI 0.70 to 0.98). There was also a reduction in suture removal in the continuous suturing groups versus interrupted (RR 0.54, 95% CI 0.45 to 0.65), but no significant differences were seen in the need for re-suturing of wounds or long-term pain.

AUTHORS' CONCLUSIONS: The continuous suturing techniques for perineal closure, compared to interrupted methods, are associated

with less short-term pain. Moreover, if the continuous technique is used for all layers (vagina, perineal muscles and skin) compared to perineal skin only, the reduction in pain is even greater.

METHODS OF REPAIR FOR OBSTETRIC ANAL SPHINCTER INJURY: overlap repair reduced faecal urgency and anal incontinence but data were limited. (Fernando R, Sultan AH, Kettle C, Thakar R, Radley S) CD002866 (in RHL 11)

BACKGROUND: Anal sphincter injury during childbirth – obstetric anal sphincter injuries (OASIS) – is associated with significant maternal morbidity including perineal pain, dyspareunia and anal incontinence. Anal incontinence affects women psychologically and physically. Many do not seek medical attention because of embarrassment. The two recognised methods for the repair of damaged external anal sphincter (EAS) are end-to-end (approximation) repair and overlap repair.

OBJECTIVES: To compare the effectiveness of overlap repair versus end-to-end repair following OASIS in reducing subsequent anal incontinence, perineal pain, dyspareunia and improving quality of life.

METHODS: Standard PCG methods (see page xvii). Search date: January 2006.

MAIN RESULTS: Three eligible trials, of grade A quality, involving 279 women, were included. There was considerable heterogeneity in the outcome measures, time points and reported results. Meta-analyses showed that there was no statistically significant difference in perineal pain (relative risk (RR) 0.08, 95% confidence interval (CI) 0.00 to 1.45, one trial, 52 women), dyspareunia (RR 0.62, 95% CI 0.11 to 3.39, one trial, 52 women), flatus incontinence (RR 0.93, 95% CI 0.26 to 3.31, one trial, 52 women) or faecal incontinence (RR 0.07, 95% CI 0.00 to 1.21, one trial, 52 women) between the two repair techniques at 12 months but showed a statistically significantly lower incidence in faecal urgency (RR 0.12, 95% CI 0.02 to 0.86, one trial, 52 women) and lower anal incontinence score (weighted mean difference −1.70, 95% CI −3.03 to −0.37) in the overlap group. Overlap technique was also associated with a statistically significant lower risk of deterioration of anal incontinence symptoms over 12 months (RR 0.26, 95% CI 0.09 to 0.79, one trial, 41 women). There was no significant difference in quality of life.

AUTHORS' CONCLUSIONS: The limited data available show that compared to immediate primary end-to-end repair of OASIS, early primary overlap repair appears to be associated with lower risks for faecal urgency and anal incontinence symptoms. As the experience of the surgeon is not addressed in the three studies reviewed, it would be inappropriate to recommend one type of repair in favour of another.

ANTIBIOTIC PROPHYLAXIS FOR FOURTH-DEGREE PERINEAL TEAR DURING VAGINAL BIRTH: no randomised trials to provide reliable evidence. (Buppasiri P, Lumbiganon P, Thinkhamrop J, Thinkhamrop B) CD005125

BACKGROUND: One to eight per cent of women suffer third-degree perineal tears (anal sphincter injury) and fourth-degree perineal tear (rectal mucosa injury) during vaginal birth, and these tears are more common after forceps delivery (28%) and midline episiotomies. Fourth-degree tears can become contaminated with bacteria from the rectum and this significantly increases the chance of perineal wound infection. Prophylactic antibiotics might have a role in preventing this infection.

OBJECTIVES: To assess the effectiveness of antibiotic prophylaxis for reducing maternal morbidity and side-effects in fourth-degree perineal tear during vaginal birth.

METHODS: Standard PCG methods (see page xvii). Search date: July 2005.

MAIN RESULTS: No randomised controlled trials were identified.

AUTHORS' CONCLUSIONS: There are insufficient data to support a policy of routine prophylactic antibiotics in fourth-degree perineal tear during vaginal birth. A well-designed randomised controlled trial is needed.

7.10   Operative vaginal birth

In 1920 De Lee argued cogently for routine forceps delivery under general anaesthesia for all nulliparous and most multiparous women. Today instrumental vaginal birth (assisted birth) is used to shorten the second stage of labour in the case of a compromised baby; for prolonged second stage; when the mother is unable to bear down; and to protect the baby's head in the case of prematurity or breech birth.

Many factors influence the choice of instrument. Forceps are needed for premature babies, breech births and face presentations. The vacuum extractor has particular advantages for small, android pelves and deflexed positions other than occipito-anterior, because it does not take up additional space in the pelvis, and can improve flexion and thus rotation of the head. The benefits and risks of these alternative methods have been evaluated in randomised trials (see below) Techniques of vacuum extraction are demonstrated in the video presentation 'Vacuum extraction': WHO reproductive Health Library, **www.rhlibrary.com.**

> **INSTRUMENTS FOR ASSISTED VAGINAL DELIVERY:** (O'Mahony F, Hofmeyr GJ, Menon V) Protocol [see page xviii] CD005455

ABRIDGED BACKGROUND: Instrumental or 'assisted' vaginal delivery is a frequently and widely practiced obstetric intervention, accounting for 11% of deliveries in the UK. There are widespread procedural variations in assisted vaginal delivery that depend on many factors. Forceps are classified according to whether traction alone or rotation of the fetal head is required. Vacuum cups may be either metal, plastic or silicone. Again they are classified according to whether rotation of the fetal head is required into posterior cups or anterior cups. The choice of instrument for assisted vaginal delivery may be limited by the clinical circumstances. For example, for face presentation and aftercoming head of the breech, forceps but not ventouse may be used. Where more than one instrument is appropriate, the choice should take into account evidence of the relative benefits and risks of the various instruments.

Another important issue in some low- and middle-income country settings is the high prevalence of HIV infections and the fact that many women do not have access to or decline to undergo testing. The potential for precipitating mother-to-child transmission of viral infections needs to be taken into account.

OBJECTIVES: The objective of this review is to answer the overall question: 'When assisted vaginal birth is needed, which instrument would be best?'. Individual vacuum devices or forceps used for assisted vaginal delivery will be reviewed in terms of maternal outcome, neonatal outcome and training requirements. The main questions concerning choice of instrument will therefore fall into three categories, namely:

1) should forceps or ventouse be used;
2) if it were forceps, which type would be best;
3) if it were ventouse, which type would be best?

☺ **VACUUM EXTRACTION VERSUS FORCEPS FOR ASSISTED VAGI-NAL DELIVERY:** was successful more frequently, with less maternal and more neonatal injury. (Johanson RB, Menon V) CD000224 (in RHL 11)

BACKGROUND: Proponents of vacuum delivery argue that it should be chosen first for assisted vaginal delivery, because it is less likely to injure the mother.

OBJECTIVES: To assess the effects of vacuum extraction compared to forceps on failure to achieve delivery and maternal and neonatal morbidity.

METHODS: Standard PCG methods (see page xvii). Search date: February 1999.

MAIN RESULTS: 10 trials were included. The trials were of reasonable quality. Use of the vacuum extractor for assisted vaginal delivery when compared to forceps delivery was associated with significantly less maternal trauma (odds ratio 0.41, 95% confidence interval 0.33 to 0.50) and with less general and regional anaesthesia. There were more deliveries with vacuum extraction (odds ratio 1.69, 95% confidence interval 1.31 to 2.19). Fewer caesarean sections were carried out in the vacuum extractor group. However the vacuum extractor was associated with an increase in neonatal cephalhaematomata and retinal haemorrhages. Serious neonatal injury was uncommon with either instrument.

AUTHORS' CONCLUSIONS: Use of the vacuum extractor rather than forceps for assisted delivery appears to reduce maternal morbidity. The reduction in cephalhaematoma and retinal haemorrhages seen with forceps may be a compensatory benefit.

RAPID VERSUS STEPWISE NEGATIVE PRESSURE APPLICATION FOR VACUUM EXTRACTION ASSISTED VAGINAL DELIVERY: (Suwannachat B, Lumbiganon P, Laopaiboon M) Protocol [see page xviii] CD006636

ABRIDGED BACKGROUND: Vacuum extraction is fast becoming the method of choice for many assisted vaginal deliveries. There is a traditional recommendation that, for vacuum cup application, the operator should gradually increase negative pressure at 0.2 kg/cm^2 every two minutes, to reach 0.8 kg/cm^2 over 8 to 10 minutes. More recently, it has been suggested that there is no significant difference in the traction force developed between stepwise and rapid application of the vacuum – that an adequate chignon forms within one to two minutes of creating the vacuum, and traction may be commenced after one minute without compromising efficiency and safety.

OBJECTIVES: To assess efficacy and safety of rapid versus stepwise negative pressure application for assisted vaginal delivery by vacuum extraction.

☺ **SOFT VERSUS RIGID VACUUM EXTRACTOR CUPS FOR ASSISTED VAGINAL DELIVERY:** reduced scalp injury, but failed more often, particularly for rotational deliveries. (Johanson R, Menon V) CD000446

BACKGROUND: The original cups used for vacuum extraction delivery of the fetus were rigid metal cups. Subsequently, soft cups of flexible materials such as silicone rubber or plastic were introduced. Soft cups are thought to have a poorer success rate than metal cups. However they are also thought to be less likely to be associated with scalp trauma and less likely to injure the mother.

OBJECTIVES: To assess the effects of soft versus rigid vacuum extractor cups on perineal injury, fetal scalp injury and success rate.

METHODS: Standard PCG methods (see page xvii). Search date: February 2000.

MAIN RESULTS: Nine trials involving 1375 women were included. The trials were of average quality. Soft cups are significantly more likely to fail to achieve vaginal delivery (odds ratio 1.65, 95% confidence interval 1.19 to 2.29). However, they were associated with less scalp injury (odds ratio 0.45, 95% confidence interval 0.15 to 0.60). There was no difference between the two groups in terms of maternal injury.

AUTHORS' CONCLUSIONS: Metal cups appear to be more suitable for 'occipito-posterior', transverse and difficult 'occipito-anterior' position deliveries. The soft cups seem to be appropriate for straightforward deliveries.

ANTIBIOTIC PROPHYLAXIS FOR OPERATIVE VAGINAL DELIVERY: not enough data to provide reliable evidence. (Liabsuetrakul T, Choobun T, Peeyananjarassri K, Islam M) CD004455

BACKGROUND: Vacuum and forceps assisted vaginal deliveries are reported to increase the incidence of postpartum infections and maternal readmission to hospital compared to spontaneous vaginal delivery. Prophylactic antibiotics are prescribed to prevent these infections. However, the benefit of antibiotic prophylaxis for operative vaginal deliveries is still unclear.

OBJECTIVES: To assess the effectiveness and safety of antibiotic prophylaxis in reducing infectious puerperal morbidities in women undergoing operative vaginal deliveries including vacuum or forceps deliveries, or both.

METHODS: Standard PCG methods (see page xvii). Search date: June 2007.

MAIN RESULTS: One trial, involving 393 women undergoing either vacuum or forceps deliveries, was included. This trial identified only two out of the nine outcomes specified in this review. It reported seven women with endomyometritis in the group given no antibiotic and none in the prophylactic antibiotic group. This difference did not reach statistical significance, but the relative risk reduction was 93% (relative risks 0.07; 95% confidence interval (CI) 0.00 to 1.21). There was no difference in the length of hospital stay between the two groups (weighted mean difference 0.09 days; 95% CI -0.23 to 0.41).

AUTHORS' CONCLUSIONS: The data were too few and of insufficient quality to make any recommendations for practice. Future research on antibiotic prophylaxis for operative vaginal delivery is needed to conclude whether it is useful for reducing postpartum morbidity.

TRIAL OF INSTRUMENTAL DELIVERY IN THEATRE VERSUS IMMEDIATE CAESAREAN SECTION FOR ANTICIPATED DIFFICULT ASSISTED BIRTHS: (Majoko F, Devenish-Meares P, Gardener G) Protocol [see page xviii] CD005545

ABRIDGED BACKGROUND: The majority of women have spontaneous vaginal birth but some women need assistance with delivery of the baby in the second stage of labour. Instrumental vaginal delivery is when obstetric forceps or the vacuum extractor is used to assist delivery of the baby. The majority of instrumental vaginal deliveries are conducted in the delivery room but in a small proportion (2% to 5%) a trial of instrumental vaginal delivery is conducted in theatre with preparations made for proceeding to caesarean section. Although all instrumental vaginal deliveries can be considered a trial, there are clinical factors such as malposition and level of presenting part that may influence the operator in deciding on delivery in the room or in theatre. Some trials of instrumental vaginal delivery fail to complete delivery by the vaginal route and caesarean section is performed. There are reports that suggest increased maternal and neonatal morbidity following failed trial of instrumental vaginal delivery and others suggesting that failed trial of instrumental vaginal delivery does not increase maternal and neonatal morbidity. Immediate caesarean section without trial of instrumental vaginal delivery may increase caesarean section rate by performing caesarean section in women who could have a successful trial of instrumental vaginal delivery.

OBJECTIVES: To determine differences in maternal and neonatal morbidity for women where a trial of anticipated difficult instrumental vaginal delivery is conducted in theatre compared to women who have immediate caesarean section in the second stage for maternal or fetal indications.

7.11   Caesarean section

In 1826 James Barry, a British military doctor, courageously performed the first known caesarean section in South Africa. The child's grandson became Prime Minister, James Barry Munnik Herzog. Dr Barry was discovered posthumously to have been a woman. It was not until the following century that caesarean section became a relatively safe procedure.

The reasons for and consequences of caesarean section are discussed elsewhere (Pages 106, 186, 195–7, 213, 223, 262, 287, 300, 302, 354).

There is considerable variation in the techniques used for caesarean section. Many doctors find it difficult to change their preferred methods in the light of evidence from systematic review of randomised trials.

Pre-operative preparation and counselling is important, including decisions regarding thromboprophylaxis (drugs given prophylactically to try to reduce the chance of a blood clot forming) and consideration of special circumstances such as low-lying or morbidly adherent placenta. In the operating theatre, the baby's lie, presentation and position are checked to plan the delivery, and the baby's heart beat confirmed. The indication for caesarean section is reviewed, as the obstetric situation may have changed since the original decision was made, such as spontaneous version of a breech, rapid progress of cervical dilation which had been slow, or death of a baby with fetal distress.

Caesarean section provides a convenient opportunity to perform tubal ligation, though concern has been expressed regarding the adequacy of decisions made by parents in the acute situation.

7.11.1 Anaesthesia

> **REGIONAL VERSUS GENERAL ANAESTHESIA FOR CAESAREAN SECTION:** not enough data to provide reliable evidence; the choice will often depend on whether the woman wishes to be awake or not during the operation. (Afolabi BB, Lesi FEA, Merah NA) CD004350 (in RHL 11)

BACKGROUND: Regional and general anaesthesia (GA) are commonly used for caesarean section (CS) and both have advantages and disadvantages. It is important to clarify what type of anaesthesia is more efficacious.

OBJECTIVES: To compare the effects of regional anaesthesia (RA) with those of GA on the outcomes of CS.

METHODS: Standard PCG methods (see page xvii). Search date: December 2005.

MAIN RESULTS: 16 studies (1586 women) were included in this review.

Women who had either epidural anaesthesia or spinal anaesthesia were found to have a significantly lower difference between pre and postoperative haematocrit (weighted mean difference (WMD) 1.70, 95% confidence interval (CI) 0.47 to 2.93, one trial, 231 women; WMD 3.10, 95% CI 1.73 to 4.47, one trial, 209 women). Compared to GA, women having either an epidural or spinal anaesthesia had a lower estimated maternal blood loss (WMD −126.98 millilitres, 95% CI −225.06 to −28.90, two trials, 256 women; WMD −84.79 millilitres, 95% CI

−126.96 to −42.63, two trials, 279 women). More women preferred to have GA for subsequent procedures when compared with epidural (odds ratio (OR) 0.56, 95% CI 0.32 to 0.96, one trial, 223 women) or spinal (OR 0.44, 95% CI 0.24 to 0.81, 221 women). The incidence of nausea was also less for this group of women compared with epidural (OR 3.17, 95% CI 1.64 to 6.14, three trials, 286 women) or spinal (OR 23.22, 95% CI 8.69 to 62.03, 209 women).

No significant difference was seen in terms of neonatal Apgar scores of six or less and of four or less at one and five minutes and need for neonatal resuscitation with oxygen.

AUTHORS' CONCLUSIONS: There is no evidence from this review to show that RA is superior to GA in terms of major maternal or neonatal outcomes. Further research to evaluate neonatal morbidity and maternal outcomes, such as satisfaction with technique, will be useful.

USE OF HYPERBARIC VERSUS ISOBARIC BUPIVACAINE FOR SPINAL ANAESTHESIA FOR CAESAREAN SECTION: (Sia ATH, Lim Y, Tan KH) Protocol [see page xviii] CD005143 (Anaesthesia Group)

ABRIDGED BACKGROUND: Both isobaric and hyperbaric bupivacaine have consistently been able to provide adequate anaesthesia for caesarean sections. The difference in density between the two forms of bupivacaine affects the diffusion patterns and distribution of the local anaesthetic when it is introduced into the subarachnoid space.
OBJECTIVES: (1) To determine the effectiveness of hyperbaric bupivacaine when compared to isobaric bupivacaine for caesarean section. (2) To determine the safety and side effects of hyperbaric bupivacaine when compared to isobaric bupivacaine for caesarean section.

SUPPLEMENTAL OXYGEN FOR CAESAREAN SECTION DURING REGIONAL ANAESTHESIA: (Chatmogkolchart S, Lee BB, Uakridathikarn T) Protocol [see page xviii] CD006161 (Anaesthesia Group)

ABRIDGED BACKGROUND: Spinal anaesthesia is recommended for caesarean section, but may lead to impaired maternal respiratory function and hypotension resulting in impaired maternal–fetal gas exchange. Many pregnant women are empirically given supplemental oxygen intraoperatively, at least until delivery of the baby. This is theoretically to provide hyperoxygenation to the fetus to enable it to better tolerate any unforeseen intra-natal and postnatal oxygen deprivation.

The benefit of administering supplemental oxygen to healthy, low-risk pregnant women during elective caesarean section under regional anaesthesia is controversial.

OBJECTIVES: Our primary objective is to compare maternal and fetal outcomes between women, with low-risk term pregnancies undergoing elective or scheduled caesarean section under regional anaesthesia with or without oxygen supplementation. Our intention is to identify adverse outcomes that might be prevented by the use of supplemental oxygen.

Our secondary objectives are to compare the maternal and fetal outcomes between women who are given oxygen at:

1. different flow rates of administration;
2. different concentrations;
3. different oxygen delivery devices.

☺ **SPINAL VERSUS EPIDURAL ANAESTHESIA FOR CAESAREAN SECTION:** spinal was effective more quickly, but caused more hypotension. (Ng K, Parsons J, Cyna AM, Middleton P) CD003765 (in RHL 11)

BACKGROUND: Regional anaesthesia (spinal or epidural anaesthesia) for caesarean section is the preferred option when balancing risks and benefits to the mother and her fetus. Spinal anaesthesia for caesarean section is thought to be advantageous due to simplicity of technique, rapid administration and onset of anaesthesia, reduced risk of systemic toxicity and increased density of spinal anaesthetic block.

OBJECTIVES: To assess the relative efficacy and side-effects of spinal versus epidural anaesthesia in women having caesarean section.

METHODS: Standard PCG methods (see page xvii). Search date: February 2003.

MAIN RESULTS: 10 trials (751 women) met our inclusion criteria. No difference was found between spinal and epidural techniques with regard to failure rate (RR 0.98, 95% CI 0.23 to 4.24; four studies), need for additional intraoperative analgesia (RR 0.88, 95% CI 0.59 to 1.32; five studies), need for conversion to general anaesthesia intraoperatively, maternal satisfaction, need for postoperative pain relief and neonatal intervention. Women receiving spinal anaesthesia for caesarean section showed reduced time from start of the anaesthetic to start of the operation (WMD 7.91 minutes less (95% CI −11.59 to −4.23; four studies), but increased need for treatment of hypotension (RR 1.23, 95% CI 1.00 to 1.51; six studies).

AUTHORS' CONCLUSIONS: Both spinal and epidural techniques are shown to provide effective anaesthesia for caesarean section. Both techniques are associated with moderate degrees of maternal satisfaction. Spinal anaesthesia has a shorter onset time, but treatment for hypotension is more likely if spinal anaesthesia is used. No conclusions can be drawn about intraoperative side-effects and postoperative complications because they were of low incidence and/or not reported.

DRUGS AT CAESAREAN SECTION FOR PREVENTING NAUSEA, VOMITING AND ASPIRATION PNEUMONITIS: (Paranjothy S, Liu E, Brown H, Thomas J) Protocol [see page xviii] CD004943

ABRIDGED BACKGROUND: Aspiration pneumonitis was first described by Mendelson in the 1940s. It occurs when gastric acid gains access to the lungs in the absence of a cough reflex. Although rare during caesarean section, aspiration pneumonitis is still a cause of maternal mortality even in well-resourced countries such as the United Kingdom. Several different types of drugs have been used to reduce the risks and effects of acid aspiration. These include antacids, H2 receptor antagonists, proton pump inhibitors and prokinetic drugs, either singly or in combination. Non-pharmacological methods (e.g., acupressure/acupuncture, herbal agents, homeopathic agents or hypnosis) have the potential to have fewer side-effects and in general there is a growing consumer demand for non-pharmacological interventions.

OBJECTIVES: 1. To determine whether antiemetics (pharmacological and non-pharmacological) given prior to having a caesarean section reduces the incidence of nausea and vomiting in healthy women with an uncomplicated pregnancy. 2. To determine whether drugs given prior to having a caesarean section reduce the incidence of aspiration pneumonitis in healthy women with an uncomplicated pregnancy.

© **TECHNIQUES FOR PREVENTING HYPOTENSION DURING SPINAL ANAESTHESIA FOR CAESAREAN SECTION:** pre-emptive crystalloid or colloid fluids, ephedrine and lower limb compression reduced the incidence of hypotension during spinal anaesthesia. (Cyna AM, Andrew M, Emmett RS, Middleton P, Simmons SW) CD002251

BACKGROUND: Maternal hypotension, the most frequent complication of spinal anaesthesia for caesarean section, can be associated with severe nausea or vomiting which can pose serious risks to the mother (unconsciousness, pulmonary aspiration) and baby (hypoxia, acidosis and neurological injury).

OBJECTIVES: To assess the effects of prophylactic interventions for hypotension following spinal anaesthesia for caesarean section.

METHODS: Standard PCG methods (see page xvii). Search date: November 2005.

MAIN RESULTS: We included 75 trials (a total of 4624 women). Crystalloids were more effective than no fluids (relative risk (RR) 0.78, 95% confidence interval (CI) 0.60 to 1.00; one trial, 140 women, sequential analysis) and colloids were more effective than crystalloids (RR 0.68, 95% CI 0.52 to 0.89; 11 trials, 698 women) in preventing hypotension following spinal anaesthesia at caesarean section. No differences were detected for different doses, rates or methods of administering colloids or crystalloids. Ephedrine was significantly more effective than control (RR 0.51, 95% CI 0.33 to 0.78; seven trials, 470 women) or crystalloid (RR 0.70, 95% CI 0.50 to 0.96; four trials, 293 women) in preventing hypotension. No significant differences in hypotension were seen between ephedrine and phenylephrine (RR 0.95, 95% CI 0.37 to 2.44; three trials, 97 women) and phenylephrine was more effective than controls (RR 0.27, 95% CI 0.16 to 0.45; two trials, 110 women). High rates or doses of ephedrine may increase hypertension and tachycardia incidence. Lower limb compression was more effective than control (no leg compression) (RR 0.69, 95% CI 0.53 to 0.90; seven trials, 399 women) in preventing hypotension, although different methods of compression appeared to vary in their effectiveness. No other comparisons between different physical methods such as position were shown to be effective, but these trials were often small and thus underpowered to detect true effects should they exist.

AUTHORS' CONCLUSIONS: While interventions such as colloids, ephedrine, phenylephrine or lower leg compression can reduce the incidence of hypotension, none have been shown to eliminate the need to treat maternal hypotension during spinal anaesthesia for caesarean section. No conclusions can be drawn regarding rare adverse effects due to the relatively small numbers of women studied.

MUSIC DURING CAESAREAN SECTION UNDER REGIONAL ANAESTHESIA FOR IMPROVING MATERNAL AND INFANT OUTCOMES: (Laopaiboon M, Lumbiganon P, Martis R, Vatanasapt P, Somchiwong B) Protocol [see page xviii] CD006914

ABRIDGED BACKGROUND: Pregnant mothers undergoing caesarean section often experience anxiety, which can increase the risk of psychological and physiological complications. Music can reduce anxiety effectively and improves the mood of medical and surgical patients, patients in intensive care units and patients undergoing procedures. Providing music to caregivers may be a cost-effective and enjoyable strategy to improve empathy, compassion and relationship-centred care while not increasing errors or interfering with technical aspects of care.

OBJECTIVES: To assess the effectiveness of music during caesarean section under regional anaesthesia on improving clinical and psychological outcomes for mothers and infants.

7.11.2   Perioperative measures for caesarean section

PREOPERATIVE SKIN ANTISEPTICS FOR PREVENTING SURGICAL WOUND INFECTIONS AFTER CLEAN SURGERY: not enough data from general surgical literature to provide reliable evidence. (Edwards PS, Lipp A, Holmes A) CD003949 (Wounds Group)

BACKGROUND: Approximately 15% of elective surgery patients and 30% of patients receiving contaminated or dirty surgery are estimated to develop post-operative wound infections. The costs of surgical wound infection can be considerable in financial as well as social terms. Preoperative skin antisepsis is performed to reduce the risk of post-operative wound infections by removing soil and transient organisms from the skin. Antiseptics are thought to be both toxic to bacteria and aid their mechanical removal. The effectiveness of preoperative skin preparation is thought to be dependent on both the antiseptic used and the method of application, however it is unclear whether preoperative skin antisepsis actually reduces post-operative wound infection and if so which antiseptic is most effective.

OBJECTIVES: To determine whether preoperative skin antisepsis reduces post-operative surgical wound infection.

SEARCH STRATEGY: We searched the Cochrane Wounds Group Specialised Trials Register and the Cochrane Central Register of Controlled Trials in April 2004. In addition, we handsearched journals, conference proceedings and bibliographies.

SELECTION CRITERIA: Randomised controlled trials evaluating the use of preoperative skin antiseptics applied immediately prior to incision in clean surgery. There were no restrictions based on language, date or publication status.

DATA COLLECTION AND ANALYSIS: Three reviewers independently undertook data extraction and assessment of study quality. Pooling was inappropriate and trials are discussed in a narrative review.

MAIN RESULTS: We identified six eligible RCTs evaluating preoperative antiseptics. There was significant heterogeneity in the comparisons and the results could not be pooled. In one study, infection rates were significantly lower when skin was prepared using chlorhexidine compared with iodine. There was no evidence of a benefit in four trials associated with the use of iodophor impregnated drapes.

AUTHORS' CONCLUSIONS: There is insufficient research examining the effects of preoperative skin antiseptics to allow conclusions to be drawn regarding their effects on post-operative surgical wound infections. Further research is needed.

PREOPERATIVE HAIR REMOVAL TO REDUCE SURGICAL SITE INFECTION: hair removal prior to surgery (not specifically caesarean section) did not reduce infections. When hair was removed, shaving caused more infections than clipping or depilatory creams. (Tanner J, Woodings D, Moncaster K) CD004122 (Wounds Group)

BACKGROUND: The preparation of people for surgery has traditionally included the routine removal of body hair from the intended surgical wound site. However, there are studies which claim that pre-operative hair removal is deleterious to patients, perhaps by causing surgical site infections (SSIs), and should not be carried out.

OBJECTIVES: The primary objective of this review was to determine if routine pre-operative hair removal results in fewer SSIs than not removing hair.

SEARCH STRATEGY: The reviewers searched the Cochrane Wounds Group Specialised Register (October 2005), The Cochrane Central Register of Controlled Trials (*The Cochrane Library* Issue 3, 2005), MEDLINE (1966 to 2005), EMBASE (1980 to 2005), CINAHL (1982 to 2005) and the ZETOC database of conference proceedings (1993 to 2005). We also contacted manufacturers of hair removal products.

SELECTION CRITERIA: Randomised controlled trials (RCTs) comparing hair removal with no hair removal, different methods of hair removal, hair removal conducted at different times prior to surgery and hair removal carried out in different settings.

DATA COLLECTION AND ANALYSIS: Three authors independently assessed the relevance and quality of each trial. Data was extracted independently by one author and cross checked for accuracy by a second author.

MAIN RESULTS: Eleven RCTs were included in this review. Three trials involving 625 people compared hair removal using either depilatory cream or razors with no hair removal and found no statistically significant difference between the groups in terms of surgical site infections. No trials were identified which compared clipping with no hair removal. Three trials involving 3193 people compared shaving with clipping and found that there were statistically significantly more SSIs when people were shaved rather than clipped (RR 2.02, 95%CI 1.21 to 3.36). Seven trials involving 1213 people compared shaving with removing hair using a depilatory cream and found that there were statistically significantly more SSIs when people were shaved than when a cream was used (RR 1.54, 95%CI 1.05 to 2.24). No trials were found that compared clipping with a depilatory cream.

One trial compared shaving on the day of surgery with shaving the day before surgery and one trial compared clipping on the day of surgery with clipping the day before surgery; neither trial found a statistically significant difference in the number of SSIs. No trials were found that compared depilatory cream at different times or that compared hair removal in different settings.

AUTHORS' CONCLUSIONS: The evidence finds no difference in SSIs among patients who have had hair removed prior to surgery and those who have not. If it is necessary to remove hair then both clipping and depilatory creams result in fewer SSIs than shaving using a razor. There is no difference in SSIs when patients are shaved or clipped one day before surgery or on the day of surgery.

PREOPERATIVE BATHING OR SHOWERING WITH SKIN ANTISEPTICS TO PREVENT SURGICAL SITE INFECTION: not enough data from general surgery literature to provide reliable evidence. (Webster J, Osborne S) CD004985 (Wounds Group)

BACKGROUND: Surgical site infections (SSIs) are wound infections that occur after invasive (surgical) procedures. Preoperative bathing or showering with an antiseptic skin wash product is a well-accepted procedure for reducing skin bacteria (microflora). It is less clear whether reducing skin microflora leads to a lower incidence of surgical site infection.

OBJECTIVES: To review the evidence for preoperative bathing or showering with antiseptics for the prevention of hospital-acquired (nosocomial) surgical site infection.

SEARCH STRATEGY: We searched the Cochrane Wounds Group Specialised Register (December 2005), the Cochrane Central Register of Controlled Trials (The Cochrane Library Issue 4, 2005), MEDLINE (January 1966 to December 2005) and reference lists of articles.

SELECTION CRITERIA: Randomised controlled trials comparing any antiseptic preparation used for preoperative full-body bathing or showering with non-antiseptic preparations in patients undergoing surgery.

DATA COLLECTION AND ANALYSIS: Two authors independently assessed studies for selection, trial quality and extracted data. Study authors were contacted for additional information.

MAIN RESULTS: Six trials involving a total of 10007 participants were included. Three of the included trials had three comparison groups. The antiseptic used in all trials was four per cent chlorhexidine gluconate (Hibiscrub). Three trials involving 7691 participants compared chlorhexidine with a placebo. Bathing with chlorhexidine compared with placebo did not result in a statistically significant reduction in SSIs; the relative risk of SSI (RR) was 0.91 (95% confidence interval (CI) 0.80 to 1.04). When only trials of high quality were included in this comparison, the RR of SSI was 0.95 (95%CI 0.82 to 1.10).

Three trials of 1443 participants compared bar soap with chlorhexidine; when combined there was no difference in the risk of SSIs (RR 1.02, 95% CI 0.57 to 1.84). Two trials of 1092 patients compared bathing with chlorhexidine with no washing one large study found a statistically significant difference in favour of bathing with chlorhexidine (RR 0.36, 95%CI 0.17 to 0.79). The second smaller study found no difference between patients who washed with chlorhexidine and those who did not wash preoperatively.

AUTHORS' CONCLUSIONS: This review provides no clear evidence of benefit for preoperative showering or bathing with chlorhexidine over other wash products to reduce surgical site infection. Efforts to reduce the incidence of nosocomial surgical site infection should focus on interventions where effect has been demonstrated.

☺ **ANTIBIOTIC PROPHYLAXIS FOR CESAREAN SECTION:** reduced postoperative fever, endometritis, wound infection, urinary tract infection and serious infection; no outcomes on the baby assessed. (Smaill F, Hofmeyr GJ) CD000933 (in RHL 11)

BACKGROUND: The single most important risk factor for postpartum maternal infection is cesarean delivery.

OBJECTIVES: To assess the effects of prophylactic antibiotic treatment on infectious complications in women undergoing cesarean delivery.

METHODS: Standard PCG methods (see page xvii). Search date: January 2002.

MAIN RESULTS: 81 trials were included. Use of prophylactic antibiotics in women undergoing cesarean section substantially reduced the incidence of episodes of fever, endometritis, wound infection, urinary tract infection and serious infection after cesarean section. The reduction in the risk of endometritis with antibiotics was similar across different patient groups: the relative risk (RR) for endometritis for elective cesarean section (number of women = 2037) was 0.38 (95% confidence interval (CI) 0.22 to 0.64); the RR for non-elective cesarean section (n = 2132) was 0.39 (95% CI 0.34 to 0.46); and the RR for all patients (n = 11937) was 0.39 (95% CI 0.31 to 0.43). Wound infections were also reduced: for elective cesarean section (n = 2015) RR 0.73 (95% CI 0.53 to 0.99); for non-elective cesarean section (n = 2780) RR 0.36 (95% CI 0.26 to 0.51); and for all patients (n = 11 142) RR 0.41 (95% CI 0.29 to 0.43).

AUTHORS' CONCLUSIONS: The reduction of endometritis by two thirds to three quarters and a decrease in wound infections justifies a policy of recommending prophylactic antibiotics to women undergoing elective or non-elective cesarean section.

ANTIBIOTIC PROPHYLAXIS REGIMENS AND DRUGS FOR CESAREAN SECTION: single dose ampicillin or first generation cephalosporins were as effective as broader spectrum antibiotics and multiple dose regimens. (Hopkins L, Smaill F) CD001136 (in RHL 11)

BACKGROUND: Prophylactic antibiotics for cesarean section have been shown to reduce the incidence of maternal postoperative infectious morbidity. Many different antibiotic regimens have been reported to be effective.

OBJECTIVES: To determine which antibiotic regimen is most effective in reducing the incidence of infectious morbidity in women undergoing cesarean section.

METHODS: Standard PCG methods (see page xvii). Search date: October 1998.

Trials that compared placebo with a single antibiotic regimen were not included as these are studies which have been analyzed in another Cochrane review.

MAIN RESULTS: 51 trials published between 1979 and 1994 were included in the review and four were excluded from the review. The following results refer to reductions in the incidence of endometritis. Both ampicillin and first generation cephalosporins have similar efficacy with an odds ratio (OR) of 1.27 (95% confidence interval (CI): 0.84–1.93). In comparing ampicillin with second or third generation cephalosporins the odds ratio was 0.83 (95% CI 0.54–1.26) and in comparing a first generation cephalosporin with a second or third generation agent the odds ratio was 1.21 (95% CI 0.97–1.51). A multiple dose regimen for prophylaxis appears to offer no added benefit over a single dose regimen: OR 0.92 (95% CI 0.70–1.23). Systemic and lavage routes of administration appear to have no difference in effect: OR 1.19 (95% CI 0.81–1.73). There was no significant heterogeneity between the trials contained in the various sub-group analyses, although confidence intervals were sometimes wide.

AUTHORS' CONCLUSIONS: Both ampicillin and first generation cephalosporins have similar efficacy in reducing postoperative

endometritis. There does not appear to be added benefit in utilizing a broader spectrum agent or a multiple dose regimen. There is a need for an appropriately designed randomized trial to test the optimal timing of administration (immediately after the cord is clamped versus pre-operative).

☺ **DOUBLE GLOVING TO REDUCE SURGICAL CROSS-INFECTION:** double gloving and other protective measures reduce inner glove perforations in general surgery. (Tanner J, Parkinson H) CD003087 (Wounds Group)

BACKGROUND: The invasive nature of surgery, with its increased exposure to blood, means that during surgery there is a high risk of transfer of pathogens. Pathogens can be transferred through contact between surgical patients and the surgical team, resulting in post-operative or blood borne infections in patients or blood borne infections in the surgical team. Both patients and the surgical team need to be protected from this risk. This risk can be reduced by implementing protective barriers such as wearing surgical gloves. Wearing two pairs of surgical gloves, triple gloves, glove liners or cloth outer gloves, as opposed to one pair, is considered to provide an additional barrier and further reduce the risk of contamination.

OBJECTIVES: The primary objective of this review was to determine if additional glove protection reduces the number of surgical site or blood borne infections in patients or the surgical team. The secondary objective was to determine if additional glove protection reduces the number of perforations to the innermost pair of surgical gloves. The innermost gloves (next to skin) compared with the outermost gloves are considered to be the last barrier between the patient and the surgical team.

SEARCH STRATEGY: We searched the Cochrane Wounds Group Specialised Register (January 2006) and the Cochrane Central Register of Controlled Trials (CENTRAL) (The Cochrane Library Issue 4, 2005). We also contacted glove manufacturing companies and professional organisations.

SELECTION CRITERIA: Randomised controlled trials involving: single gloving, double gloving, triple gloving, glove liners, knitted outer gloves, steel weave outer gloves and perforation indicator systems.

DATA COLLECTION AND ANALYSIS: Both authors independently assessed the relevance and quality of each trial. Data was extracted by one author and cross checked for accuracy by the second author.

MAIN RESULTS: Two trials were found which addressed the primary outcome, namely, surgical site infections in patients. Both trials reported no infections.

Thirty one randomised controlled trials measuring glove perforations were identified and included in the review.

Fourteen trials of double gloving (wearing two pairs of surgical latex gloves) were pooled and showed that there were significantly more perforations to the single glove than the innermost of the double gloves (OR 4.10, 95% CI 3.30 to 5.09).

Eight trials of indicator gloves (coloured latex gloves worn underneath latex gloves to more rapidly alert the team to perforations) showed that significantly fewer perforations were detected with single gloves compared with indicator gloves (OR 0.10, 95% CI 0.06 to 0.16) or with standard double glove compared with indicator gloves (OR 0.08, 95% CI 0.04 to 0.17).

Two trials of glove liners (a glove knitted with cloth or polymers worn between two pairs of latex gloves)(OR 26.36, 95% CI 7.91 to 87.82), three trials of knitted gloves (knitted glove worn on top of latex surgical gloves)(OR 5.76, 95% CI 3.25 to 10.20) and one trial of triple gloving (three pairs of latex surgical gloves)(OR 69.41, 95% CI 3.89 to 1239.18), all compared with standard double gloves, showed that there were significantly more perforations to the innermost glove of a standard double glove in all comparisons.

AUTHORS' CONCLUSIONS: There is no direct evidence that additional glove protection worn by the surgical team reduces surgical site infections in patients; however the review has insufficient power for this outcome. The addition of a second pair of surgical gloves significantly reduces perforations to innermost gloves. Triple gloving, knitted outer gloves and glove liners also significantly reduce perforations to the innermost glove. Perforation indicator systems result in significantly more innermost glove perforations being detected during surgery.

DISPOSABLE SURGICAL FACE MASKS FOR PREVENTING SURGICAL WOUND INFECTION IN CLEAN SURGERY: not enough data from general surgery literature to provide reliable evidence. (Lipp A, Edwards P) CD002929 (Wounds Group)

BACKGROUND: Surgical face masks were originally developed to contain and filter droplets containing microorganisms expelled from the mouth and nasopharynx of healthcare workers during surgery, thereby providing protection for the patient. However there are several ways in which surgical face masks could potentially contribute to contamination of the surgical wound, e.g. by incorrect wear, by leaking air from the side of the mask due to poor string tension.

OBJECTIVES: To identify and review all randomised controlled trials evaluating disposable surgical face masks worn by the surgical team during clean surgery to prevent post-operative surgical wound infection.

SEARCH STRATEGY: All relevant publications about disposable surgical face masks were sought through the Cochrane Wounds Group Specialised Register (February 2006) and the Cochrane Central Register of Controlled Trials (Issue 1, 2006). Manufacturers and distributors of disposable surgical masks as well as professional organisations including the National Association of Theatre Nurses and the American Operating Room Nurses Association were contacted for details of unpublished and ongoing studies.

SELECTION CRITERIA: Randomised controlled trials (RCTs) and quasi-randomised controlled trials comparing the use of disposable surgical masks with the use of no mask were included.

DATA COLLECTION AND ANALYSIS: Data were extracted independently by two reviewers.

MAIN RESULTS: No new trials were included in this update. Two randomised controlled trials were included involving a total of 1453 participants. In one small trial there was a trend towards masks being associated with fewer infections, whereas in one large trial there was no statistically significant difference in infection rates between the masked and unmasked group.

AUTHORS' CONCLUSIONS: From the limited results it is unclear whether wearing surgical face masks results in any harm or benefit to the patient undergoing clean surgery.

7.11.3 Surgical techniques

In recent years, several time-honoured details of caesarean section technique have been challenged, and considerable evidence from randomised trials is available to guide choice of the most effective procedure. For a demonstration of newer, evidence-based techniques, see the video presentation: 'Caesarean section: evidence based technique': WHO Reproductive Health Library, **www.rhlibrary.com**.

☺ **TECHNIQUES FOR CAESAREAN SECTION:** 'Joel Cohen based' methods have short term advantages; long term effects uncertain. (Hofmeyr GJ, Mathai M, Shah A, Novikova N) CD004662

BACKGROUND: Rates of caesarean section (CS) have been rising globally. It is important to use the most effective and safe technique.

OBJECTIVES: To compare the effects of complete methods of caesarean section; and to summarise the findings of reviews of individual aspects of caesarean section technique.

METHODS: Standard PCG methods (see page xvii). Search date: August 2007.

MAIN RESULTS: 'Joel-Cohen based' compared with Pfannenstiel CS was associated with:

- less blood loss (five trials, 481 women; weighted mean difference (WMD) −64.45 ml; 95% confidence interval (CI) −91.34 to −37.56 ml);
- shorter operating time (five trials, 581 women; WMD −18.65 minutes; 95% CI −24.84 to −12.45 minutes);
- postoperatively, reduced time to oral intake (five trials, 481 women; WMD −3.92 hours; 95% CI −7.13 to −0.71 hours);
- less fever (eight trials, 1412 women; relative risk (RR) 0.47; 95% CI 0.28 to 0.81);
- shorter duration of postoperative pain (two comparisons from one trial, 172 women; WMD −14.18 hours; 95% CI −18.31 to −10.04 hours);
- fewer analgesic injections (two trials, 151 women; WMD −0.92; 95% CI −1.20 to −0.63); and
- shorter time from skin incision to birth of the baby (five trials, 575 women; WMD −3.84 minutes; 95% CI −5.41 to −2.27 minutes).

Serious complications and blood transfusions were too few for analysis. Misgav-Ladach compared with the traditional method (lower midline abdominal incision) was associated with reduced:

- blood loss (339 women; WMD −93.00; 95% CI −132.72 to −53.28 ml);
- operating time (339 women; WMD−7.30; 95% CI −8.32 to −6.28 minutes);
- time to mobilisation (339 women; WMD −16.06; 95% CI −18.22 to −13.90 hours); and
- length of postoperative stay for the mother (339 women; WMD −0.82; 95% CI −1.08 to −0.56 days).

Misgav-Ladach compared with modified Misgav-Ladach methods was associated with a longer time from skin incision to birth of the baby (116 women; WMD 2.10; 95% CI 1.10 to 3.10 minutes).

AUTHORS' CONCLUSIONS: 'Joel-Cohen based' methods have advantages compared to Pfannenstiel and to traditional (lower midline) CS techniques, which could translate to savings for the health system. However, these trials do not provide information on mortality and serious or long-term morbidity such as morbidly adherent placenta and scar rupture.

ABDOMINAL SURGICAL INCISIONS FOR CAESAREAN SECTION:
The Joel-Cohen incision was associated with less fever, pain, analgesic, and blood loss; no information on severe or long-term morbidity and mortality. (Mathai M, Hofmeyr GJ) CD004453

BACKGROUND: Caesarean section is the commonest major operation performed on women worldwide. Operative techniques, including abdominal incisions, vary. Some of these techniques have been evaluated through randomised trials.

OBJECTIVES: To determine the benefits and risks of alternative methods of abdominal surgical incisions for caesarean section.

METHODS: Standard PCG methods (see page xvii). Search date: April 2006.

MAIN RESULTS: Four studies were included in this review.

Two studies (411 participants) compared the Joel-Cohen incision with the Pfannenstiel incision. Overall, there was a 65% reduction in reported postoperative morbidity (relative risk (RR) 0.35, 95% confidence interval (CI) 0.14 to 0.87) with the Joel-Cohen incision. One of the trials reported reduced postoperative analgesic requirements (RR 0.55, 95% CI 0.40 to 0.76); operating time (weighted mean difference (WMD) −11.40, 95% CI −16.55 to −6.25 minutes); delivery time (WMD −1.90, 95% CI −2.53 to −1.27); total dose of analgesia in the first 24 hours (WMD −0.89, 95% CI −1.19 to −0.59); estimated blood loss (WMD −58.00, 95% CI −108.51 to −7.49 ml); postoperative hospital stay for the mother (WMD −1.50, 95% CI −2.16 to −0.84); and increased time to the first dose of analgesia (WMD 0.80, 95% CI 0.12 to 1.48) compared to the Pfannenstiel group. No other significant differences were found in either trial.

Two studies compared muscle cutting incisions with the Pfannenstiel incision. One study (68 women) comparing the Mouchel incision with the Pfannenstiel incision did not contribute data to this review. The other study (97 participants) comparing the Maylard muscle-cutting incision with the Pfannenstiel incision reported no difference in febrile morbidity (RR 1.26, 95% CI 0.08 to 19.50); need for blood transfusion (RR 0.42, 95% CI 0.02 to 9.98); wound infection (RR 1.26, 95% CI 0.27 to 5.91); physical tests on muscle strength at three months' postoperative and postoperative hospital stay (WMD 0.40 days, 95% CI −0.34 to 1.14).

AUTHORS' CONCLUSIONS: The Joel-Cohen incision has advantages compared to the Pfannenstiel incision. These are less fever, pain and analgesic requirements; less blood loss; shorter duration of surgery and hospital stay. These advantages for the mother could be extrapolated to savings for the health system. However, these trials do not provide information on severe or long-term morbidity and mortality.

> **SURGICAL TECHNIQUES INVOLVING THE UTERUS AT THE TIME OF CAESAREAN SECTION:** (Dodd JM, Anderson ER, Gates S) Protocol [see page xviii] CD004732

ABRIDGED BACKGROUND: There are many possible ways of performing a caesarean section operation, and operative techniques vary widely. This review will specifically assess surgical techniques involving the uterus at the time at caesarean section, and will include:

(1) the type of uterine incision (lower transverse uterine incision versus other types of uterine incision);
(2) methods of performing the uterine incision ('sharp' uterine entry versus 'blunt' uterine entry);

(3) suturing materials and techniques for the uterus at caesarean section; and

(4) single versus double layer suturing for closing the uterine incision at caesarean section.

OBJECTIVES: To compare, using the best available evidence, the effects of:

(1) different types of uterine incision;
(2) different methods of performing the uterine incision;
(3) different materials and techniques for closure of the uterine incision; and
(4) single versus double layer closure of the uterine incision on maternal and/or infant health and health care resource use.

⊗ **CLOSURE VERSUS NON-CLOSURE OF THE PERITONEUM AT CAESAREAN SECTION:** increased operating time, postoperative fever and hospital stay; no good data on long term outcomes as yet. (Bamigboye AA, Hofmeyr GJ) CD000163 (in RHL 11)

BACKGROUND: Caesarean section is a very common surgical procedure worldwide. Suturing the peritoneal layers at caesarean section may or may not confer benefit, hence the need to evaluate whether this step should be omitted or not.

OBJECTIVES: To assess the effects of non-closure as an alternative to closure of the peritoneum at caesarean section on intraoperative, immediate and long-term postoperative and long-term outcomes.

METHODS: Standard PCG methods (see page xvii). Search date: October 2006.

MAIN RESULTS: 14 trials, involving 2908 women, were included and analysed. The methodological quality of the trials was variable. Non-closure of the peritoneum reduced operating time whether both or either layer was not sutured. For both layers, the operating time was reduced by 6.05 minutes, 95% confidence interval (CI) −6.74 to −5.37. There was significantly less postoperative fever and reduced postoperative stay in hospital for visceral peritoneum and for both layer non-closure. The number of postoperative analgesic doses was reduced in the peritoneal non-closure group (weighted mean difference −0.20, 95% CI −0.33 to −0.08). There were no other statistically significant differences. The trend for wound infection tended to favour non-closure, while endometritis results were variable. Long-term follow up in one trial showed no significant differences. The power of the study to show differences was low.

AUTHORS' CONCLUSIONS: There was improved short-term postoperative outcome if the peritoneum was not closed. This in itself can support those who opt not to close the peritoneum. Long-term studies following caesarean section are limited; there is therefore no overall evidence for non-closure until long-term data become available.

☺ **EXTRA-ABDOMINAL VERSUS INTRA-ABDOMINAL REPAIR OF THE UTERINE INCISION AT CAESAREAN SECTION:** reduced febrile morbidity; increased hospital stay. (Jacobs-Jokhan D, Hofmeyr GJ) CD000085 (in RHL 11)

BACKGROUND: Different techniques have been described to reduce morbidity during caesarean section. After the baby has been born by caesarean section and the placenta has been extracted, temporary removal of the uterus from the abdominal cavity (exteriorisation of the uterus) to facilitate repair of the uterine incision has been postulated as a valuable technique. This is particularly so when exposure of the incision is difficult and when there are problems with haemostasis. Several clinical trials have been done, with varying results, including substantial reduction in the rate of postoperative infection and morbidity with extra-abdominal closure of the uterine incision, and less associated peri-operative haemorrhage. Subsequent studies suggest that the method of placental removal rather than method of closure of the uterine incision influences peri-operative morbidity.

OBJECTIVES: To evaluate the effects of extra-abdominal repair of the uterine incision compared to intra-abdominal repair.

METHODS: Standard PCG methods (see page xvii). Search date: September 2003.

MAIN RESULTS: Six studies were included, with 1294 women randomised overall, and 1221 women included in the analysis. There were no statistically significant differences between the groups in most of the outcomes identified, except for febrile morbidity and length of hospital stay. With extra-abdominal closure of the uterine incision, febrile morbidity was lower (relative risk 0.41, 95% confidence interval (CI) 0.17 to 0.97), and the hospital stay was longer (weighted mean difference 0.24 days, 95% CI 0.08 to 0.39).

AUTHORS' CONCLUSIONS: There is no evidence from this review to make definitive conclusions about which method of uterine closure offers greater advantages, if any. However, these results are based on too few and too small studies to detect differences in rare, but severe, complications.

INDWELLING BLADDER CATHETERIZATION AS PART OF POST-OPERATIVE CARE FOR CAESAREAN SECTION: (Page G, Buntinx F, Hanssens M) Protocol [see page xviii] CD004354

ABRIDGED BACKGROUND: Peri-operative bladder injury, urinary retention and urinary tract infection are well known factors of maternal morbidity after caesarean section. Bladder catheterization is thought to avoid bladder injury during surgery by facilitating surgery on the lower uterine segment. The review is aimed to look for postoperative bladder care since the introduction of an indwelling catheter is thought to prevent urinary retention, another important aspect of maternal morbidity associated with caesarean section. The role of caesarean section in postpartum retention is difficult to discern; after a caesarean section, women generally have an indwelling catheter for at least 24 hours postoperatively and the effects of surgery and anaesthesia complicate postpartum bladder changes. Acute retention without obstruction can be dealt with by intermittent catheterization once or twice, resorting to indwelling catheter if it becomes necessary to catheterize the woman more than twice. Although catheterization of the bladder is often considered a harmless procedure, development of urinary tract infection following this procedure has been reported in a considerable number of women after vaginal or abdominal delivery.

OBJECTIVES: To assess a policy of routine indwelling bladder catheterization compared with no and/or intermittent (routine or ad hoc) bladder drainage in women undergoing caesarean section with the main aim to avoid urinary retention.

METHODS OF DELIVERING THE PLACENTA AT CAESAREAN SECTION: (Anorlu R, Maholwana B) Protocol [see page xviii] CD004737

ABRIDGED BACKGROUND: Worldwide, caesarean section is the most common major operation performed on women. Some of the reported short-term morbidities include haemorrhage, need for blood transfusion, postoperative fever and endometritis (infection of the lining of the uterus). There are many possible ways of performing a caesarean section operation and variations in the techniques used may increase some of the complications mentioned. Different methods for the delivery of the placenta at caesarean section have been described: (1) placental drainage with spontaneous delivery, (2) cord traction and (3) manual removal.

OBJECTIVES: To compare, using the best available evidence, the effects of manual removal of placenta compared with cord traction at caesarean section.

TECHNIQUES AND MATERIALS FOR CLOSURE OF THE ABDOMINAL WALL IN CAESAREAN SECTION: closure of the subcutaneous fat layer reduced wound complications; no evidence was found for other techniques. (Anderson ER, Gates S) CD004663 (in RHL 11)

BACKGROUND: There is a variety of techniques for closing the abdominal wall during caesarean section. Some methods may be better in terms of postoperative recovery and other important outcomes.

OBJECTIVES: To compare the effects of alternative techniques for closure of the rectus sheath and subcutaneous fat on maternal health and healthcare resource use.

METHODS: Standard PCG methods (see page xvii). Search date:September 2003.

(a) any suturing technique or material used for closure of the rectus sheath versus any other;
(b) closure versus non-closure of subcutaneous fat;
(c) any suturing technique or material used for closure of the subcutaneous fat versus any other;
(d) any type of needle for repair of the abdominal wall in caesarean section versus any other;
(e) any other comparison of methods of abdominal wall closure.

MAIN RESULTS: Seven studies involving 2056 women were included. The risk of haematoma or seroma was reduced with fat closure compared with non-closure (relative risk (RR) 0.52, 95% confidence interval (CI) 0.33 to 0.82), as was the risk of 'wound complication' (haematoma, seroma, wound infection or wound separation) (RR 0.68,

95% CI 0.52 to 0.88). No difference in the risk of wound infection alone or other short-term outcomes was found. No long-term outcomes were reported. There was no difference in the risk of wound infection between blunt needles and sharp needles in one small study. No studies were found examining suture techniques or materials for closure of the rectus sheath or subcutaneous fat.

AUTHORS' CONCLUSIONS: *Implications for practice*: **Closure of the subcutaneous fat may reduce wound complications but it is unclear to what extent these differences affect the well-being and satisfaction of the women concerned.**

Implications for research: **Further trials are justified to investigate whether the apparent increased risk of haematoma or seroma with non-closure of the subcutaneous fat is real. These should use a broader range of short- and long-term outcomes, and ensure that they are adequately powered to detect clinically important differences. Further research comparing blunt and sharp needles is justified, as are trials evaluating suturing materials and suturing techniques for the rectus sheath.**

TECHNIQUES AND MATERIALS FOR SKIN CLOSURE IN CAESAREAN SECTION: Skin staples had poorer outcomes (except speed); no evidence was found for other methods. (Alderdice F, McKenna D, Dornan J) CD003577

BACKGROUND: Caesarean section is a common operation with no agreed standard on operative techniques and materials to use. The skin layer can be repaired by sub-cuticular stitch immediately below the skin layer, an interrupted stitch or with skin staples. A great variety of materials and techniques are used for skin closure after caesarean section and there is a need to identify which provide the best outcomes for women.

OBJECTIVES: To compare the effects of skin closure techniques and materials on maternal outcomes and time taken to perform a caesarean section.

METHODS: Standard PCG methods (see page xvii). Search date: May 2004.

MAIN RESULTS: Only one small randomised controlled trial, involving 66 women, was included in the review. Frishman et al compared staples with absorbable sub-cuticular suture for closure following caesarean section. While operating time was significantly shorter when using staples, the use of absorbable sub-cuticular suture resulted in less postoperative pain and yielded a better cosmetic result at the post-operative visit.

AUTHORS' CONCLUSIONS: There is no conclusive evidence about how the skin should be closed after caesarean section. Questions regarding the best closure technique and material and the outcomes associated with each remain unanswered. The appearance and strength of the scar following caesarean section is important to women and the choice of technique and materials should be made by women in consultation with their obstetrician based on the limited information currently available.

WOUND DRAINAGE FOR CAESAREAN SECTION: took time; did not show benefits as a routine procedure. (Gates S, Anderson ER) CD004549 (Wounds Group)

BACKGROUND: Subcutaneous and sub rectussheath wound drains are sometimes used in women who have undergone caesarean section. The indications for using drains vary by clinician.

OBJECTIVES: To compare the effects of using a wound drain with not using a wound drain at caesarean section, and of different types of drain, on maternal health and healthcare resource use.

SEARCH STRATEGY: This review draws on the search strategy developed for the Cochrane Wounds Group as a whole. Electronic databases (MEDLINE, EMBASE, Cinahl and CAB Health) and the reference lists of included articles were also searched up to June 2004

SELECTION CRITERIA: Studies were included if they allocated women to groups at random and they compared any type of wound drain with no wound drainage, or with any other type of drain, in women undergoing caesarean section.

DATA COLLECTION AND ANALYSIS: Trials were evaluated for appropriateness for inclusion and methodological quality without consideration of their results. This was done by two reviewers according to pre-stated eligibility criteria.

MAIN RESULTS: Seven trials (1993 women) were included in the review. Meta-analysis found no difference in the risk of wound infection, other wound complications, febrile morbidity or endometritis in women who had wound drains compared with those who did not. There was some evidence that caesarean sections may be about five minutes shorter and that blood loss may be slightly lower when drains were not used.

AUTHORS' CONCLUSIONS: There is no evidence in the seven small trials included to suggest that the routine use of wound drains at caesarean section confers any benefit on the women involved.

These trials do not answer the question of whether wound drainage is of benefit when haemostasis is not felt to be adequate.

Further large trials are justified using blinded outcome assessment to examine the role of different types of wound drain at caesarean section. Comparing the use of drains in women with different degrees of obesity and in women having first or repeat caesareans and intrapartum or prelabour caesarean sections would be of interest. Women's views and experience of drains have not been studied in these trials.

TOCOLYSIS FOR ASSISTING DELIVERY AT CAESAREAN SECTION: not enough data to provide reliable evidence. (Dodd JM, Reid K) CD004944

BACKGROUND: Caesarean section involves making an incision in the woman's abdomen and cutting through the uterine muscle. The baby is then delivered through that incision. Difficult caesarean birth may result in injury for the infant. Medication that relaxes the uterus (tocolytic medication) may facilitate the birth of the baby at caesarean section.

OBJECTIVES: To compare the use of tocolysis (routine or selective use) with no use of tocolysis or placebo at the time of caesarean section for outcomes of infant birth trauma, maternal complications (particularly postpartum haemorrhage requiring blood transfusion) and long-term measures of infant and childhood morbidity.

METHODS: Standard PCG methods (see page xvii). Search date: January 2006.

MAIN RESULTS: A single randomised trial involving 97 women was identified and included in the review. Maternal and infant health outcomes were not reported.

AUTHORS' CONCLUSIONS: There is currently insufficient information available from randomised trials to support or refute the routine or selective use of tocolytic agents to facilitate infant birth at the time of caesarean section.

7.11.4 Post-operative care

> ☺ **EARLY COMPARED WITH DELAYED ORAL FLUIDS AND FOOD AFTER CAESAREAN SECTION:** improved postoperative outcomes.
> (Mangesi L, Hofmeyr GJ) CD003516 (in RHL 11)

BACKGROUND: It is customary for fluids and/or food to be withheld for a period of time after abdominal operations. After caesarean section, practices vary considerably. These discrepancies raise concern as to the bases of different practices.

OBJECTIVES: To assess the effect of early versus delayed introduction of fluids and/or food after caesarean section.

METHODS: Standard PCG methods (see page xvii). Search date: January 2002. The criteria for 'early' feeding were as defined by the individual trial authors – usually within six to eight hours of surgery.

MAIN RESULTS: Of 12 studies considered, six were included in this review. Four were excluded and two are pending further information. The methodological quality of the studies was variable. Only one to three studies contributed usable data to each outcome. Three studies were limited to surgery under regional analgesia, while three included both regional analgesia and general anaesthesia.

Early oral fluids or food were associated with: reduced time to first food intake (one study, 118 women; the intervention was a slush diet and food was introduced according to clinical parameters; weighted mean difference −7.20 hours, 95% confidence interval −13.26 to −1.14); reduced time to return of bowel sounds (one study, 118 women; −4.30 hours, −6.78 to −1.82); reduced postoperative hospital stay following surgery under regional analgesia (two studies, 220 women; −0.75 days, −1.37 to −0.12; random effects model); and a trend to reduced abdominal distension (three studies, 369 women; relative risk 0.78, 95% confidence interval 0.55 to 1.11). No significant differences were identified with respect to nausea, vomiting, time to bowel action/ passing flatus, paralytic ileus and number of analgesic doses.

AUTHORS' CONCLUSIONS: There was no evidence, from the limited randomised trials reviewed, to justify a policy of withholding oral fluids after uncomplicated caesarean section. Further research is justified.

DRESSINGS AND TOPICAL AGENTS FOR SURGICAL WOUNDS HEALING BY SECONDARY INTENTION: not enough data from general surgery literature to provide reliable evidence. (Vermeulen H, Ubbink D, Goossens A, de Vos R, Legemate D) CD001836 (Wounds Group)

BACKGROUND: Many different wound dressings and topical applications are used to cover surgical wounds healing by secondary intention. It is not known whether these dressings heal wounds at different rates.

OBJECTIVES: To assess the effectiveness of dressings and topical agents on surgical wounds healing by secondary intention.

SEARCH STRATEGY: We sought relevant trials from the Cochrane Central Register of Controlled Trials, Cochrane Wounds Group Specialised Trials Register, MEDLINE, EMBASE and CINAHL databases in March 2002.

SELECTION CRITERIA: All randomised controlled trials (RCTs) evaluating the effectiveness of dressings and topical agents for surgical wounds healing by secondary intention.

DATA COLLECTION AND ANALYSIS: Eligibility for inclusion was confirmed by two reviewers who independently judged the methodological quality of the trials according to the Dutch Cochrane Centre list of factors relating to internal and external validity. Two reviewers summarised data from eligible studies using a data extraction sheet, any disagreements were referred to a third reviewer.

MAIN RESULTS: Fourteen reports of 13 RCTs on dressings or topical agents for postoperative wounds healing by secondary intention were identified.

Wound healing: Whilst a single small trial of aloe vera supplementation vs gauze suggests delayed healing with aloe vera, the results of this trial are uninterpretable since there was a large differential loss to follow up. A plaster cast applied to an amputation stump accelerated wound healing compared with elastic compression (WMD −25.60 days, 95% CI −49.08 to −2.12 days; one trial). There were no statistically significant differences in healing for other dressing comparisons (e.g. gauze, foam, alginate; 11 trials).

Pain: Gauze was associated with significantly more pain for patients than other dressings (four trials).

Patient satisfaction: Patients treated with gauze were less satisfied compared with those receiving alternative dressings (three trials).

Costs: Gauze is inexpensive but its use is associated with the use of significantly more nursing time than foam (two trials).

Length of hospital stay: Four trials showed no difference in length of hospital stay. One trial found shorter hospital stay in people after amputation when plaster casts were applied compared with elastic compression (WMD −30.10 days; 95% CI −49.82 to −10.38).

AUTHORS' CONCLUSIONS: We found only small, poor quality trials; the evidence is therefore insufficient to determine whether the choice of dressing or topical agent affects the healing of surgical wounds by secondary intention. Foam is best studied as an alternative for gauze and appears to be preferable as to pain reduction, patient satisfaction and nursing time.

7.12   Pregnancy following caesarean section

Caesarean section places women at risk for problems in a subsequent pregnancy, including placenta praevia, morbidly adherent placenta and rupture of the uterine scar. The aphorism 'Once a caesarean, always a caesarean', referred to the classical caesarean section, which has a considerably higher risk of rupture than the lower segment caesarean section. For pregnancy following lower segment caesarean sections, the small risk of uterine rupture must be weighed against the risks of repeat caesarean section.

PLANNED ELECTIVE REPEAT CAESAREAN SECTION VERSUS PLANNED VAGINAL BIRTH FOR WOMEN WITH A PREVIOUS CAESAREAN BIRTH: no randomised trials to provide reliable evidence. (Dodd JM, Crowther CA, Huertas E, Guise JM, Horey D) CD004224

BACKGROUND: When a woman has had a previous caesarean birth, there are two options for her care in a subsequent pregnancy: planned elective repeat caesarean or planned vaginal birth. While there are risks and benefits for both planned elective repeat caesarean birth and planned vaginal birth after caesarean, current sources of information are limited to non-randomised cohort studies. Studies designed in this way have significant potential for bias and consequently conclusions based on these results are limited in their reliability and should be interpreted with caution.

OBJECTIVES: To assess, using the best available evidence, the benefits and harms of a policy of planned elective repeat caesarean section with a policy of planned vaginal birth after caesarean section for women with a previous caesarean birth.

METHODS: Standard PCG methods (see page xvii). Search date: June 2004.

MAIN RESULTS: There were no randomised controlled trials identified.

AUTHORS' CONCLUSIONS: Planned elective repeat caesarean section and planned vaginal birth after caesarean section for women with a prior caesarean birth are both associated with benefits and harms. Evidence for these care practices is drawn from non-randomised studies, associated with potential bias. Any results and conclusions must therefore be interpreted with caution. Randomised controlled trials are required to provide the most reliable evidence regarding the benefits and harms of both planned elective repeat caesarean section and planned vaginal birth for women with a previous caesarean birth.

LOCAL ANAESTHETIC WOUND INFILTRATION AND ABDOMINAL NERVES BLOCK DURING CAESAREAN SECTION FOR POSTOPERATIVE PAIN RELIEF: (Bamigboye AA, **HOFMEYR** GJ) Protocol [see page xviii] CD006954

ABRIDGED BACKGROUND: Prompt and adequate postoperative pain relief can make the immediate postdelivery period less discomforting and more emotionally gratifying. Several studies have given reports on pre-emptive local anaesthetics (local anaesthetic given during operation to prevent or reduce pain after operation) to relieve postoperative pain. There may be effects on wound healing, either enhancing it or delaying the physiological process of wound healing. The local anaesthetic agent eventually gets absorbed systemically. It is secreted in breastmilk, and side effects on breastfed babies have not yet been documented.

OBJECTIVES: To assess the effects of local anaesthetic agent wound infiltration or abdominal nerve blocks, or both, on postcaesarean section pain and on the mother's ability to meet the physical, psychological and nutritional needs of the baby.

RECTAL ANALGESIA FOR PAIN RELIEF AFTER CAESAREAN SECTION: (Pearce EM, Dodd JM) Protocol [see page xviii] CD004738

ABRIDGED BACKGROUND: Caesarean section involves the birth of a baby through the incision in the mother's abdomen. After this operation, women experience pain from the wound and a longer recovery period than is associated with vaginal birth. Pain relief can be given orally, by injection into a vein (intravenous) or a muscle (intramuscular), or by rectal suppository. Potential advantages of using medication rectally rather than orally include better bioavailability and a reduction in side-effects (such as gastric irritation) and an ability to provide adequate pain relief when a woman may not tolerate oral medication (for example due to nausea or vomiting).

OBJECTIVES:

1 To assess the effects of analgesic rectal suppositories for relief of pain in women following caesarean section.

2 To assess the need for additional analgesia when analgesic rectal suppositories are used.

3 To compare the cost of analgesic rectal suppositories with other types of analgesia for pain relief after caesarean section.

4 To assess women's satisfaction with treatment and its effects on emotional well-being and quality of life.

CORTICOSTEROIDS FOR PREVENTING NEONATAL RESPIRATORY MORBIDITY AFTER ELECTIVE CAESAREAN SECTION AT TERM: (Sotiriadis A, Makrdimas G, Ioannidis JPA) Protocol [see page xviii] CD006614

ABRIDGED BACKGROUND: Caesarean section is a risk factor for the development of neonatal respiratory complications, mostly respiratory distress syndrome (RDS) and transient tachypnoea of the newborn, both in term and preterm infants. Infants born at term by caesarean delivery are more likely to develop respiratory morbidity than infants born vaginally, and this risk increases furthermore for the subgroup of children born after elective caesarean section, i.e. before onset of labour, with potentially severe implications. Prophylactic corticosteroids in singleton preterm pregnancies accelerate lung maturation and reduce the incidence of RDS, and administration of steroids is currently recommended between 24 and 34 weeks in cases of threatened preterm labour, antepartum haemorrhage, preterm rupture of membranes or in any condition requiring elective preterm delivery.

The evidence for administration of corticosteroids at or after 36 weeks is more controversial.

OBJECTIVES: The objective of this review is to assess the maternal and neonatal benefits and side-effects from prophylactic administration of corticosteroids in term elective caesarean section.

7.13 Extrauterine pregnancy

Advanced extrauterine pregnancy may be surprisingly difficult to diagnose. Chronic abdominal pain and unusual position of the baby may draw attention to the diagnosis. In early pregnancy, operative removal without delay is recommended. Some women decline intervention, and may carry the pregnancy to viability, though serious intra-abdominal bleeding is a risk. Sometimes the diagnosis is made only in late pregnancy. The baby is delivered by laparotomy. If removal of the placenta appears hazardous (for example, attachment to large vessels, bowel, spleen or liver) the option of leaving the placenta undisturbed, to resorb over several months, arises, as does the option of using methotrexate to promote absorption.

There are no Cochrane reviews of this topic.

7.14 Postpartum haemorrhage and retained placenta

Primary postpartum haemorrhage (defined as blood loss > 500 ml in the first 24 hours, with blood loss > 1000 ml considered a more appropriate measure for morbidity) may occur because of poor contraction of the uterus, retained products of conception, tears of the uterus, cervix or vagina, or coagulopathy. Secondary haemorrhage (24 hours or more after birth) may be due to infection or retained products of conception.

The comparatively low mortality from postpartum haemorrhage in well-resourced facilities suggests that overall, modern methods of treatment are effective. These include resuscitation, intravascular fluid volume replacement, uterotonic drugs, blood transfusion, medical anti-shock garments, evacuation of the uterus, repair of genital tract tears, methods to compress or interrupt the blood supply to bleeding sites, and hysterectomy. Key features are a systematic approach and speed. However, surprisingly little direct evidence of effectiveness of specific treatment strategies is available.

> **TREATMENT FOR PRIMARY POSTPARTUM HAEMORRHAGE:** there is limited evidence that misoprostol may be effective; there were no randomised trials to provide reliable evidence on other treatments. (Mousa HA, Alfirevic Z) CD003249 (in RHL 11)

BACKGROUND: Primary postpartum haemorrhage (PPH) is one of the top five causes of maternal mortality in both developed and developing countries.

OBJECTIVES: To assess the effectiveness and safety of pharmacological, surgical and radiological interventions used for the treatment of primary PPH.

METHODS: Standard PCG methods (see page xvii). Search date: October 2006.

MAIN RESULTS: Three studies (462 participants) were included. Two placebo-controlled randomised trials compared misoprostol (dose 600 to 1000 mcg) with placebo and showed that misoprostol use was not associated with any significant reduction of maternal mortality (two trials, 398 women; relative risk (RR) 7.24, 95% confidence interval (CI) 0.38 to 138.6), hysterectomy (two trials, 398 women; RR 1.24, 95% CI 0.04 to 40.78), the additional use of uterotonics (two trials, 398 women; RR 0.98, 95% CI 0.78 to 1.24), blood transfusion (two trials, 394 women; RR 1.33, 95% CI 0.81 to 2.18) or evacuation of retained products (one trial, 238 women; RR 5.17, 95% CI 0.25 to 107). Misoprostol use was associated with a significant increase of maternal pyrexia (two trials, 392 women; RR 6.40, 95% CI 1.71 to 23.96) and shivering (two trials, 394 women; RR 2.31, 95% CI 1.68 to 3.18).

One unblinded trial showed better clinical response to rectal misoprostol compared with a combination of syntometrine and oxytocin. We did not identify any trial dealing with surgical techniques, radiological interventions or haemostatic drugs for women with primary PPH unresponsive to uterotonics.

AUTHORS' CONCLUSIONS: There is insufficient evidence to show that the addition of misoprostol is superior to the combination of oxytocin and ergometrine alone for the treatment of primary PPH. Large multi-centre, double-blind, randomised controlled trials are required to identify the best drug combinations, route and dose of uterotonics for the treatment of primary PPH. Further work is required to assess

the best way of managing women who fail to respond to uterotonics therapy.

TREATMENTS FOR SECONDARY POSTPARTUM HAEMORRHAGE: no randomised trials to provide reliable evidence. (Alexander J, Thomas P, Sanghera J) CD002867

BACKGROUND: Secondary postpartum haemorrhage is any abnormal or excessive bleeding from the birth canal occurring between 24 hours and 12 weeks postnatally. In developed countries, two per cent of postnatal women are admitted to hospital with this condition, half of them undergoing uterine surgical evacuation. Data are not available from developing countries.

OBJECTIVES: To evaluate the relative effectiveness and safety of the treatments used for secondary postpartum haemorrhage.

METHODS: Standard PCG methods (see page xvii). Search date: January 2007.

MAIN RESULTS: Of the 46 papers identified, none met the inclusion criteria.

AUTHORS' CONCLUSIONS: No information is available from randomised controlled trials to inform the management of women with secondary postpartum haemorrhage. This topic may have received little attention because it is perceived as being associated with maternal morbidity rather than mortality in developed countries; it is only recently that the extent and importance of postnatal maternal morbidity has been recognised. A well-designed randomised controlled trial comparing the various therapies for women with secondary postpartum haemorrhage against each other and against placebo or no treatment groups is needed.

☺ **UMBILICAL VEIN INJECTION FOR MANAGEMENT OF RETAINED PLACENTA:** using oxytocin or prostaglandins in saline reduced the need for manual removal of the placenta. (Carroli G, Bergel E) CD001337 (in RHL 11)

BACKGROUND: If a retained placenta is left untreated, there is a high risk of maternal death. However, manual removal of the placenta is an invasive procedure with its own serious complications of haemorrhage, infection or genital tract trauma.

OBJECTIVES: To assess the use of umbilical vein injection of saline solution alone or with oxytocin in comparison either with expectant management or with an alternative solution or other uterotonic agent for retained placenta. The main comparisons include the following agents: saline solution alone, saline solution plus oxytocin, saline solution plus prostaglandin and plasma

METHODS: Standard PCG methods (see page xvii). Search date: March 2001.

MAIN RESULTS: 12 trials were included. The trials were of variable quality. Compared with expectant management, umbilical vein injection of saline solution alone did not show any significant difference in the incidence of manual removal of the placenta (relative risk (RR): 0.97; 95% confidence interval (CI): 0.83 to 1.14). Umbilical vein injection of saline solution plus oxytocin compared with expectant management showed a reduction in manual removal, although this was not statistically significant (RR: 0.86; 95% CI: 0.72 to 1.01). Saline solution with oxytocin compared with saline solution alone showed a significant reduction in manual removal of the placenta (RR: 0.79; 95% CI: 0.69 to 0.91) (number needed to treat: 8; 95% CI: 5 to 20). No discernible difference was detected in length of third stage of labour, blood loss, haemorrhage, haemoglobin, blood transfusion, curettage, infection, hospital stay, fever, abdominal pain and oxytocin augmentation. Umbilical vein injection of saline solution plus oxytocin compared with umbilical vein injection of plasma expander showed higher, but not statistically significant, incidence of manual removal of placenta (RR: 1.34; 95% CI: 0.97 to 1.85) and no difference in blood loss but there is only one small trial contributing to this comparison. Saline solution plus prostaglandin, compared with saline solution alone, was associated with a statistically significant lower incidence in manual removal of placenta (RR: 0.05; 95% CI: 0.00 to 0.73) but no difference was observed in blood loss, fever, abdominal pain, or oxytocin augmentation but there is only one small trial contributing to these results. There were no significant differences between saline solution plus prostaglandin and saline solution plus oxytocin (RR: 0.10; 95% CI: 0.01 to 1.59) but again there is only one small trial contributing to this meta-analysis.

AUTHORS' CONCLUSIONS: Umbilical vein injection of saline solution plus oxytocin appears to be effective in the management of retained placenta. Saline solution alone does not appear be more effective than expectant management. Further research into umbilical vein injection of oxytocin, prostaglandins or plasma expander is warranted.

PROPHYLACTIC ANTIBIOTICS FOR MANUAL REMOVAL OF RETAINED PLACENTA IN VAGINAL BIRTH: no randomised trials to provide reliable evidence. (Chongsomchai C, Lumbiganon P, Laopaiboon M) CD004904

BACKGROUND: Retained placenta is a potentially life-threatening condition because of its association with postpartum haemorrhage. Manual removal of placenta increases the likelihood of bacterial contamination in the uterine cavity.

OBJECTIVES: To compare the effectiveness and side-effects of routine antibiotic use for manual removal of placenta in vaginal birth in women who received antibiotic prophylaxis and those who did not, and to identify the appropriate regimen of antibiotic prophylaxis for this procedure.

METHODS: Standard PCG methods (see page xvii). Search date: November 2005.

MAIN RESULTS: No studies that met the inclusion criteria were identified.

AUTHORS' CONCLUSIONS: There are no randomised controlled trials to evaluate the effectiveness of antibiotic prophylaxis to prevent endometritis after manual removal of placenta in vaginal birth.

7.14.1 Morbidly adherent placenta

Increasing caesarean section rates have resulted in increased cases of morbidly adherent placenta related to the previous scar. Whether the technique of closure of the uterus affects this risk is not known. Failure to separate a morbidly adherent placenta from the uterine wall may necessitate hysterectomy. More recently with antenatal ultrasound diagnosis of morbidly adherent placenta, the option of leaving the placenta in place and awaiting spontaneous absorption has evolved.

There are no Cochrane reviews of this topic.

7.15   Inversion of the uterus

Inability to feel the fundus of the uterus in the lower abdomen after birth alerts one to the likelihood of inversion of the uterus. Methods used to reduce the inversion include manual replacement and the hydrostatic method (saline is run into the vagina under gravity to push the uterus back into position; an inflated Foley catheter bulb or a soft vacuum extraction cup may be used to help seal the vagina).

There are no Cochrane reviews of this topic.

CHAPTER 8: CARE AFTER CHILDBIRTH

Following the anticipation of pregnancy and the drama of birth, attention paid to care after birth may be less than is warranted. This is a time of major adjustment for the new family. Common problems which arise in the puerperium include perineal discomfort and dysfunction, breastfeeding difficulties, adjustment problems, depression and psychosis. Occasionally dangerous conditions arise, including haemorrhage, infection, thromboembolism (blood clots) and cardiomyopathy (heart muscle dysfunction).

Care during labour which increases a mother's sense of satisfaction (for example continuous support, see page 255) may facilitate her adaptation to parenthood.

8.1 Basic care of mother and baby

Many previously entrenched hospital routines have been challenged in recent decades. These include separation of mothers and their babies, strict breastfeeding schedules and a 'lying-in' period of seven days.

> **POSTNATAL PARENTAL EDUCATION FOR IMPROVING FAMILY HEALTH** (Gagnon AJ, Barkun L) Protocol [see page xviii] CD004068

ABRIDGED BACKGROUND: Birth takes place in the home for the vast majority of women in many parts of the world, and much of the related education regarding care of self and of the newborn is provided by an informal structure consisting of mother, sister, grandmother, aunt and other extended relatives. This informal informational structure exists in all societies and is relied upon to various degrees by virtually all women, including those giving birth in hospitals.

A Cochrane Pocketbook: Pregnancy and Childbirth G.J. Hofmeyr et al.
Copyright © 2008, Z. Alfiervic, C. A. Crowther, L. Duley, A. M. Gulmezoglu, G. ML. Gyte , E. D. Hodnett, G. J. Hofmeyr, J. P. Neilson

In many developed countries, birth takes place in institutions (hospitals or birth centres) and educational interventions are provided by professionals such as nurses, midwives and physicians. The content and emphasis placed on this education varies. Literature on postnatal education suggests that families be assessed for knowledge in several areas of physical, emotional and developmental health and be offered the necessary related information through any of a number of formats available through hospital or community services.

OBJECTIVES: The primary objective is to assess the effects of structured postnatal education delivered by an educator to an individual or group on maternal/paternal and infant outcomes and health services use.

A secondary objective is to determine whether the effects of structured postnatal education vary by length or type of intervention and by population.

☺ **EARLY SKIN-TO-SKIN CONTACT FOR MOTHERS AND THEIR HEALTHY NEWBORN INFANTS:** improved breastfeeding and early attachment. (Moore E, Anderson GC, Bergman N) CD003519 (in RHL 11)

BACKGROUND: Mother–infant separation postbirth is common in Western culture. Early skin-to-skin contact (SSC) begins ideally at birth and involves placing the naked baby, covered across the back with a warm blanket, prone on the mother's bare chest. According to mammalian neuroscience, the intimate contact inherent in this place (habitat) evokes neurobehaviors ensuring fulfillment of basic biological needs. This time may represent a psychophysiologically 'sensitive period' for programming future behavior.

OBJECTIVES: To assess the effects of early SSC on breastfeeding, behavior, and physiological adaptation in healthy mother–newborn dyads.

METHODS: Standard PCG methods (see page xvii). Search date: August 2006.

MAIN RESULTS: 30 studies involving 1925 participants (mother–infant dyads) were included. Data from more than two trials were available for only 8-of-64 outcome measures. We found statistically significant and positive effects of early SSC on breastfeeding at one to four months postbirth (10 trials; 552 participants) (odds ratio (OR) 1.82, 95% confidence interval (CI) 1.08 to 3.07), and breastfeeding duration (seven trials; 324 participants) (weighted mean difference (WMD) 42.55, 95% CI −1.69 to 86.79). Trends were found for improved summary scores for maternal affectionate love/touch during observed breastfeeding (four trials; 314 participants) (standardized mean difference (SMD) 0.52, 95% CI 0.07 to 0.98) and maternal attachment behavior (six trials; 396 participants) (SMD 0.52, 95% CI 0.31 to 0.72) with early SSC. SSC infants cried for a shorter length of time (one trial; 44 participants) (WMD −8.01, 95% CI −8.98 to −7.04). Late preterm infants had better cardio-respiratory stability with early SSC (one trial; 35 participants) (WMD 2.88, 95% CI 0.53 to 5.23). No adverse effects were found.

AUTHORS' CONCLUSIONS: Limitations included methodological quality, variations in intervention implementation, and outcome variability. The intervention may benefit breastfeeding outcomes, early mother–infant attachment, infant crying and cardio-respiratory stability, and has no apparent short or long-term negative effects. Further investigation is recommended. To facilitate meta-analysis, future research should be done using outcome measures consistent with those in the studies included here. Published reports should clearly indicate if the intervention was SSC and include means, standard deviations, exact probability values, and data to measure intervention dose.

> **EARLY POSTNATAL DISCHARGE FROM HOSPITAL FOR HEALTHY MOTHERS AND TERM INFANTS:** not enough data to provide reliable evidence. (Brown S, Small R, Faber B, Krastev A, Davis P) CD002958 (in RHL 11)

BACKGROUND: Length of postnatal hospital stay has declined dramatically in the past thirty years. There is ongoing controversy concerning whether or not staying less time in hospital is harmful or beneficial.

OBJECTIVES: To assess the safety, impact and effectiveness of a policy of early discharge for healthy mothers and term infants, with respect to the health and well-being of mothers and babies, satisfaction with postnatal care, overall costs of health care and broader impacts on families.

METHODS: Standard PCG methods (see page xvii). Search date: April 2002.

MAIN RESULTS: Eight trials were identified involving 3600 women. There was substantial variation in the definition of 'early discharge', and the extent of antenatal preparation and midwife home care following discharge offered to women in intervention and control groups.

Five trials recruited and randomized women in pregnancy; three randomized women following childbirth. Post randomization exclusions were high. Protocol violations occurred in both directions.

No statistically significant differences in infant or maternal readmissions were found in six trials reporting data on these outcomes. Three trials had mixed results showing either no significant difference or results favouring early discharge for the outcome of maternal depression although none used a well-validated standardized instrument. The results of six trials showed that early discharge had no impact on breastfeeding although significant heterogeneity was present between studies.

AUTHORS' CONCLUSIONS: The findings are inconclusive. There is no evidence of adverse outcomes associated with policies of early postnatal discharge, but methodological limitations of included studies mean that adverse outcomes cannot be ruled out. It remains unclear how important midwifery support at home is to the safety and acceptability of early discharge.

Large well-designed trials of early discharge programs incorporating process evaluation to assess the uptake of co-interventions, and using standardized approaches to outcome assessment, are needed.

☺ **DIET OR EXERCISE, OR BOTH, FOR WEIGHT REDUCTION IN WOMEN AFTER CHILDBIRTH:** diet and exercise help reduce weight; more research is needed. (Amorim AR, Linne YM, Lourenco PMC) CD0005627

BACKGROUND: Weight retention after pregnancy may contribute to obesity. It is known that diet and exercise are recommended components of any weight loss programme in the general population. However, strategies to achieve healthy body weight among postpartum women have not been adequately evaluated.

OBJECTIVES: The objectives of this review were to evaluate the effect of diet, exercise or both for weight reduction in women after childbirth, and to assess the impact of these interventions on maternal body composition, cardiorespiratory fitness, breastfeeding performance and other child and maternal outcomes.

METHODS: Standard PCG methods (see page xvii). Search date: September 2006.

MAIN RESULTS: Six trials involving 245 women were included. Women who exercised did not lose significantly more weight than women in the usual care group (one trial; n = 33; WMD 0.00 kg; 95% confidence interval (CI) −8.63 to 8.63). Women who took part in a diet (one trial; n = 45;

WMD −1.70 kg; 95% CI −2.08 to −1.32), or diet plus exercise programme (four trials; n = 169; WMD −2.89 kg; 95% CI −4.83 to −0.95), lost significantly more weight than women in the usual care. There was no difference in the magnitude of weight loss between diet and diet plus exercise group (one trial; n = 43; WMD 0.30 kg; 95% CI −0.60 to 0.66). The interventions seemed not to affect breastfeeding performance adversely.

AUTHORS' CONCLUSIONS: Preliminary evidence from this review suggests that dieting and exercise together appear to be more effective than diet alone at helping women to lose weight after childbirth, because the former improves maternal cardiorespiratory fitness level and preserves fat-free mass, while diet alone reduces fat-free mass. For women who are breastfeeding, more evidence is required to confirm whether diet or exercise, or both, is not detrimental for either mother or baby. Due to insufficient available data, additional research, with larger sample size, is needed to confirm the results.

MATERNAL DIETARY ANTIGEN AVOIDANCE DURING PREGNANCY OR LACTATION, OR BOTH, FOR PREVENTING OR TREATING ATOPIC DISEASE IN THE CHILD: during pregnancy was not effective; during lactation there was limited evidence of effectiveness. (Kramer MS, Kakuma R) CD000133

BACKGROUND: Some breastfed infants with atopic eczema benefit from elimination of cows milk, egg, or other antigens from their mother's diet. Maternal dietary antigens are also known to cross the placenta.

OBJECTIVES: To assess the effects of prescribing an antigen avoidance diet during pregnancy or lactation, or both, on maternal and infant nutrition and on the prevention or treatment of atopic disease in the child.

METHODS: Standard PCG methods (see page xvii). Search date: March 2006. All randomized or quasi-randomized comparisons of maternal dietary antigen avoidance prescribed to pregnant or lactating women. We excluded trials of multimodal interventions that included manipulation of the infant's diet other than breast milk or of nondietary aspects of the infant's environment.

MAIN RESULTS: The evidence from four trials, involving 334 participants, does not suggest a protective effect of maternal dietary antigen avoidance during pregnancy on the incidence of atopic eczema during the first 18 months of life. Data on allergic rhinitis or conjunctivitis, or both, and urticaria are limited to a single trial each and are insufficient to draw meaningful inferences. Longer-term atopic outcomes have not been reported. The restricted diet during pregnancy was associated with a slightly but statistically significantly lower mean gestational weight gain, a nonsignificantly higher risk of preterm birth, and a nonsignificant reduction in mean birthweight.

The evidence from one trial, involving 26 participants, did not observe a significant protective effect of maternal antigen avoidance during lactation on the incidence of atopic eczema during the first 18 months.

One crossover trial involving 17 lactating mothers of infants with established atopic eczema found that maternal dietary antigen avoidance was associated with a nonsignificant reduction in eczema severity.

AUTHORS' CONCLUSIONS: Prescription of an antigen avoidance diet to a high-risk woman during pregnancy is unlikely to reduce substantially her child's risk of atopic diseases, and such a diet may adversely affect maternal or fetal nutrition, or both. Prescription of an antigen avoidance diet to a high-risk woman during lactation may reduce her child's risk of developing atopic eczema, but better trials are needed. Dietary antigen avoidance by lactating mothers of infants with atopic eczema may reduce the severity of the eczema, but larger trials are needed.

8.2 Perineal pain

> **RECTAL ANALGESIA FOR PAIN FROM PERINEAL TRAUMA FOLLOWING CHILDBIRTH:** was effective in reducing the incidence of pain in the first 24 hours; no data on long-term outcomes, nor women's satisfaction. (Hedayati H, Parsons J, Crowther CA) CD003931

BACKGROUND: Perineal pain from a tear and/or surgical cut (episiotomy) is a common problem following vaginal birth. Strategies to reduce perineal trauma and the appropriate repair of any perineal damage sustained are important for avoiding and alleviating pain. Where pain is present, numerous treatments are used in clinical practice, such as local anaesthetics, oral analgesics, therapeutic ultrasound, antiseptics and non-pharmacological applications such as ice packs and baths. This review assesses the evidence for using rectal analgesia for pain relief following perineal trauma.

OBJECTIVES: To assess the effectiveness of analgesic rectal suppositories for pain from perineal trauma following childbirth.

METHODS: Standard PCG methods (see page xvii). Search date: July 2002.

MAIN RESULTS: Three trials involving 249 women met the inclusion criteria. Only two of the trials identified for inclusion in this review had data that could be entered in a meta-analysis, with the third not providing data in a useable format. Women were less likely to experience pain at or close to 24 hours after birth if they received non-steroidal anti-inflammatory drug (NSAID) suppositories compared with placebo (relative risk (RR) 0.37, 95% confidence interval (CI) 0.10 to 1.38, two trials, 150 women). Women in the NSAID suppositories group compared with women in the placebo group required less additional analgesia in the first 24 hours' after birth (RR 0.31, 95% CI 0.17 to 0.54, one trial, 89 women) and this effect was still evident at 48 hours postpartum (RR 0.63, 95% CI 0.45 to 0.89, one trial, 89 women). No information was available on pain experienced more than 72 hours after birth or other outcomes of importance to women such as the impact on daily activities, resumption of sexual intercourse and the impact on the mother–baby relationship.

AUTHORS' CONCLUSIONS: NSAID rectal suppositories are associated with less pain up to 24 hours after birth, and less additional analgesia is required. More research is required regarding long-term effects and maternal satisfaction with the treatment.

> **THERAPEUTIC ULTRASOUND FOR POSTPARTUM PERINEAL PAIN AND DYSPAREUNIA:** not enough data to provide reliable evidence. (Hay-Smith EJC) CD000495

BACKGROUND: Proponents of therapeutic ultrasound suggest it can decrease pain by resolution of inflammation processes and reducing the pressure on pain sensitive structures by haematoma and oedema.

OBJECTIVES: To assess the effects of therapeutic ultrasound for treating acute perineal pain, persistent perineal pain or dyspareunia, or both, following childbirth.

METHODS: Standard PCG methods (see page xvii). Search date: April 2006.

Randomised and quasi-randomised trials comparing active therapeutic ultrasound with no treatment, placebo ultrasound or any other
'standard' or active treatment for women with acute or persistent perineal pain or dyspareunia, or both, following childbirth.

MAIN RESULTS: Four trials involving 659 women were included.
The trials were of variable quality. Based on two placebo controlled trials, women treated with active ultrasound for acute perineal
pain were more likely to report improvement in pain with treatment (odds ratio (OR) 0.37, 95% confidence interval (CI) 0.19 to
0.69). No other outcome reached significance. In one trial comparing pulsed electromagnetic energy with ultrasound for acute perineal pain, women treated with ultrasound were more likely to have
bruising post-treatment (OR 1.64, 95% CI 1.04 to 2.60). However,
those treated with ultrasound were less likely to have experienced
perineal pain within the last 24 hours at 10 days (OR 0.56, 95%
CI 0.34 to 0.92) and pain within the last week at three months
(OR 0.43, 95% CI 0.22 to 0.84). No other outcome reached significance. Based on one trial, women treated with ultrasound for
persistent perineal pain or dyspareunia, or both, were less likely
to report pain with sexual intercourse compared with the placebo
group (OR 0.31, 95% CI 0.11 to 0.84). None of the other outcomes
measured reached significance.

**AUTHORS' CONCLUSIONS: There is not enough evidence to evaluate
the use of ultrasound in treating perineal pain or dyspareunia, or
both, following childbirth.**

**LOCAL COOLING FOR RELIEVING PAIN FROM PERINEAL TRAUMA
SUSTAINED DURING CHILDBIRTH:** there was limited evidence for
pain relief; was less effective than pulsed electromagnetic energy. (East
CE, Begg L, Henshall NE, Marchant P, Wallace K) CD006304

BACKGROUND: Perineal trauma is common during childbirth and may
be painful. Contemporary maternity practice includes offering women
numerous forms of pain relief, including the local application of cooling
treatments.

OBJECTIVES: To evaluate the effectiveness and side effects of localised
cooling treatments compared with no treatment, other forms of cooling
treatments and non-cooling treatments.

METHODS: Standard PCG methods (see page xvii). Search date: January 2007.

MAIN RESULTS: Seven published RCTs were included, comparing local cooling treatments (ice packs, cold gel pads or cold/iced baths) with no treatment, hamamelis water (witch hazel), pulsed electromagnetic energy (PET), hydrocortisone/pramoxine foam (Epifoam) or warm baths. The RCTs reported on a total of 859 women. Ice packs provided improved pain relief 24 to 72 hours after birth compared with no treatment (risk ratio (RR) 0.61, 95% confidence interval (CI) 0.41 to 0.91). Women preferred the utility of the gel pads compared with ice packs or no treatment, although no differences in pain relief were detected between the treatments. None of our comparisons of treatments resulted in differences detected in perineal oedema or bruising. Women reported more pain (RR 5.60, 95% CI 2.35 to 13.33) and used more additional analgesia (RR 4.00, 95% CI 1.44 to 11.13) following the application of ice packs compared with PET.

AUTHORS' CONCLUSIONS: There is only limited evidence to support the effectiveness of local cooling treatments (ice packs, cold gel pads, cold/iced baths) applied to the perineum following childbirth to relieve pain.

TOPICALLY APPLIED ANAESTHETICS FOR TREATING PERINEAL PAIN AFTER CHILDBIRTH: not enough data to provide reliable evidence. (Hedayati H, Parsons J, Crowther CA) CD004223

BACKGROUND: Perineal trauma is a major problem affecting millions of women around the world each year. The degree of perineal pain and discomfort associated with perineal trauma is often underestimated. Pain often interferes with basic daily activities for the woman such as walking, sitting and passing urine and also negatively impacts on motherhood experiences.

OBJECTIVES: To assess the effects of topically applied anaesthetics for relief of perineal pain following childbirth whilst in hospital and following discharge.

METHODS: Standard PCG methods (see page xvii). Search date: June 2007.

MAIN RESULTS: Eight trials made up of 976 women were included in the review. Five of these trials measured pain experienced up to

24 hours after birth but different methods to assess pain were used in each of the studies. All five trials showed no difference in pain relief when the topical anaesthetic was compared with placebo. One of these studies looked at topical anaesthetics compared with indomethacin vaginal suppositories but there was no significant difference in mean pain scores. All trials reported only short-term follow up (up to four days). Two trials looked at additional analgesia taken for perineal pain, with one trial finding that less additional analgesia was required with epifoam use in comparison with placebo (relative risk (RR) 0.58, 95% confidence interval (CI) 0.40 to 0.84, one trial, 97 women). However, lignocaine/lidocaine showed no difference with regard to additional analgesia use. Adverse effects were not formally measured in the studies; however, some studies commented that there were no side-effects severe enough to discontinue treatment. One study found that the women in the treatment group were more satisfied than the placebo group (RR 0.09, 95% CI 0.01 to 0.65, one trial, 103 women).

AUTHORS' CONCLUSIONS: Evidence for the effectiveness of topically applied local anaesthetics for treating perineal pain is not compelling. There has been no evaluation for the long-term effects of topically applied local anaesthetics.

8.3   Family planning

The possibility of becoming pregnant again may be the last thing on the mind of women adjusting to motherhood, particularly if no menstruation occurs while breastfeeding. Breastfeeding reduces fertility, but not reliably. The question of postpartum contraception needs to be discussed specifically with pregnant women, preferably before the birth

---

EDUCATION FOR CONTRACEPTIVE USE BY WOMEN AFTER CHILD-BIRTH: no randomised trials to provide reliable evidence. (Hiller JE, Griffith E, Jenner F) CD001863 (in RHL 11) (Fertility Regulation Group)

BACKGROUND: In 1966, the Population Council (a non-profit, non-government organisation which aims to foster reproductive health around the world) sponsored demonstration projects (known as the 'International Postpartum Programme') on postpartum family planning, focussing primarily on developing countries and including 25 hospitals in 14 countries (Zatuchni, 1970). These projects were based on the assumptions that women are receptive to family planning education in the postpartum period, and that they will not return to health centres for contraception once they have been discharged from hospital. The demonstration projects were declared a success given their ability to reach large numbers of women, and they were expanded to include hospitals in 21 countries (Winikoff et al, 1991). Randomised controlled trials were not used to assess the effectiveness of the program.

The provision of education on contraceptive use to postpartum mothers has come to be considered a standard component of postnatal care, with up to 84% of women noting that a discussion on contraception took place with a midwife on the postnatal floor (Glasier et al, 1996). Although education frequently is provided as an integral component of discharge planning, many women experience this as a perfunctory discussion included as part of a checklist of topics (Glasier et al, 1996). Midwifery and obstetric texts routinely refer to the provision of such education as a responsibility in the provision of postpartum care; however, the effectiveness of this intervention is seldom questioned (Keith et al, 1980; Semeraro 1996). Questions have been raised about the assumptions that are the basis for such programmes, e.g. that postpartum women are motivated to use contraception and that they will not return to a health centre for family planning advice (Winikoff et al, 1991). In addition surveys conducted postpartum indicate that women may wish to discuss contraception antenatally and post hospital discharge, preferably in the context of general education about maternal and child health (Ozvaris, 1997).

OBJECTIVES: Postpartum education on contraceptive use is a routine component of discharge planning in many different countries with a wide variety of health care systems. This education is based on assumptions concerning women's receptivity to contraceptive education during the postpartum period and their presumed lack of access to such education after that time. The objective of this review is to assess the effects of education about contraceptive use to postpartum mothers.

SEARCH STRATEGY: We searched the Cochrane Controlled Trials Register, MEDLINE, EMBASE, CINAHL, Psychlit, Popline, citations indexes and reference lists of relevant articles. We contacted subject experts to locate additional research, in addition to the Group's Specialised

Register of Controlled Trials. Date of the most recent search: March 2001.

SELECTION CRITERIA: Trials using random or quasi-random methods of allocation which evaluated the effectiveness of postpartum education about contraceptive use.

DATA COLLECTION AND ANALYSIS: Two independent reviewers abstracted data on trial characteristics and results.

MAIN RESULTS: No new trials were identified since this review was updated in 1999.

Three trials were identified with 5438 women. These trials were conducted in Lebanon, Peru and Nepal. None of the trials examined all major prespecified endpoints.

Postpartum education about contraceptive use influenced short-term use assessed between 40 days' and three months' postpartum. Women in the intervention groups were less likely to be non-users than women in the comparison groups (Odds Ratio (OR) = 0.47, 95% Confidence Interval (CI) 0.39 to 0.58). This benefit was not apparent following analysis of data from better quality studies (OR = 0.67, 95% CI 0.41 to 1.13). An apparent benefit on contraceptive use at six months' postpartum (OR = 0.52, 95% CI 0.37 to 0.74) was not apparent following sensitivity analyses (OR = 0.59, 95% CI 0.33 to 1.06). Data are inadequate to assess the impact on cessation of breast feeding and non-attendance at family planning clinics. Unplanned pregnancies, knowledge about contraception and satisfaction with care were not assessed in any trial.

AUTHORS' CONCLUSIONS: The effectiveness of postpartum education about contraceptive use has not yet been established in randomised controlled trials. Such education may be effective in increasing the short-term use of contraception. However, there are only limited data examining a more-important longer-term effect on the prevention of unplanned pregnancies. Research needs to be undertaken to assess the effectiveness of the minimalist education provided in more developed countries and the variety of programmes provided in less developed regions. Such research should examine the content, timing, range and organisation of postpartum education on contraceptive use, including lactational amenorrhoea, as well as its impact on breast feeding rates.

IMMEDIATE POST-PARTUM INSERTION OF INTRAUTERINE
DEVICES: no randomized trials to provide reliable evidence. (Grimes
DA, Schulz KF, Van Vliet H, Stanwood N, Lopez LM). CD003036
(in RHL 11) (Cochrane Fertility Regulation Group)

BACKGROUND: Insertion of an intrauterine device (IUD) immediately
after delivery is appealing for several reasons. The woman is known
not to be pregnant, her motivation for contraception may be high, and
the setting may be convenient for both the woman and her provider.
However, the risk of spontaneous expulsion may be unacceptably high.

OBJECTIVES: To assess the efficacy and feasibility of IUD insertion immediately after expulsion of the placenta. Our a priori hypothesis was
that this practice is safe but associated with higher expulsion rates than
interval IUD insertion.

SEARCH STRATEGY: We used MEDLINE, POPLINE, EMBASE, and CEN-
TRAL computer searches, supplemented by review articles and contact
with investigators.

SELECTION CRITERIA: We sought all randomized controlled trials that
had at least one treatment arm that involved immediate post-partum
(within ten minutes of placental expulsion) insertion of an IUD. Comparisons could include different IUDs, different insertion techniques,
immediate versus delayed post-partum insertion, or immediate versus
interval insertion (unrelated to pregnancy). Studies could include either
vaginal or cesarean deliveries.

DATA COLLECTION AND ANALYSIS: We evaluated the methodological
quality of each report and sought to identify duplicate reporting of data
from multicenter trials. We abstracted data onto data collection forms.
Principal outcome measures included pregnancy, expulsion, and continuation rates. Because the trials did not have uniform interventions,
we were unable to aggregate them in a meta-analysis.

MAIN RESULTS: We found no randomized controlled trials that directly
compared immediate post-partum insertion with either delayed postpartum or interval insertion. Modifications of existing devices, such as
adding absorbable sutures or additional appendages, did not appear
beneficial. Most studies showed no important differences between insertions done by hand or by instruments. Lippes Loop and Progestasert
devices did not perform as well as did copper devices.

AUTHORS' CONCLUSIONS: Immediate post-partum insertion of IUDs appeared safe and effective, though direct comparisons with other insertion times were lacking. Advantages of immediate post-partum insertion include high motivation, assurance that the woman is not pregnant, and convenience. However, expulsion rates appear to be higher than with interval insertion. The popularity of immediate post-partum IUD insertion in countries as diverse as China, Mexico, and Egypt support the feasibility of this approach. Early follow-up may be important in identifying spontaneous IUD expulsions.

8.4 Perinatal death

As for miscarriage, many women who experience a perinatal loss are anxious for answers to three questions, though they may not be verbalised: 'What was the cause? Was it my fault? And will it happen again?'

SUPPORT FOR MOTHERS, FATHERS AND FAMILIES AFTER PERINATAL DEATH: no randomised trials to provide reliable evidence. (Flenady V, Wilson T) CD000452

BACKGROUND: Provision of an empathetic caring environment, and strategies to enable the mother, father and family to accept the reality of perinatal death, are now an accepted part of standard nursing and social support in most of the developed world. Provision of interventions such as psychological support or counselling, or both, has been suggested to improve outcomes for families after a perinatal death.

OBJECTIVES: The objective of this review was to assess the effects of the provision of any form of medical, nursing, social or psychological support or counselling, or both, to mother, father and families after perinatal death.

METHODS: Standard PCG methods (see page xvii). Search date: 30 October 2007.

MAIN RESULTS: No trials were included.

AUTHORS' CONCLUSIONS: There is currently insufficient information available from randomised trials to indicate whether there is or is not a benefit from interventions which aim to provide psychological support or counselling for mothers, fathers or families after perinatal death. Methodologically rigorous trials are needed.

8.5 Medical conditions after childbirth

> **ANALGESIA FOR RELIEF OF PAIN DUE TO UTERINE CRAMPING/ INVOLUTION AFTER BIRTH:** (Deussen A, Ashwood PJ, Agett SA) Protocol [*see* page xviii] CD004908

ABRIDGED BACKGROUND: Women may experience differing types of pain and discomfort following the birth of their baby. These can include incisional pain after a caesarean section, perineal pain following perineal trauma or episiotomy during vaginal delivery, nipple pain from breastfeeding and cramping after-birth pains associated with involution of the uterus.

The incidence and severity of after-birth pains is not widely reported. Endogenous oxytocin released during breastfeeding stimulates the uterus to contract and increases the severity of after-birth pain felt by the mother. Many women prefer not to use pharmacological agents for pain relief during the postnatal period due to concerns about the potential presence of these agents in breast milk. However, it has been documented that some women consider their after-birth pain to be a major burden requiring powerful analgesia.

OBJECTIVES: To assess the effectiveness and safety of analgesia (pharmacological, by any route, or non-pharmacological) for relief of after-birth pains.

> **ANTIBIOTIC REGIMENS FOR ENDOMETRITIS AFTER DELIVERY:** clindamycin and once-daily gentamycin were more effective than other regimens; continued oral treatment after response, was unnecessary. (French LM, Smaill FM) CD001067 (in RHL 11)

BACKGROUND: Postpartum endometritis, which is more common after cesarean section, occurs when vaginal organisms invade the endometrial cavity during labor and birth. Antibiotic treatment is warranted.

OBJECTIVES: The effect of different antibiotic regimens for the treatment of postpartum endometritis on failure of therapy and complications was systematically reviewed.

METHODS: Standard PCG methods (see page xvii). Search date: January 2007.

MAIN RESULTS: Thirty-nine trials with 4221 participants were included. Fifteen studies comparing clindamycin and an aminoglycoside with another regimen showed more treatment failures with the other regimen (relative risk (RR) 1.44; 95% confidence interval (CI) 1.15 to 1.80). Failures of those regimens with poor activity against penicillin resistant anaerobic bacteria were more likely (RR 1.94; 95% CI 1.38 to 2.72). In three studies that compared continued oral antibiotic therapy after intravenous therapy with no oral therapy, no differences were found in recurrent endometritis or other outcomes. In four studies comparing once daily with thrice daily dosing of gentamicin there were fewer failures with once daily dosing. There was no evidence of difference in incidence of allergic reactions. Cephalosporins were associated with less diarrhea.

AUTHORS' CONCLUSIONS: The combination of gentamicin and clindamycin is appropriate for the treatment of endometritis. Regimens with activity against penicillin-resistant anaerobic bacteria are better than those without. There is no evidence that any one regimen is associated with fewer side-effects. Once uncomplicated endometritis has clinically improved with intravenous therapy, oral therapy is not needed.

8.6   Unhappiness after childbirth

Depression is common in the months following childbirth. The distress caused is compounded by failure of women, their families and caregivers to recognise it as a clinical problem. Routine screening tools such as the Edinburgh Postnatal Depression Inventory have been developed to help identify women with significant depression.

> **ANTENATAL PSYCHOSOCIAL SCREENING FOR PREVENTION OF ANTENATAL AND POSTNATAL ANXIETY AND DEPRESSION:** (Priest SR, Austin MP, Sullivan E) Protocol [see page xviii] CD005124

ABRIDGED BACKGROUND: Perinatal mental health problems associated with pregnancy, childbirth and the first postnatal year are recognised as a major public health issue with 15% to 25% of childbearing women likely to develop a clinically significant mental health disorder in the interval between conception and the end of the first postpartum year. Suicide is the leading cause of death following severe maternal psychiatric illness.

Antenatal psychosocial screening is a public health policy initiative set within a primary prevention framework that is being trialed in many centres in conjunction with prevention, early intervention, and treatment programmes with the objective of reducing high morbidity and mortality rates. Screening programmes are designed to identify women who show early symptoms of disorders, and/or have risk factors known to be associated with clinical onset of mental health problems so that they can be linked in with appropriate services.

OBJECTIVES: *Primary aims*: To evaluate the effectiveness of antenatal psychosocial screening during pregnancy and the early postnatal period.
Secondary aims: (1) To evaluate psychosocial measures used to screen pregnant women. (2) To review the criteria used to determine risk status. (3) To examine the methods used to diagnose anxiety and depression.

PSYCHOSOCIAL AND PSYCHOLOGICAL INTERVENTIONS FOR PREVENTING POSTPARTUM DEPRESSION: depression was reduced by intensive professional postpartum support, identifying mothers at risk and individual interventions focussed on the postnatal period; however, overall psychosocial interventions did not reduce depression significantly. (Dennis C-L, Creedy D) CD001134 (in RHL 11)

BACKGROUND: The cause of postpartum depression remains unclear, with extensive research suggesting a multi-factorial aetiology. However, epidemiological studies and meta-analyses of predictive studies have consistently demonstrated the importance of psychosocial and psychological variables. While interventions based on these variables may be effective treatment strategies, theoretically they may also be used in pregnancy and the early postpartum period to prevent postpartum depression.

OBJECTIVES: Primary: to assess the effect of diverse psychosocial and psychological interventions compared with usual antepartum, intrapartum or postpartum care to reduce the risk of developing postpartum depression. Secondary: to examine (1) the effectiveness of specific types of psychosocial and psychological interventions, (2) the effectiveness of individual versus group-based interventions, (3) the effects of intervention onset and duration, and (4) whether interventions are more effective in women selected with specific risk factors.

METHODS: Standard PCG methods (see page xvii). Search date: January 2004.

MAIN RESULTS: 15 trials, involving over 7600 women, were included. Overall, women who received a psychosocial intervention were equally likely to develop postpartum depression as those receiving standard care (relative risk (RR) 0.81, 95% confidence interval (CI) 0.65 to 1.02). One promising intervention appears to be the provision of intensive postpartum support provided by public health nurses or midwives (RR 0.68, 95% CI 0.55 to 0.84). Identifying mothers 'at-risk' assisted the prevention of postpartum depression (RR 0.67, 95% CI 0.51 to 0.89). Interventions with only a postnatal component appeared to be more beneficial (RR 0.76, 95% CI 0.58 to 0.98) than interventions that also incorporated an antenatal component. While individually-based interventions may be more effective (RR 0.76, 95% CI 0.59 to 1.00) than those that are group-based, women who received multiple-contact intervention were just as likely to experience postpartum depression as those who received a single-contact intervention.

AUTHORS' CONCLUSIONS: Overall psychosocial interventions do not reduce the numbers of women who develop postpartum depression. However, a promising intervention is the provision of intensive, professionally-based postpartum support.

OESTROGENS AND PROGESTINS FOR PREVENTING AND TREATING POSTPARTUM DEPRESSION: oestrogen treatment improved depression; norethisterone enantate increased depression; insufficient evidence was found for natural progestogens. (Dennis CL, Ross LE, Herxheimer A) CD001690

BACKGROUND: Postpartum depression is a common complication of childbirth, affecting approximately 13% of women. A hormonal aetiology has long been hypothesised due to the sudden and substantial fluctuations in concentrations of steroid hormones associated with pregnancy and the immediate postpartum period. There is also convincing evidence that oestrogens, progestins and related compounds have important central nervous system activity at physiological concentrations.

OBJECTIVES: The primary objective of this review was to assess the effects of oestrogens and progestins, including natural progesterone and synthetic progestogens, compared with placebo or usual antepartum, intrapartum or postpartum care in the prevention and treatment of postpartum depression.

METHODS: Standard PCG methods (see page xvii). Search date: June 2004.

All published and unpublished randomised controlled trials comparing an oestrogen and progestin intervention with a placebo or usual antepartum, intrapartum or postpartum care among pregnant women or new mothers recruited within the first year postpartum.

MAIN RESULTS: Two trials, involving 229 women, met the selection criteria. Norethisterone enanthate, a synthetic progestogen, administered within 48 hours of delivery was associated with a significantly higher risk of developing postpartum depression. Oestrogen therapy was associated with a greater improvement in depression scores than placebo among women with severe depression.

AUTHORS' CONCLUSIONS: Synthetic progestogens should be used with significant caution in the postpartum period. The role of natural progesterone in the prevention and treatment of postpartum depression has yet to be evaluated in a randomised, placebo-controlled trial. Oestrogen therapy may be of modest value for the treatment of severe postpartum depression. Its role in the prevention of recurrent postpartum depression has not been rigorously evaluated. Further research is warranted.

ANTIDEPRESSANT PREVENTION OF POSTNATAL DEPRESSION: not enough data to provide reliable evidence. (Howard LM, Hoffbrand S, Henshaw C, Boath L, Bradley E) CD004363 (Depression, Anxiety and Neurosis Group)

BACKGROUND: Postnatal depression is a common and important complication of childbearing. Untreated depression can lead to potentially negative effects on the foetus and infant, in addition to serious morbidity for the mother. The use of antidepressants during pregnancy for prevention of postnatal depression is unclear, due to the possibility of adverse effects on the mother and developing foetus, and the difficulty of reliably identifying the women who would go on to develop postnatal depression.

OBJECTIVES: To evaluate the effectiveness of different antidepressant drugs in addition to standard clinical care in the prevention of postnatal depression.

To compare the effectiveness of different antidepressant drugs and with any other form of intervention for postnatal depression, i.e. hormonal, psychological or social support.

To assess any adverse effects of antidepressant drugs in either the mother or the foetus/infant.

SEARCH STRATEGY: The register of clinical trials maintained and updated by the Cochrane Depression, Anxiety and Neurosis Group and the Cochrane Pregnancy and Childbirth Group were searched.

SELECTION CRITERIA: Randomised studies of antidepressants alone or in combination with another treatment, compared with placebo or a psychosocial intervention in non-depressed pregnant women or women who had given birth in the previous six weeks (i.e. women at risk of postnatal depression)

DATA COLLECTION AND ANALYSIS: Data were extracted independently from the trial reports by the authors. Missing information was requested from investigators wherever possible. Data were sought to allow an 'intention to treat' analysis.

MAIN RESULTS: Two trials fulfilled the inclusion criteria for this review. Both looked at women with a past history of postpartum depression. Nortriptyline (n=26) (Wisner, 2001) did not show any benefit over placebo (n=25). Sertraline (n=14) (Wisner, 2004) reduced the recurrence of postnatal depression and the time to recurrence when compared with placebo (n=8). Intention to treat analyses were not carried out in either trial.

AUTHORS' CONCLUSIONS: It is not possible to draw any clear conclusions about the effectiveness of antidepressants given immediately postpartum in preventing postnatal depression and, therefore, they cannot be recommended for prophylaxis of postnatal depression, due to the lack of clear evidence. Larger trials are needed which also include comparisons of antidepressant drugs with other prophylactic treatments to reflect clinical practice, and examine adverse effects for the foetus and infant, as well as assess women's attitudes to the use of antidepressants at this time.

ANTIDEPRESSANT TREATMENT FOR POST-NATAL DEPRESSION: not enough data to provide reliable evidence. (Hoffbrand S, Howard L, Crawley H) CD002018 (Depression, Anxiety and Neurosis Group)

BACKGROUND: Postnatal depression is a common disorder which can have profound short and long term effects on maternal morbidity, the new infant and the family as a whole. Social factors appear to be particularly important in the aetiology and prognosis of postnatal depression and treatment is often largely by social support and psychological interventions. It is not known whether antidepressants are an effective and safe choice for treatment of this disorder.

OBJECTIVES: To evaluate the effectiveness of different antidepressant drugs and compare their effectiveness with other forms of treatment.

To assess any adverse effects of antidepressants in the mother or the nursing baby.

SEARCH STRATEGY: The registers of clinical trials maintained and updated by the Cochrane Depression, Anxiety and Neurosis Group and the Cochrane Pregnancy and Childbirth Group were searched. Contact was made with pharmaceutical companies and experts in the field.

SELECTION CRITERIA: All trials were considered in which women with depression in the first six months postpartum were randomised to receive antidepressants alone or in combination with another treatment, or to receive any other treatment including placebo.

DATA COLLECTION AND ANALYSIS: Data was extracted independently from the trial reports by the reviewers. Missing information was requested from investigators wherever possible. Data was sought to allow an 'intention to treat' analysis.

MAIN RESULTS: Only one trial (Appleby, 1997) could be included in this review, leaving all the objectives of the review unfulfilled. The authors reported that fluoxetine was, after an initial session of counselling, as effective as a full course of cognitive-behavioural counselling in the treatment of postnatal depression. The clinical interview schedule (CIS-R) geometric mean score at 12 weeks for fluoxetine plus one session of counselling was 11.1 (95% confidence interval (C.I) 6.9–17.6) and for placebo plus six sessions of counselling was 13.0 (95% C.I 9.2–18.1).

AUTHORS' CONCLUSIONS: It is not possible to make any recommendations for antidepressant treatment in postnatal depression from this single small trial. More trials are needed, with larger sample sizes and longer follow-up periods, to compare different antidepressants in the treatment of postnatal depression, to compare antidepressant treatment with psychosocial interventions and to assess adverse effects of antidepressants. Treatment of postnatal depression is an area that has been neglected despite the large public health impact described above.

ANTIPSYCHOTIC DRUGS FOR NON-AFFECTIVE PSYCHOSIS DURING PREGNANCY AND POSTPARTUM: no randomised trials to provide reliable evidence. (Webb RT, Howard L, Abel KM) CD004411 (Schizophrenia Group)

BACKGROUND: Antipsychotics are commonly prescribed for women suffering psychotic illnesses during pregnancy and the postpartum period. The potential adverse consequences of these different options are multiple and complex, impacting on the foetus, neonate, infant and early development of the child as well as the woman herself.

OBJECTIVES: To establish whether the benefits of taking antipsychotic drugs outweigh the risks for pregnant or postpartum women.

SEARCH STRATEGY: The Cochrane Schizophrenia Group's Register (January 2003) was searched in order to identify all published trials of women during pregnancy or the postpartum period. We inspected all references of all identified studies. If any studies had been found, the first authors of each included study would have been contacted.

SELECTION CRITERIA: Randomised controlled clinical trials investigating the effects of any type of antipsychotic drug compared with any other treatment option (including standard psychosocial care, any other antipsychotic drug, or an alternative therapy such as electro-convulsive therapy or cognitive behavioural therapy) and involving pregnant women and/or women during the postpartum period diagnosed with a non-affective psychotic disorder.

DATA COLLECTION AND ANALYSIS: Citations and, where possible, abstracts were independently inspected by reviewers and the papers ordered were scrutinised and quality assessed. Data would have been extracted independently by at least two reviewers. Binary outcomes were to have been analysed using Relative Risks (RR) and their 95% Confidence Intervals (CI).

MAIN RESULTS: We found no trials that met the broad inclusion criteria.

AUTHORS' CONCLUSIONS: Current guidelines and clinical practice for the use of antipsychotic drugs in women with non-affective disorders during pregnancy and postpartum are not based on evidence from randomised controlled trials. Although ethical concerns have to date precluded the use of randomised controlled trials to address this research topic, the continued use of antipsychotic drugs in this group

of women in itself poses significant clinical and ethical problems. Evidence is required from large pragmatic trials that reflect routine clinical practice, examine a broad range of outcomes and accurately quantify risks and benefits to both mothers and their offspring, so that comparison between different treatment options can be made.

MOTHER AND BABY UNITS FOR SCHIZOPHRENIA: no randomised trials to provide reliable evidence. (Joy CB, Saylan M) CD006333 (Schizophrenia Group)

BACKGROUND: Mother and baby units (MBUs) are recommended, in the UK, as an optimal site for treating post partum psychoses. Naturalistic studies suggest poor outcomes for mothers and their children if admission is needed during the first year after birth, but the evidence for the effectiveness of MBUs in addressing the problems faced by both mothers with mental illness and their babies is unclear.

OBJECTIVES: To review the effects of mother and baby units for mothers with schizophrenia or psychoses needing admission during the first year after giving birth, and their children, in comparison to standard care on a ward without a mother and baby unit.

SEARCH STRATEGY: We undertook electronic searches of the Cochrane Schizophrenia Group's Register (June 2006).

SELECTION CRITERIA: We included all randomised clinical trials comparing placement on a mother and baby unit compared to any other standard care without attachment to such a unit.

DATA COLLECTION AND ANALYSIS: If data were available we would have independently extracted data and analysed on an intention-to-treat basis; calculated the relative risk (RR) and 95% confidence intervals (CI) of homogeneous dichotomous data using a random effects model, and where possible calculated the number needed to treat (NNT); calculated weighted mean differences (WMD) for continuous data.

MAIN RESULTS: Unfortunately, we did not find any relevant studies to include. One non-randomised trial, published in 1961, suggested beneficial effects for those admitted to mother and baby units. For the experimental group, more women were able to care for their baby on their own and experienced fewer early relapses on their return home compared with standard care. Care practices for people with schizophrenia have changed dramatically over the past 40 years and a sensitively designed pragmatic trial is possible and justified.

AUTHORS' CONCLUSIONS: Mother and by units are reportedly common in the UK but less common in other countries and rare or non-existent in the developing world. However, there does not appear to be any trial-based evidence for the effectiveness of these units. This lack of data is of concern as descriptive studies have found poor outcomes such as anxious attachment and poor development for children of mothers with schizophrenia and a greater risk of the children being placed under supervised or foster care. Effective care of both mothers and babies during this critical time may be crucial to prevent poor clinical and parenting outcomes. Good, relevant research is urgently needed.

8.7 Breastfeeding

The benefits of breastfeeding have been recognised for many centuries: '… those children who are nourished by their mothers' milk enjoy the most appropriate and natural food.' Galen C. *Hygiene*. Springfield, Illinois: Charles C Thomas, 1951. Recent research has identified benefits for the baby including nutritional, immunological, developmental and intellectual. In communities without access to safe water supplies and adequate replacement formula, babies who are not breastfed are at risk of malnutrition and death from diarrhoeal disease. Aggressive marketing of breast milk substitutes has been held responsible for childhood morbidity and mortality on an enormous scale.

Today, education about breastfeeding has been complicated by the HIV epidemic. Women who are HIV infected are advised not to breast-feed, unless they are not in a position to provide safe alternative feeding, in which case the risks of morbidity and mortality from unsafe feeding practices may outweigh the risk of HIV transmission in breast milk. There is also a danger that mixed messages about breastfeeding may compromise attempts to encourage HIV uninfected women to breastfeed.

8.7.1 Antenatal preparation for breastfeeding

Antenatal preparation for breastfeeding may include education as well as physical measures to prepare the breasts.

INTERVENTIONS FOR PROMOTING THE INITIATION OF BREAST-
FEEDING: breastfeeding education increased breastfeeding initiation
rates. (Dyson L, McCormick F, Renfrew MJ) CD001688 (in RHL 11)

BACKGROUND: Despite the widely documented health benefits of
breastfeeding, initiation rates remain relatively low in many high-income
countries, particularly among women in lower income groups.

OBJECTIVES: To evaluate the effectiveness of interventions which aim to
encourage women to breastfeed in terms of changes in the number of
women who start to breastfeed.

METHODS: Standard PCG methods (see page xvii). Search date:
May 2006. Randomised controlled trials, with or without blinding, of any
breastfeeding promotion intervention in any population group except
women and infants with a specific health problem.

MAIN RESULTS: Seven trials involving 1388 women were included.
Five trials involving 582 women on low incomes in the USA showed
breastfeeding education had a significant effect on increasing initiation
rates compared to routine care (relative risk (RR) 1.53, 95% confidence
interval (CI) 1.25 to 1.88).

**AUTHORS' CONCLUSIONS: Evidence from this review shows that the
forms of breastfeeding education evaluated were effective at increasing breastfeeding initiation rates among women on low incomes in
the USA.**

ANTENATAL BREASTFEEDING EDUCATION FOR INCREASING
BREASTFEEDING DURATION: (Lumbiganon P, Martis R, Laopiboon
M, Festin MR, Ho JJ, Hakimi M) Protocol [see page xviii] CD006425

ABRIDGED BACKGROUND: Another Cochrane systematic review provides evidence that various forms of breastfeeding education are effective at increasing rates of breastfeeding initiation among women on
low incomes in the USA and will, therefore, not be discussed in this review. The impact of antenatal breastfeeding education on the duration
of breastfeeding, however, has not been widely reported. Antenatal
breastfeeding education is defined as breastfeeding information being
imparted during the pregnancy in a variety of forms.

OBJECTIVES: (1) To assess the effectiveness of antenatal breastfeeding education for increasing breastfeeding duration. (2) To compare the effectiveness of various forms of antenatal education: for example, peer support, educational programme, didactic teaching session, workshop, booklets, etc, or a combination of these interventions for increasing breastfeeding duration.

> **ANTENATAL BREAST EXAMINATION FOR PROMOTING BREAST-FEEDING:** (Lee SJ, Thomas J) Protocol [*see* page xviii] CD006064

ABRIDGED BACKGROUND: Breast examination during pregnancy may be performed by a healthcare provider or by the pregnant woman herself. The rationale for antenatal breast examination has included the need to determine whether any problems with breastfeeding could be anticipated, using the time during examination as an opportunity for the healthcare provider to introduce and discuss the importance of breastfeeding, and for the detection of breast cancer during pregnancy. Despite these purported benefits of antenatal breast examination, whether there is evidence that it should be recommended for all pregnant women remains unclear.

OBJECTIVES: The main objective of this review is to determine the effect of antenatal breast examination(s) on the initiation of breastfeeding.

The secondary objectives of this review are to assess other potential effects of antenatal breast examination, such as providing opportunities to discuss breastfeeding with women and the detection of breast abnormalities.

8.7.2 Supporting breastfeeding mothers

> ☺ **SUPPORT FOR BREASTFEEDING MOTHERS:** prolonged the duration of breastfeeding. (Britton C, McCormick FM, Renfrew MJ, Wade A, King SE) CD001141 (IN RHL 11)

BACKGROUND: There is extensive evidence of the benefits of breastfeeding for infants and mothers. In 2003, the World Health Organization (WHO) recommended infants be fed exclusively on breast milk until six months of age. However, breastfeeding rates in many developed countries continue to be resistant to change.

OBJECTIVES: To assess the effectiveness of support for breastfeeding mothers.

METHODS: Standard PCG methods (see page xvii). Search date: January 2006.

MAIN RESULTS: We have included 34 trials (29 385 mother–infant pairs) from 14 countries. All forms of extra support analysed together showed an increase in duration of 'any breastfeeding' (includes partial and exclusive breastfeeding) (relative risk (RR) for stopping any breastfeeding before six months 0.91, 95% confidence interval (CI) 0.86 to 0.96). All forms of extra support together had a larger effect on duration of exclusive breast-feeding than on any breastfeeding (RR 0.81, 95% CI 0.74 to 0.89). Lay and professional support together extended duration of any breastfeed-ing significantly (RR before four–six weeks 0.65, 95% 0.51 to 0.82; RR before two months 0.74, 95% CI 0.66 to 0.83). Exclusive breastfeeding was significantly prolonged with use of WHO/UNICEF training (RR 0.69, 95% CI 0.52 to 0.91). Maternal satisfaction was poorly reported.

AUTHORS' CONCLUSIONS: Additional professional support was effective in prolonging any breastfeeding, but its effects on exclusive breastfeeding were less clear. WHO/UNICEF training courses ap-peared to be effective for professional training. Additional lay sup-port was effective in prolonging exclusive breastfeeding, while its effects on duration of any breastfeeding were uncertain. Effective support offered by professionals and lay people together was spe-cific to breastfeeding and was offered to women who had decided to breastfeed. Further trials are required to assess the effectiveness (including cost-effectiveness) of both lay and professional support in different settings, particularly those with low rates of breastfeeding initiation, and for women who wish to breastfeed for longer than three months. Trials should consider timing and delivery of support interventions and relative effectiveness of intervention components, and should report women's views. Research into appropriate train-ing for supporters (whether lay or professional) of breastfeeding mothers is also needed.

INTERVENTIONS FOR PREVENTING AND TREATING NIPPLE PAIN IN BREASTFEEDING MOTHERS: (McCormick FM, Renfrew MJ) Protocol [see page xviii] CD004657

ABRIDGED BACKGROUND: Studies from around the world have reported painful breasts or nipples as the second most common reason for discontinuing breastfeeding. Factors causing breast pain and nipple pain might differ, and the aetiology of breast pain is not well understood. The focus of this review is the prevention and treatment of nipple pain.

Evidence-based interventions to support women learning to position their babies at the breast and enable pain free, effective feeding have been devised, notably as one of the Ten Steps to Successful Breast-feeding adopted by WHO/UNICEF in the international Baby Friendly Hospital Initiative.

OBJECTIVES: To evaluate interventions to prevent or treat nipple pain in terms of numbers of mothers who stop breastfeeding.

To assess the impact of the interventions on other outcomes, such as reported nipple pain, nipple trauma, nipple infections and mastitis, duration of breastfeeding and maternal satisfaction.

INTERVENTIONS IN THE WORKPLACE TO SUPPORT BREAST-FEEDING FOR WOMEN IN EMPLOYMENT: no randomised trials to provide reliable evidence. (Abdulwadud OA, Snow ME) CD006177

BACKGROUND: In recent years there has been a rise in the participation rate of women in employment. Some may become pregnant while in employment and subsequently deliver their babies. Most may decide to return early to work after giving birth for various reasons. Unless these mothers get support from their employers and fellow employees, they might give up breastfeeding when they return to work. As a result, the duration and exclusivity of breastfeeding to the recommended age of the babies would be affected.

Workplace environment can play a positive role to promote breast-feeding. For women going back to work, various types of workplace support interventions are available and this should not be ignored by employers. Notably, promoting breastfeeding in a workplace may have benefits for the women, the baby and also the employer.

OBJECTIVES: To assess the effectiveness of workplace interventions to support and promote breastfeeding among women returning to paid work after the birth of their children, and its impact on process outcomes pertinent to employees and employers.

METHODS: Standard PCG methods (see page xvii). Search date: November 2006.

MAIN RESULTS: There were no randomised controlled trials or quasi-randomised controlled trials identified.

AUTHORS' CONCLUSIONS: No trials have evaluated the effectiveness of workplace interventions in promoting breastfeeding among women returning to paid work after the birth of their child. The impact of such intervention on process outcomes is also unknown. Randomised controlled trials are required to establish the benefits of various types of workplace interventions to support, encourage and promote breastfeeding among working mothers.

SEPARATE CARE FOR NEW MOTHER AND INFANT VERSUS ROOMING-IN FOR INCREASING THE DURATION OF BREASTFEED-ING: (Sharifah H, Lee KS, Ho JJ) Protocol [see page xviii] CD006641

ABRIDGED BACKGROUND: Babies born at home may remain together with their mother after birth or, in some cultures, the traditional practice is to provide separate care for the mother and baby. Increased levels of stress hormones during childbirth have been shown to affect the onset of copious breast-milk production that might lead to early breastfeeding failure. Thus, placing the infants in the hospital nursery after birth might be beneficial for both the mother and infant as it allows the mother to sleep and rest without having to worry about the care of her infant. On the other hand, mother–infant rooming-in, as recommended by the WHO/UNICEF Baby Friendly Hospital Initiative in the ten steps to successful breastfeeding, is believed to be the most favorable arrangement for optimal breast-milk production.
OBJECTIVES: To assess the effect of mother–infant separation versus rooming-in on the duration of breastfeeding (exclusive and total duration of breastfeeding).

MEDICATIONS FOR INCREASING MILK SUPPLY IN MOTHERS EXPRESSING BREASTMILK FOR THEIR HOSPITALISED INFANTS: (Donovan T, Buchanan K) Protocol [see page xviii] CD005544

ABRIDGED BACKGROUND: Infants who are born preterm, or otherwise ill, are dependent on expressed breastmilk for a substantial period of their hospitalisation. These mothers often have difficulty supporting lactation when milk production is solely maintained by breast expression.

Interventions reported to increase breastmilk supply have included hand and mechanical breast expression, enhanced maternal support, galactagogue medications and complementary medicines. Galactagogue medications have included medications thought to improve breastmilk supply by increasing milk production and/or milk release from the breast during expression or suckling.

This review will focus on randomised controlled trials that have assessed the use of medications or herbal preparations for improving breastmilk supply in mothers of hospitalised infants.

OBJECTIVES: *Primary objective:* To assess the effect of medication taken by mothers to augment the breastfeeding of their preterm or hospitalised infants on the outcome of breastmilk supply (breastmilk volume and duration of breastfeeding). Trials of breastmilk augmenting medications that are compared with placebo or with other augmenting medications are to be considered.

Secondary objective: To assess maternal and infant adverse effects from medications taken to augment breastfeeding, when compared with placebo.

METHODS OF MILK EXPRESSION FOR LACTATING WOMEN:
(Becker GE, Renfrew MJ) Protocol [*see* page xviii] CD006170

ABRIDGED BACKGROUND: Not all babies are able to feed at the breast due to illness or abnormalities, prematurity, separation, and other reasons. Expressed milk is needed for these babies. The Baby Friendly Hospital Initiative, a global project of WHO/UNICEF, requires that mothers be assisted to learn the skill of hand expression before discharge from maternity services. However, there is limited research on the best way of learning this skill.

The ability to express milk may improve the eventual breastfeeding of premature or ill infants and assist in sustaining breastfeeding..

OBJECTIVES: The main objectives of this review are to assess acceptability, effectiveness, safety, effect on milk composition, bacterial contamination and cost implications of a range of methods of milk expression, including hand expression, manual, battery and electric pumps.

ANTIBIOTICS FOR MASTITIS IN BREASTFEEDING WOMEN:
(Ng C, Jahanfar S, Teng CL) Protocol [*see* page xviii] CD005458

ABRIDGED BACKGROUND: Mastitis is an inflammatory condition of the breast, usually associated with lactation. The primary cause of mastitis is milk stasis, which may or may not be associated with infection. Delayed, inappropriate or inadequate treatment may result in unnecessary discontinuation of breastfeeding, breast tissue damage, relapse and substantial cost.

The principles of treating mastitis include supportive counselling and supportive therapy (bed rest, increased fluids), milk removal, symptomatic treatment (pain medication, use of inflammatory agents) and antibiotic therapy. There is little consensus on which patients should receive antibiotics, the most appropriate antibiotic to use, when is the best time to begin treatment and how long the treatment should continue.

OBJECTIVES: The objective of this review is to examine the effectiveness of antibiotic therapies in relieving symptoms for breastfeeding women who have mastitis.

EARLY ADDITIONAL FOOD AND FLUIDS FOR HEALTHY BREASTFED FULL-TERM INFANTS: (Remmington S, Remmington T) Protocol [see page xviii] CD006462

ABRIDGED BACKGROUND: The World Health Organization's Global Strategy for Young Child Feeding recommends exclusive breastfeeding for the first six months of life, followed by the introduction of complementary foods from six months, and continued breastfeeding for up to at least two years of age. Yet few of the 129 million babies born annually receive such optimal breastfeeding and some are not breastfed at all. Early cessation of breastfeeding in favour of commercial breast milk substitutes and unnecessary supplementation are still common.

Exclusive breastfeeding should be considered as the normative model against which all alternative feeding methods should be measured with regard to growth, health and short- and long-term outcomes.

OBJECTIVES: The main objective of the review will be to assess the benefits and harms of additional foods and fluids for full-term healthy breastfed infants. We also aim to determine what impact the timing of supplementation (during early phase of initiation of breastfeeding versus later on for maintenance) and type of supplementation have on these infants.

VITAMIN A SUPPLEMENTATION FOR BREASTFEEDING MOTHERS: (Oliveira JM, Bergamaschi DP, East CE, Pai M) Protocol [see page xviii] CD005944

ABRIDGED BACKGROUND: Vitamin A is a generic term for a group of fat-soluble substances that carry out similar biological activity in the human metabolism. It plays an important role in normal vision, gene expression, growth and physical development, maintenance and proliferation of epithelial cells, and immune function, at all stages of life, particularly during pregnancy and lactation, given fetal and newborn requirements.

WHO, UNICEF and the International Vitamin A Consultative Group recommend that in areas of endemic vitamin A deficiency high doses of supplementary vitamin A should be given to breastfeeding women during the postpartum period (four to six weeks after childbirth), as a strategy to improve mothers' and infants' stores of this micronutrient. Since the real effects of vitamin A supplementation on mothers' and newborns' health are unclear, a systematic review is called for.

OBJECTIVES: To assess the effects of vitamin A supplementation, alone or in combination with other micronutrients (e.g. iron, folic acid, vitamin E), in mothers during the postpartum period, on maternal and infant health. Specific objectives are to compare the effects of vitamin A supplementation (alone or in combination with other micronutrients) with placebo or no supplementation on:

(1) the duration and occurrence of maternal morbidity (xerophthalmia, infection) or illness symptoms (night blindness, fever, nausea, vomiting);
(2) the duration and occurrence of neonatal or infant morbidity (respiratory tract infection, diarrhoea, measles) or illness symptoms (fever, nausea, vomiting);
(3) maternal serum retinol concentration;
(4) infant serum retinol concentration;
(5) breast milk retinol concentration; and
(6) maternal satisfaction.

8.7.3 Breastfeeding difficulties

Breastfeeding success appears to be influenced by the mother's sense of confidence and positive interaction with her baby, as well as with correct breastfeeding technique and the support she receives from health professionals and family. Health professionals and parents may worry whether mothers are producing adequate milk. Reassurance, with or without technical breastfeeding support, may be all that is needed, though care should be taken not to miss rare cases of true lack of milk production. Short-term treatment with dopamine receptor antagonists has been used both for perceived lack of milk production and to initiate lactation in women who have not been breastfeeding for some time.

> **TREATMENTS FOR BREAST ENGORGEMENT DURING LACTATION:** (Mangesi L, Muzonzini G) Protocol [see page xviii] CD006946

ABRIDGED BACKGROUND: Breast engorgement is the overfilling of breast milk that causes discomfort and pain to the mother. Inadequate emptying of breasts results in problems such as breast engorgement, plugged milk duct, breast infection and insufficient milk supply. Many methods of treating breastfeeding engorgement have been introduced.
OBJECTIVES: To identify the best forms of treatment for women who experience breast engorgement.

8.7.4 Duration of breastfeeding

> **OPTIMAL DURATION OF EXCLUSIVE BREASTFEEDING:** exclusive breastfeeding for six months rather than three to four months reduced gastrointestinal infections without measurable adverse effects. (Kramer MS, Kakuma R) CD003517 (in RHL 11)

BACKGROUND: Although the health benefits of breastfeeding are widely acknowledged, opinions and recommendations are strongly divided on the optimal duration of exclusive breastfeeding. Much of the debate has centered on the so-called 'weanling's dilemma' in developing countries: the choice between the known protective effect of exclusive breastfeeding against infectious morbidity and the (theoretical) insufficiency of breast milk alone to satisfy the infant's energy and micronutrient requirements beyond four months of age.
OBJECTIVES: To assess the effects on child health, growth, and development, and on maternal health, of exclusive breastfeeding for six months versus exclusive breastfeeding for three to four months with mixed breastfeeding (introduction of complementary liquid or solid foods with continued breastfeeding) thereafter through six months.
METHODS: Standard PCG methods (see page xvii). Search date: December 2006. We selected all internally-controlled clinical trials and observational studies comparing child or maternal health outcomes

with exclusive breastfeeding for six or more months versus exclusive breastfeeding for at least three to four months with continued mixed breastfeeding until at least six months. Studies were stratified according to study design (controlled trials versus observational studies), provenance (developing versus developed countries), and timing of compared feeding groups (three to seven months versus later).

MAIN RESULTS: We identified 22 independent studies meeting the selection criteria: 11 from developing countries (two of which were controlled trials in Honduras) and 11 from developed countries (all observational studies). Definitions of exclusive breastfeeding varied considerably across studies. Neither the trials nor the observational studies suggest that infants who continue to be exclusively breastfed for six months show deficits in weight or length gain, although larger sample sizes would be required to rule out modest differences in risk of undernutrition. In developing-country settings where newborn iron stores may be suboptimal, the evidence suggests that exclusive breastfeeding without iron supplementation through six months may compromise hematologic status. Based on studies from Belarus, Iran, and Nigeria, infants who continue exclusive breastfeeding for six months or more appear to have a significantly reduced risk of gastrointestinal and (in the Iranian and Nigerian studies) respiratory infection. No significant reduction in risk of atopic eczema, asthma, or other atopic outcomes has been demonstrated in studies from Finland, Australia, and Belarus. Data from the two Honduran trials and from observational studies from Bangladesh and Senegal suggest that exclusive breastfeeding through six months is associated with delayed resumption of menses and, in the Honduran trials, more rapid postpartum weight loss in the mother.

AUTHORS' CONCLUSIONS: We found no objective evidence of a 'weanling's dilemma'. Infants who are exclusively breastfed for six months experience less morbidity from gastrointestinal infection than those who are mixed breastfed as of three or four months, and no deficits have been demonstrated in growth among infants from either developing or developed countries who are exclusively breastfed for six months or longer. Moreover, the mothers of such infants have more prolonged lactational amenorrhea. Although infants should still be managed individually so that insufficient growth or other adverse outcomes are not ignored and appropriate interventions are provided, the available evidence demonstrates no apparent risks in

recommending, as a general policy, exclusive breastfeeding for the first six months of life in both developing and developed-country settings. Large randomized trials are recommended in both types of setting to rule out small effects on growth and to confirm the reported health benefits of exclusive breastfeeding for six months or beyond.

8.7.5   Suppressing lactation and breast symptoms in women who are not breastfeeding

Physical methods are suggested to suppress the production of milk in women who do not intend to breastfeed. These include binding the breasts; advice to avoid expressing milk (unless to relieve painful engorgement); and advice to reduce feeding or express milk slowly to avoid painful engorgement. To suppress lactation dopamine agonists are also used.

There are no Cochrane reviews of this topic.

> **TREATMENTS FOR SUPPRESSION OF LACTATION:** (Oladapo OT, Fawole B) Protocol [see page xviii] CD005937

ABRIDGED BACKGROUND: In spite of the well-known advantages of breastfeeding (for example, infant protection against diarrheal morbidity and mortality), there are instances when the wellbeing of the mother or infant requires suppression of lactation. Although physiologic cessation of lactation eventually occurs in the absence of physical stimulus such as infant suckling, a variable proportion of women experience moderate to severe milk leakage and discomfort, before lactation ceases. Interventions to suppress lactation in nonbreastfeeding women have evolved for centuries. Before the 20th century, these approaches included breast binding or strapping, emptying of the breast by massage, fluid and diet restrictions and application of external products such as belladonna ointment to the breast and nipples. Later, the avoidance of tactile breast stimulation and application of external agents such as cabbage leaves, jasmine flower and ice packs were included.. After it was demonstrated that postpartum lactation depends primarily on pituitary prolactin secretion, the synthetic dopamine agonist and strong prolactin inhibitor bromocriptine was introduced in 1972. Since then, many other drugs have been used for suppression of lactation, including those with recognised prolactin-lowering activity and those with uncertain mechanism of action. These include different preparations of estrogens, estrogen in combination with androgens or progestogens, or both, clomiphene, pyridoxine, prostaglandin E2, other dopamine agonists (cabergoline and lisuride) and serotonin antagonists (cyproheptadine, methysergide and methergoline).

OBJECTIVES: The objective of this review is to evaluate the effectiveness and safety of interventions used for suppression of lactation in puerperal women to determine which approach has the greatest comparative benefits with least risk.

CHAPTER 9: ROGUES' GALLERY

Intuitively beneficial interventions which randomised trials found to be harmful.

⊗ **OESTROGEN SUPPLEMENTATION, MAINLY DIETHYLSTILBES-TROL, FOR PREVENTING MISCARRIAGES AND OTHER ADVERSE PREGNANCY OUTCOMES:** was ineffective, with multiple long-term complications for the offspring. (Bamigboye AA, Morris J) CD004353

⊗ **THYROTROPIN-RELEASING HORMONE ADDED TO CORTI-COSTEROIDS FOR WOMEN AT RISK OF PRETERM BIRTH FOR PREVENTING NEONATAL RESPIRATORY DISEASE:** increased adverse outcomes. (Crowther CA, Alfirevic Z, Haslam RR) CD000019

⊗ **MAGNESIUM SULPHATE FOR PREVENTING PRETERM BIRTH IN THREATENED PRETERM LABOUR:** was ineffective at delaying birth or preventing preterm birth; increases adverse outcomes for the baby. (Crowther CA, Hiller JE, Doyle LW) CD001060

⊗ **ROUTINE PERINEAL SHAVING ON ADMISSION IN LABOUR:** was associated with more bacterial colonisation and no benefits. (Basevi V, Lavender T) CD001236

⊗ **EPISIOTOMY FOR VAGINAL BIRTH:** a liberal episiotomy policy increased perineal trauma, suturing and complications; reduced anterior vaginal trauma. (Carroli G, Belizan J) CD000081

⊗ **EARLY VERSUS DELAYED UMBILICAL CORD CLAMPING IN PRE-TERM INFANTS:** increased neonatal blood transfusions and intraventricular haemorrhage. (Rabe H, Reynolds G, Diaz-Rossello J) CD003248

⊗ **PELVIMETRY FOR FETAL CEPHALIC PRESENTATIONS AT OR NEAR TERM:** x-ray pelvimetry increased caesarean section rates. (Pattinson RC, Farrell E) CD000161

⊗ **CLOSURE VERSUS NON-CLOSURE OF THE PERITONEUM AT CAESAREAN SECTION:** increased operating time, postoperative fever and hospital stay but no good data on long term outcomes as yet. (Bamigboye AA, Hofmeyr GJ) CD000163

Index

3TC *see* lamivudine
abdominal
  decompression   140–1
  incisions   343–4, 348–9
  nerves block   355
  stretch marks   35–6
abnormal presentation *see*
  presentation
abortions *see* termination
absorbable synthetic
  sutures   319–20
acquired immunodeficiency
  syndrome (AIDS)   102
activated charcoal   120
active management   263, 268–9, 289
acupressure   280–1
acupuncture
  induction   225, 244–5
  pain during labour   280–1
  symptoms during
    pregnancy   34–5, 37–8
acyclovir   203–4
advanced extrauterine
  pregnancies   357
advice during pregnancy   13–22
  see also counselling
aerobic exercise
  advice during pregnancy   21–2
  diabetes mellitus   90–1
  hypertension   59–60
  weight retention   366–7
AFV *see* amniotic fluid volume
age assessment   128–9

AIDS *see* acquired
  immunodeficiency syndrome
albuterol   179
alcohol   17–20
alloimmune thrombocytopenia   95
alloimmunisation   147–9
aloe vera   353–4
ambulatory blood pressure
  monitoring   69–70
amino acid supplements   144
amniocentesis   129–30
amnioinfusion   155, 310, 313–15
amnionitis   153
amniotic fluid volume (AFV)   138, 146
amniotomy
  induction   229–31, 238, 240–1
  slow progress during
    labour   287–9
amoxicillin   200, 201–2
ampicillin   211, 338–9
anaemia   85–9
  malaria   114–18
  maternal   29–30
  prevention   86–7
  treatment   87–9
anaesthesia
  caesarean section   328–33, 355
  general   328–9
  labour   261, 263–4, 266–7
  local   355
  postnatal care   371–2
  regional   328–33
  topical   371–2

parasitic 214–16
preterm births 160–1, 165–7, 181–2, 199, 201
screening 207, 216
urinary tract infections 207–10
vaccination 213–17
see also human immunodeficiency virus
influenza 114
inherited coagulation defects 95
insecticide-treated nets (ITNs) 117–18
instrumental births *see* operative vaginal births
insulin 90, 93–4, 222
intermittent auscultation 308
interrupted sutures 320–1
intra-abdominal repair 346–7
intra-amniotic infection 210–11
intracervical prostaglandins 226–7, 228, 231
intracranial haemorrhage 70
intrapartum
fetal distress 311–12, 315–16
fetal scalp lactate sampling 308–9
intrauterine devices (IUDs) 374–6
intrauterine fetal death 91, 220–1
intrauterine growth restriction (IUGR)
antenatal care 13, 29–30
hypertension 63–4, 69
intrauterine pressure catheters (IUPC) 289–90
intravaginal prostaglandins 225–6, 228, 231
intravenous immunoglobulin 44–5, 46
intravenous prostaglandins 237–8
inversion of the uterus 362
iodine deficiency 120–1
iron supplementation 32–3, 86–9
iron-deficiency anaemia 85–9
isobaric bupivacaine 329
isoimmunisation 150–1
isosorbide mononitrate 248

isotonic hydration 146
isradipine 74
itching 35
ITNs *see* insecticide-treated nets
IUDs *see* intrauterine devices
IUGR *see* intrauterine growth restriction
IUPC *see* intrauterine pressure catheters

jaundice 150–1
Joel-Cohen incisions 342–4

ketanserin 80–1
ketosis 260–1
Kristellar manoeuver 291

labetalol 80–1
labour 251–362
anaesthesia 261, 263–4, 266–7
assessment programs 254–5
caregivers 251–3, 255–6
compromised fetal condition 302–17
cord prolapse 317
episiotomy 264–8, 399
extrauterine pregnancies 357
first stage 257–8
infections 261–2, 279–80, 399
inversion of the uterus 362
maternal positions/mobility 257–8, 266–7
normal birth 264–80
operative vaginal births 315, 322–7
pain 280–7
perineal trauma 317–22
place of birth 251, 252–3
postpartum haemorrhage 268–71, 272–4, 276–8, 357–61
presentation 290–2, 294–302
retained placenta 359–61
routine care 253–80
second stage 264–8
shoulder dystocia 292–4